CAMBRIDGE LIBRARY COLLECTION

Books of enduring scholarly value

History of Medicine

It is sobering to realise that as recently as the year in which *On the Origin of Species* was published, learned opinion was that diseases such as typhus and cholera were spread by a 'miasma', and suggestions that doctors should wash their hands before examining patients were greeted with mockery by the profession. The Cambridge Library Collection reissues milestone publications in the history of Western medicine as well as studies of other medical traditions. Its coverage ranges from Galen on anatomical procedures to Florence Nightingale's common-sense advice to nurses, and includes early research into genetics and mental health, colonial reports on tropical diseases, documents on public health and military medicine, and publications on spa culture and medicinal plants.

The Works of John Hunter, F.R.S.

The surgeon and anatomist John Hunter (1728–93) left a famous legacy in the Hunterian Museum of medical specimens now in the Royal College of Surgeons, and in this collection of his writings, edited by James Palmer, with a biography by Drewry Ottley, published between 1835 and 1837. The first four volumes are of text, and the larger Volume 5 contains plates. Hunter had begun his career as a demonstrator in the anatomy classes of his brother William, before qualifying as a surgeon. He regarded surgery as evidence of failure – the mutilation of a patient who could not be cured by other means – and his studies of anatomy and natural history were driven by his belief that it was necessary to understand the normal physiological processes before attempting to cure the abnormal ones. Volume 2 discusses diseases of jaws, teeth and gums, at a time when dental surgery was rudimentary.

Cambridge University Press has long been a pioneer in the reissuing of out-of-print titles from its own backlist, producing digital reprints of books that are still sought after by scholars and students but could not be reprinted economically using traditional technology. The Cambridge Library Collection extends this activity to a wider range of books which are still of importance to researchers and professionals, either for the source material they contain, or as landmarks in the history of their academic discipline.

Drawing from the world-renowned collections in the Cambridge University Library and other partner libraries, and guided by the advice of experts in each subject area, Cambridge University Press is using state-of-the-art scanning machines in its own Printing House to capture the content of each book selected for inclusion. The files are processed to give a consistently clear, crisp image, and the books finished to the high quality standard for which the Press is recognised around the world. The latest print-on-demand technology ensures that the books will remain available indefinitely, and that orders for single or multiple copies can quickly be supplied.

The Cambridge Library Collection brings back to life books of enduring scholarly value (including out-of-copyright works originally issued by other publishers) across a wide range of disciplines in the humanities and social sciences and in science and technology.

The Works of
John Hunter, F.R.S.

VOLUME 2

EDITED BY JAMES F. PALMER

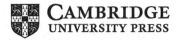
CAMBRIDGE
UNIVERSITY PRESS

CAMBRIDGE
UNIVERSITY PRESS

University Printing House, Cambridge, CB2 8BS, United Kingdom

Cambridge University Press is part of the University of Cambridge.

It furthers the University's mission by disseminating knowledge in the pursuit of
education, learning and research at the highest international levels of excellence.

www.cambridge.org
Information on this title: www.cambridge.org/9781108079587

© in this compilation Cambridge University Press 2015

This edition first published 1835
This digitally printed version 2015

ISBN 978-1-108-07958-7 Paperback

This book reproduces the text of the original edition. The content and language reflect
the beliefs, practices and terminology of their time, and have not been updated.

Cambridge University Press wishes to make clear that the book, unless originally published
by Cambridge, is not being republished by, in association or collaboration with,
or with the endorsement or approval of, the original publisher or its successors in title.

THE

WORKS

OF

JOHN HUNTER, F.R.S.

WITH

NOTES.

EDITED BY

JAMES F. PALMER,

SENIOR SURGEON TO THE ST. GEORGE'S AND ST. JAMES'S DISPENSARY; FELLOW
OF THE ROYAL MEDICAL AND CHIRURGICAL SOCIETY OF LONDON, ETC.

IN FOUR VOLUMES.

ILLUSTRATED BY A VOLUME OF PLATES, IN QUARTO.

VOL. II.

LONDON:

PUBLISHED BY

LONGMAN, REES, ORME, BROWN, GREEN, AND LONGMAN,

PATERNOSTER-ROW.

1835.

PRINTED BY RICHARD TAYLOR,
RED LION COURT, FLEET STREET.

CONTENTS OF VOL. II.

TREATISE

ON THE

NATURAL HISTORY AND DISEASES

OF THE

HUMAN TEETH,

EXPLAINING THEIR STRUCTURE, USE, FORMATION, GROWTH, AND DISEASES.

IN TWO PARTS.

BY

JOHN HUNTER, F.R.S.

WITH NOTES

BY

THOMAS BELL, F.R.S.,

FELLOW OF THE LINNEAN SOCIETY; FELLOW OF THE GEOLOGICAL SOCIETY; FELLOW OF THE ROYAL MEDICAL AND CHIRURGICAL SOCIETY OF LONDON; CORRESPONDING MEMBER OF THE SOCIETY OF NATURAL HISTORY OF PARIS; LECTURER ON COMPARATIVE ANATOMY AT GUY'S HOSPITAL, &C.

CONTENTS.

PART I.

PART II.

INTRODUCTION.

CHAP. I.

OF THE DISEASES OF THE TEETH, AND THE CONSEQUENCES OF THEM.

PREFACE.

THE state of Dental Surgery at the period when Hunter wrote the following work was perhaps lower than that of any department of professional science or practice. The treatment of the teeth was still consigned to the hands of the ignorant mechanic, whose knowledge was limited to the forcible extraction of aching teeth, the manufacture of substitutes for those which were lost, and some rude methods of filling the cavities produced by decay. That this state of a branch of practice, as susceptible of a connexion with physiological and pathological science, and as improveable by such a connexion as any other, should have early attracted the attention of a man preeminently qualified for detecting and supplying such deficiencies, and whose labours, unparalleled as they are for their scientific importance, are not less valuable from the immense influence they have since exerted upon the practice both of medicine and surgery, might have been anticipated, from the peculiar character of his mind, which was too truly great to think any subject unworthy of his anxious attention which involved the improvement of the

art of healing, or the extension of our knowledge of
Nature's operations. If it may be stated that the work
in question is perhaps the least felicitous effort of this
extraordinary genius, and that of which the errors are
the most obvious and striking, some apology may be
found even for these, in the confined nature of the
subject, and especially in the obscure and anomalous
structure of the organs of which it treats; whilst the
basis which his experiments and observations have laid
for subsequent improvements in our knowledge, both
of the physiology and pathology of the teeth as well as
in the treatment of their diseases, constitutes a never-
ceasing claim to the gratitude and admiration of every
scientific practitioner of dental surgery. If, therefore,
it may with truth be said that he was the father of
scientific surgery; if he may claim the high distinction
of having placed the practice of surgery upon the only
solid foundation, that of physiological science, it is no
less true of this humble department than of those more
important branches of the art, in which are involved
the knowledge and treatment of diseases which stand
in immediate connexion with vital organs and functions.

It is not uninteresting, even in this work, to trace the
peculiarities of his genius, and to watch the workings
of his mind in his search after truth, which he pursued
with an ingenuousness and candour which have never
been surpassed, and rarely, if ever, equalled. It is, indeed, amongst the remarkable characteristics of his
reasonings and conclusions,—and this must be the case,

too, with all who follow truth with equal zeal and sin-
gleness of purpose,—that even his errors arise from that
inviolable love of truth, that single aim at establishing,
not the dogmas of a favourite theory, but the simple
laws of Nature herself, which constitutes one principal
charm of his greatest and most important discoveries.
This is shown in a very striking point of view by the
error, and even inconsistency into which he falls when
reasoning on the structure of the teeth. His observations and experiments had shown him that these organs
differ in many important respects from the other bones;
that the phenomena which these two organs present
under comparative circumstances, whether of disease
or of experiment, differ in many important respects;
that the teeth are not susceptible of artificial injection;
that they cannot restore lost parts; and many other
peculiarities, which led him too hastily to infer that
" they are to be considered as extraneous bodies with
respect to a circulation through their substance,"
though the same candour obliges him to confess, in
the same sentence, that " they have most certainly a
living principle, by means of which they make part of
the body, and are capable of uniting with any part of
a living body," although the experiments on which he
founds the latter proposition, if they prove anything,
prove that this union with a living body is effected by
means of a vascular continuity.   Here, then, is an example of a love of truth for her own sake, so pure, so
invulnerable, that not even to avoid the dilemma into
which his imperfect reasoning upon these two incon-

sistent propositions must necessarily force him, will he
sacrifice, or modify, or gloss over one tittle of the facts
on which they are founded.

Whatever errors, however, may have crept into this
work from the causes already alluded to, it forms the
basis of all that has since been done to improve the
knowledge of this branch of practice, and still more
remarkably has it proved the foundation of all that is
now known on the physiology of the teeth. It must, on
the other hand, be conceded to his immediate follower
Dr. Blake, that if he received from Hunter the hints
from which his own discoveries were deduced, he has
so clearly elucidated what in the former was obscure,
so judiciously supplied what was deficient, and so satisfactorily harmonized what appeared to be incompatible or inconsistent, that he well deserves the praise
of having contributed more to the right understanding
of the subject than any other writer that has ever
treated on it either before or since ; and his inaugural
dissertation (the work, it must be remembered, of a
pupil,) contains opinions and statements on the structure, the formation, the growth, and the relations of
these organs, which most subsequent writers have done
well to copy, and all experimental physiologists have
only been able to confirm.

The late Joseph Fox, with far less of original talent
than his precursor, brought to the practice of his profession a mind well prepared for a diligent, correct, and
rational discharge of its duties. If, therefore, his in-
tellectual character were such as precluded him from

distinguishing himself in the field of original investigation and discovery, the sober reflective habits of his mind, joined to a regular professional education, enabled him to obtain from an extensive practice such a knowledge of the diseases of these organs, and such well-grounded principles of their treatment, as to render his work a very valuable acquisition, not to the professed dentist only, but particularly to the general practitioner ; a class of the profession to which his labours were especially devoted, as he lectured on this subject for many years in the theatre of Guy's Hospital.

It is, then, to the writers just mentioned that the profession is principally indebted for the knowledge it at present possesses of the anatomy, physiology, and diseases of the teeth. It would be useless here to notice the numerous books which have from time to time appeared, chiefly derived, as they are, from these sources, the merits of which may generally be stated to be in the inverse ratio of their originality. Equally unnecessary is it to enter into an elaborate consideration of the hypotheses which are entertained on the nature of these organs by some of the most distinguished French physiologists. The object of the author in the annotations affixed to the following Treatise has been rather to avail himself of such means as lay before him, to elucidate the text where it is obscure, to correct its errors where subsequent investigations have proved errors to exist, and to add such information on subjects imperfectly treated on as the observations and experience of others, or his own, have enabled him to obtain. He

has entered upon the task with a degree of diffidence
commensurate with the respect which the name of
Hunter commands, and with a sacred regard to the
same object of general utility as formed the guiding
star to the great Original whose work he thus humbly
endeavours to illustrate.

T. BELL.

New Broad Street,
February 1835.

N.B. The Editor's Notes are distinguished from the Author's by being
placed below the line, within brackets. They are also further distinguished by initial letters instead of the usual marks of reference.

THE NATURAL HISTORY

OF

THE HUMAN TEETH.

PART I.

Of the Upper Jaw.

BEFORE we enter into a description of the teeth themselves, it will be necessary to give an account of the upper and lower jaw-bones, in which they are inserted; insisting minutely on those parts which are connected with the teeth, or serve for their motion and action, and passing over the others slightly.

The upper jaw is composed of two bones, which generally remain distinct through life. They are very irregular at their posterior and upper parts, sending upwards and backwards a great many processes, that are connected with the bones of the face and skull*. The lower and anterior parts of the upper jaw are more uniform, making a kind of circular sweep from side to side, the convexity of which is turned forwards; the lower part terminates in a thick edge, full of sockets for the teeth. This edge is called in each bone the alveolar process†. Behind the alveolar processes there are two horizontal lamellæ, which uniting together, form part of the roof of the mouth, which is the partition between the mouth and the nose‡.

This plate, or partition, is situated about half an inch higher than the lower edge of the alveolar process; and this gives the roof of the mouth a considerable hollowness.

The use of the upper jaw is to form part of the parietes of the mouth, nose, and orbits; to give a basis, or supply the alveolar process, for the

---

superior row of teeth, and to counteract the lower jaw; but it has no
motion itself upon the bones of the head and face.

Of the Lower Jaw.

As the lower jaw is extremely moveable, and its motion is indispen-
sably necessary in all the various operations of the teeth, it requires to
be more particularly described. It is much more simple in its form than
the upper, having fewer processes, and these not so irregular. Its anterior circular part is placed directly under that of the upper jaw; but its
other parts extend further backwards*.

This jaw is at first composed of two distinct bones†; but these, soon
after birth, unite into one, at the middle of the chin. This union is
called the symphysis of the jaw. Upon the upper edge of the body of
the bone is placed the alveolar process, a good deal similar to that of
the upper jaw. The alveolar process extends all round the upper part
of the bone, from the coronoid process of one side to that of the
other‡. In both jaws they are everywhere relatively proportional
to the teeth, being thicker behind, where the teeth are larger and
more irregular, upon account of the more numerous fangs inserted into
them. The teeth that are situated backwards in the upper jaw, have
more fangs than those that correspond with them in the lower, and the
sockets are accordingly more irregular. The alveolar process of the
upper jaw is a section of a larger circle than that of the lower, especially
when the teeth are in the sockets. This arises chiefly from the anterior
teeth in the upper jaw being broader and flatter than those in the lower§.
The posterior part of the bone on each side rises almost perpendicularly,
and terminates above in two processes‖; the anterior of which is the
highest, is thin and pointed, and is called the coronoid process¶. The
anterior edge of this process forms a ridge, which goes obliquely downward and forward on the jaw, upon the outside of the posterior sockets**.
To this process the temporal muscle is attached; and as it rises above
the centre of motion, that muscle acts with nearly equal advantage in
all the different situations of the jaw.

The posterior process, which is made for a moveable articulation with
the head, runs upward, and a little backward; is narrower, thicker, and
shorter than the anterior; and terminates in an oblong rounded head,
or condyle††, whose longest axis is nearly transverse. The condyle is

* Pl. II. f. 1 & 2.   † Pl. VI. f. 1, 4, & 6.   ‡ Pl. I. f. 2.
§ Pl. II. f. 1.   ‖ Pl. II. f. 2. e & d; and Pl. III. f. 2. e & f.
¶ Pl. III. e, e.   ** Pl. II. f. 2, b.   †† Pl. III. f. 2. f.

bent a little forward; is rounded, or convex, from the fore to the back part; and likewise a little rounded from one end to the other, or from right to left. Its external end is turned a little forward, and its internal a little backward ; so that the axes of the two condyles are neither in the same straight line, nor parallel to each other; but the axis of each condyle, if continued backwards, would meet, and form an angle of about one hundred and forty-six degrees ; and lines drawn from the symphysis of the chin to the middle of the condyle would intersect their longest axis at nearly right angles *. There are, however, some exceptions, for in a lower jaw of which I have a drawing, the angle formed by the supposed continuation of the two axes, instead of being an angle of one hundred and forty-six degrees, is of one hundred and ten only. The lower jaw serves for a base to support the teeth in the alveolar process during their action on those of the upper jaw in mastication, and to give origin to some muscles that belong to other parts.

Of the Alveolar Processes.

The alveolar processes are composed of two thin bony plates, one external† and the other internal‡. These two plates are at a greater distance from each other at their posterior ends, than at the anterior, or middle part of the jaw. They are united together by thin bony partitions going across, which divide the processes at the anterior part into just as many distinct sockets as there are teeth§ ; but at the posterior part, where the teeth have more than one root or fang, there are distinct cells or sockets for every root‖. These transverse partitions are more protuberant than the alveolar plates, and thus add laterally to the depth of the cells, particularly at the anterior part of the jaw. At each partition the external plate of the alveolar process is depressed, so as to form a fluting¶ round the cells or cavities for the roots of the teeth. This is observable in the whole length of the alveolar process of the upper jaw, and in the fore part particularly of the lower jaw. The alveolar processes of each jaw form about one half of a circular, or rather of an elliptical**, figure ; and at the fore part in the lower jaw they are perpendicular, but project inwards at the posterior part, and describe a smaller circle than the body of the bone upon which they stand††, as we shall observe more particularly hereafter, when we come to treat of the jaws of old people.

* Pl. I. f. 2., or Pl. III. f. 2.
‡ Pl. I. f. 1. b, b, b.
‖ Pl. I. f. 1. d, d, and f. 2. b.
** Pl. I. f. 1, 2.

† Pl. I. f. 1. a, a, a, a, a.
§ Pl. I. f. 1. c, c, and f. 2. a.
¶ Pl. II. f. 2. f, f, f, f.
†† Pl. I. f. 2.

The alveolar processes of both jaws should rather be considered as belonging to the teeth than as parts of the jaws; for they begin to be formed with the teeth, keep pace with them in their growth, and decay and entirely disappear when the teeth fall out ; so that if we had no teeth, it is likely we should not only have no sockets, but not even these processes in which the sockets are formed ; for the jaws can perform their motions, and give origin to muscles, without either the teeth or alveolar processes. In short, there is such a mutual dependence of the teeth and alveolar processes on each other, that the destruction of the one seems to be always attended with that of the other[a].

In the head of a young subject which I examined, I found that the two first incisor teeth in the upper jaw had not cut the gum, nor had they any root or fang, excepting so much as was necessary to fasten them to the gum, on their upper surface ; and on examining the jaw, I found there was no alveolar process nor sockets in that part. What had been the cause of this I will not pretend to say ; whether it was owing to the teeth forming not in the jaw but in the gum, or to the wasting of the fangs. The appearance of the tooth favoured the first supposition, for it was not like those whose fangs are decayed in young subjects, preparatory to the shedding of the teeth ; and as it did not cut the gum, it is reasonable to think it never had any fang. That end from which the fang should have grown was formed into two round and smooth points, having each a small hole leading into the body of the tooth, which was pretty well formed.

Of the Articulation of the Lower Jaw.

Just under the beginning of the zygomatic process of each temporal bone, before the external meatus auditorius, an oblong cavity may be observed, in direction, length, and breadth in some measure corresponding with the condyle of the lower jaw*. Before and adjoining to this cavity, there is an oblong eminence, placed in the same direction, convex upon the top, in the direction of its shorter axis, which runs from behind forwards ; and a little concave in the direction of its longer axis, which runs from within outwards. It is a little broader at

* Pl. I. f. 3. c.

---

a [This observation is strictly correct: however rapidly the gum becomes absorbed, whether from indigestion, the use of mercury, the accumulation of calculous matter, or that affection which is vulgarly termed scurvy in the gum, the alveolar process never becomes exposed (unless it be a dead portion exfoliating), but absorption of the bone always keeps pace with that of the gum.]

its outer extremity, as the outer corresponding end of the condyle describes a larger circle in its motion than the inner*. The surface of
the cavity and eminence is covered with one continued smooth cartilaginous crust, which is somewhat ligamentous, for by putrefaction it
peels off, like a membrane, with the common periosteum. Both the
cavity and eminence serve for the motion of the condyle of the lower
jaw. The surface of the cavity is directed downward; that of the
eminence downward and backward, in such a manner that a transverse
section of both would represent the italic letter S†. Though the eminence may, on a first view of it, appear to project considerably below
the cavity, yet a line drawn from the bottom of the cavity to the most
depending part of the eminence is almost horizontal, and therefore
nearly parallel with the line made by the grinding surfaces of the teeth
in the upper jaw : and when we consider the articulation further, we
shall find that these two lines are so nearly parallel that the condyle
moves almost directly forwards in passing from the cavity to the eminence; and the parallelism of the motion is also preserved by the shape
of an intermediate cartilage.

In this joint there is a moveable cartilage, which, though common to
both condyle and cavity, ought to be considered rather as an appendage
of the former than of the latter, being more closely connected with it,
so as to accompany it in its motion along the common surface of both
the cavity and eminence. This cartilage is nearly of the same dimen-
sions with the condyle, which it covers, and is hollowed out on its inferior
surface, to receive the condyle. On its upper surface it is more unequal,
being moulded to the cavity and eminence of the articulating surface
of the temporal bone, though it is considerably less, and is therefore
capable of being moved with the condyle, from one part of that surface
to another‡. Its texture is ligamento-cartilagineous. This moveable
cartilage is connected with both the condyle of the jaw and the articulating surface of the temporal bone, by distinct ligaments, arising from
its edges all round. That by which it is attached to the temporal bone
is the most free and loose ; though both ligaments will allow an easy
motion of the cartilage on the respective surfaces of the condyle and
temporal bone. These attachments of the cartilage are strengthened, and the whole articulation secured, by an external ligament,
which is common to both, and which is fixed to the temporal bone, and
to the neck of the condyle. On the inner surface of the ligament
which attaches the cartilage to the temporal bone, and backwards, in
the cavity, is placed what is commonly called the gland of the joint ; at

---

* Pl. I. f. 3. *d*.　　　† Pl. I. f. 3. *c, d*.　　　‡ Pl. I. f. 3. *c*.

least the ligament is there much more vascular than at any other part.

Of the Motion in the Joint of the Lower Jaw.

The lower jaw, from the manner of its articulation, is susceptible of a great many motions. The whole jaw may be brought horizontally forwards, by the condyles sliding from the cavity towards the eminences on each side. This motion is performed chiefly when the teeth of the lower jaw are brought directly under those of the upper, in order to bite or hold anything very fast between them.

Or, the condyles only may be brought forwards, while the rest of the jaw is tilted backwards, as is the case when the mouth is open; for on that occasion the angle of the jaw is tilted backwards, and the chin moves downwards, and a little backwards also. In this last motion the condyle turns its face a little forwards; and the centre of motion lies a little below the condyle, in the line between it and the angle of the jaw. By such an advancement of the condyles forwards, together with the rotation mentioned, the aperture of the mouth may be considerably enlarged; a circumstance necessary on many obvious occasions.

The condyles may also slide alternately backwards and forwards, from the cavity to the eminence, and vice versâ; so that while one condyle advances, the other moves backwards, turning the body of the jaw from side to side, and thus grinding between the teeth the morsel separated from the larger mass by the motion first described. In this case the centre of motion lies exactly in the middle between the two condyles. And it is to be observed, that in these slidings of the condyles forwards and backwards, the moveable cartilages do not accompany the condyles in the whole extent of their motion, but only so far as to adapt their surfaces to the different inequalities of the temporal bone: for as these cartilages are hollow on their lower surfaces where they receive the condyle, and on their opposite upper surfaces are convex where they lie in the cavity, but anteriorly, at the root of the eminence, are a little hollowed, if they accompanied the condyles through the whole extent of their motion, the eminences would be applied to the eminences, the cavities would not be filled up, and the whole articulation would be rendered very insecure.

This account of the motion of the lower jaw and its cartilages clearly demonstrates the principal use of these cartilages, namely, the security of the articulation, the surfaces of the cartilage accommodating themselves to the different inequalities, in the various and free motions of this joint. This cartilage is also very serviceable for preventing the parts from being hurt by the friction; a circumstance necessary to be guarded against where there is so much motion. Accordingly I find this cartilage in the different tribes of carnivorous animals, where there is no eminence and cavity, nor other apparatus for grinding, and where the motion is of the true ginglymus kind only.

In the lower jaw, as in all the joints of the body, when the motion is carried to its greatest extent, in any direction, the muscles and ligaments are strained and the person made uneasy. The state, therefore, into which every joint most naturally falls, especially when we are asleep, is nearly in the middle state between the extremes of motion; by which means all the muscles and ligaments are equally relaxed. Thence it is that commonly and naturally the teeth of the two jaws are not in contact, nor are the condyles of the lower jaw so far back in the temporal cavities as they can go.

Of the Muscles of the Lower Jaw.

Having described the figure, articulation, motion, and use of the lower jaw, it will be necessary in the next place to give some account of the muscles that are the causes of its motion.

There are five pairs of muscles, each of them capable of producing various motions, according to the situation of the lower jaw, whether they act singly or in conjunction with others. Two or more of them may be so situated as to be capable of moving the jaw in the same direction; but every motion is produced by the action of more than one muscle at a time. Thus, if the jaw be depressed, and brought to one side, either the masseter, temporal, or pterygoideus internus of the opposite side will not only raise the jaw but bring it to its middle state. It will be necessary in the description of each muscle to give its use in the different situations of the jaw, by which means, after they are all described, their compound actions will be better understood. I shall first describe those which raise the jaw; then those which give it the lateral motion; and lastly, those which depress it; proceeding in the order in which they present themselves in dissection.

The most superficial is the masseter: it is situated upon the posterior and lower part of the face, between the cheek-bone and angle of the lower jaw, directly before the lower part of the ear. It is a thick, short, complex muscle, and a little flattened: it appears to have two distinct origins, an anterior and outer and a posterior and inner; but that is owing only to its outer edge at its origin being slit, or double, and the fibres of these two edges having a different course, decussating each other a little. The anterior and outer portion of the muscle begins to rise from a small part of the lower edge of the malar process of the maxillary bone, adjoining to the os malæ; and continues its origin all along the lower horizontal edge of this last bone to the angle where its zygomatic process turns up to join that of the temporal bone. The external layer of fibres in this portion is tendinous at its beginning, while the internal is fleshy.

The posterior and inner portion of this muscle begins to rise, partly tendinous and partly fleshy, from the same lower edge of the os malæ: not where the origin of the other portion terminates, but a little further forwards; and this origin is continued along the lower edge of the zygomatic process of the temporal bone, as far backwards as the eminence belonging to the articulation of the lower jaw.

From this extent of its origin the muscle passes downwards to its insertion into the lower jaw. The anterior external portion is broader at its insertion than at its origin; for it occupies a triangular space of the lower jaw; which, above the angle and on the outside, is about an inch in breadth, but below about an inch and a half, from the angle towards the chin. In consequence of this extent of insertion, the fibres of this portion divaricate very considerably. They are mostly fleshy at their insertion, a few only being tendinous, particularly those that are inserted backwards. The posterior and inner portion of the masseter is narrower at its insertion than at its origin; its posterior fibres running forwards as well as downwards, while its anterior run almost directly downwards. It occupies in its insertion the remaining part of the scabrous surface above the angle of the lower jaw, which lies between the anterior portion and the two upper processes, viz. the condyle and coronoid. As the anterior fibres of this portion rise on the inside of the posterior fibres of the other portion, and as its posterior fibres run forwards as well as downwards, and its anterior run almost directly downwards, while the fibres of the other portion radiate both forwards and backwards; these two portions in some measure decussate, or cross one another. The anterior fibres, which run furthest and lowest down, are tendinous at their insertion, while the posterior and shortest are fleshy.

The use of the whole muscle is to raise the lower jaw; and when it is brought forwards, the posterior and inner portion will assist in bringing it a little back: so that this muscle becomes a rotator, if the jaw happens to be turned to the opposite side.

We may observe that this muscle is intermixed with a number of tendinous portions, both at its origin and its insertion; which give rise to a greater number of fleshy fibres, and thereby add to the strength of the muscle.

Of the Temporal Muscle.

The temporal muscle is situated on the side of the head, above and a little before the ear. It is a flat and radiated muscle; broad and thin at its origin; narrow and thick at its insertion; and covered with a pretty strong fascia above the jugum.

This fascia is fixed to the bones round the whole circumference of the origin of the muscle. Above, it is fixed to a smooth white line, which is observable upon the skull, extending from a little ridge on the lateral part of the os frontis, continued across the parietal bone, and making a turn towards the mammillary process. It is fixed below to the ridge where the zygomatic process begins, just above the meatus auditorius; then to the upper edge of the zygomatic process itself, and anteriorly to the os malæ. This adhesion above, before and behind, describes, as it were, the circumference of the origin of the temporal muscle.

This muscle arises from all the bones of the side of the head that are within the line for insertion of the tendinous fascia, viz. from the lower and lateral part of the parietal bone, from all the squamous portion of the temporal bone, from the lower and lateral part of the os frontis, from the temporal process of the os sphenoides, often from a process at the lower part of this surface, (which portion, however, is often common to this muscle and the pterygoideus externus,) and from the posterior surface of the os malæ: outwardly, it arises from the inner surface of the jugum, and from the whole inner surface of the fascia. At this origin from the jugum it is not to be distinguished from the masseter, being there in fact one and the same muscle; and indeed the masseter is no more than a continuation of the same origin under the edge of the jugum, and might properly enough be reckoned the same, both as to its origin and insertion, and in some measure in its use also.

The origin is principally fleshy, and the muscle passes from thence downwards and a little forwards, converging, and forming a thin middle tendon: after which the muscle runs downwards on the inside of the jugum, and is inserted into the coronoid process of the lower jaw, on both sides tendinous and fleshy, but principally tendinous. It reaches further down upon the inside of the coronoid process than upon the outside, the insertion being continued as low down as the body of the bone.

The posterior and inferior edge of this muscle passes over the root of the zygomatic process of the temporal bone as over a pulley, which confines the action of the muscle to that of raising the lower jaw more than if its fibres had passed in a direct course from their origin to their insertion.

The use of the temporal muscle, in general, is to raise the lower jaw; and as it passes a little forwards to its insertion, it must bring the condyle at the same time backwards, and so counteract the pterygoideus externus of the opposite side; and if both muscles act, they counteract both the pterygoidei, by bringing back the whole of the jaw.

Of the Internal Pterygoid Muscle.

The internal pterygoid muscle is situated upon the inside of the lower jaw, opposite to the masseter. It is a strong short muscle, a little flattened, especially at its insertion. It arises tendinous and fleshy from the whole internal surface of the external ala of the sphenoid bone; from the external surface of the internal ala, near its bottom; from that process of the os palati that makes part of the fossa pterygoidea; likewise from the anterior rounded surface of that process where it is connected to the os maxillare superius. From thence the muscle passes downwards, a little outwards and backwards, and is inserted, tendinous and fleshy, into the inside of the lower jaw, from the angle up almost to the groove for the admission of the maxillary nerve, where the surface of the bone is remarkably scabrous.

The use of this muscle is to raise the lower jaw; and from its direction, one would suspect that it would bring the condyle a little forwards; but this motion is contrary to that of the lower jaw, for it is naturally brought back when raised.

Of the External Pterygoid Muscle.

The external pterygoid muscle is situated immediately between the external surface of the external ala of the pterygoid process and the condyle of the lower jaw, lying, as it were, horizontally along the basis of the skull. It is somewhat radiated in some bodies; broad at the origin, and small at the insertion; but the greater part of it forms a round strong fleshy belly, so that the part that makes it of the radiated kind is thin.

The thick and ordinary portion of it arises, tendinous and fleshy, from almost the whole external surface of the external ala of the pterygoid process of the sphenoid bone, excepting a little bit of the root at the posterior edge; and towards the lower part it arises a little from the inner surface of that ala. The thin portion arises from a ridge of the sphenoid that is continued from the process towards the temple, just behind the foramen lacerum inferius, which terminates in a little protuberance. This origin is sometimes wanting, and in that case the temporal muscle arises from that protuberance; and very often this origin is common to both. These two origins of this muscle are sometimes so much separated as to make it a biceps.

From these origins the muscle passes outwards and a little backwards, converging; that is, the superior fibres passing outwards and backwards, and a little downwards; while the inferior or larger portion of it passes a little upward.

It is inserted, tendinous and fleshy, into a depression on the anterior part of the condyle and neck of the lower jaw, upon the inside of that ridge which is continued from the coronoid process; a little portion is likewise inserted into the anterior part of the moveable cartilage of the joint.

When this muscle acts singly, it is a rotator; for it brings the condyle of the jaw forwards, and likewise the moveable cartilage, which throws the chin to the opposite side; but if it acts in conjunction with its fellow of the opposite side, instead of being turned to one side, the whole jaw is brought forwards, and thus these counteract the temporal, &c.

These two muscles generally act alternately; and when they do so, one acts at the time of depression, the other at the time of elevation; so that these muscles act both when the lower jaw is raised and when it is depressed; although they do not assist in this act.

Of the Superior Digastric Muscle.

The digastricus is situated immediately under and a little upon the inside of the lower jaw, and exterior to the fauces, extending from the mastoid process to the chin, nearly along the angle made by the neck and chin, or face*. The name of this muscle expresses its general shape, as it has two fleshy bellies, and of course a middle tendon. Yet some of its anterior belly does not arise from the tendon of the posterior, but from the fascia which binds it to the os hyoides. These two fleshy bellies do not run in the same line, but form an angle, just where the tendon runs into the anterior belly; so that this tendon seems rather to belong to the posterior, which is the thickest and longest.

This muscle arises from the sulcus made by the inside of the mastoid process, and a ridge upon the temporal bone, where it is united with the os occipitis. The extent of this origin is about an inch; it is fleshy

---

* Pl. I. f. 3. g.

upon its outer part, viz. that from the mastoid process, and tendinous on the inside from the ridge. From its origin it passes forwards, downwards, and a little inwards, much in the direction of the posterior edge of the mammillary process, and forms a round tendon, first in its centre and upper surface. This tendon passes on in the same direction; and when got near the os hyoides, commonly perforates the anterior end of the stylo-hyoideus muscle. From the lower edge of this tendon some fibres seem to go off, which degenerate into a kind of fascia, which binds it to the os hyoides; while some go across the lower part of the mylo-hyoideus, and joining their fellows on the opposite side, bind the os hyoides by a kind of belt. At this part the tendon becomes a little broader, makes a turn upwards, inwards, and forwards, and giving origin to the anterior belly, passes on, in the same direction, to the lower part of the chin, where it is inserted, tendinous and fleshy, into a slight depression on the under and a little on the posterior part of the lower jaw, almost contiguous to its fellow. Besides the attachment of the middle tendon to the os hyoides, there is a ligamentous binding, which serves in some measure as a pulley. This is more marked in some subjects than in others; and this depends on the strength of the tendinous expansion which binds the tendon of the digastricus to the os hyoides.

When we say that these parts are attached to the os hyoides, we do not mean that they can be traced quite into it, like some other tendons in the body; but the os hyoides seems to be the most fixed point of attachment. Very often we find two anterior bellies to each muscle: the uncommon one, which is the smallest, does not pass to the chin, but joins with a similar portion of the other side, in a middle tendon, which is often fixed to the os hyoides. At other times we find such a portion on one side only, in which case it is commonly fixed to the middle tendon of the mylo-hyoideus.

The use of these muscles with regard to the lower jaw is principally to depress it; but according as one acts a little more forcibly than the other, it thereby gives the jaw a small rotation, and becomes in that respect a kind of antagonist to the pterygoideus externus. Besides depressing the lower jaw, when we examine the dead body, they would appear to raise the larynx. But although they have this effect, a proper attention to what happens in the living body will probably show that their principal action is to depress the lower jaw, and that they are the muscles commonly employed for this purpose. Let a finger be placed on the upper part of the sterno-mastoideus muscle, just behind the posterior edge of the mastoid process, about its middle, touching that edge a little with the finger; then depress the lower jaw; and the posterior head of the digastricus will be felt to swell very consi-derably, so as to point out the direction of the muscle. In this there can be no deception, for there is no other muscle in this part that has the same direction; and those who are of opinion that the digastricus does not depress the lower jaw will more readily allow this when they are told that we find the same head of the muscle act in deglutition; but not with a force equal to that which it exerts in depressing the lower jaw. Further, if the sterno-hyoidei, sterno-thyroidei, and costo-hyoidei, acting at the same time with the mylo-hyoidei and genio-hyoidei, as-sisted in depressing the jaw, the os hyoides and thyroid cartilage would probably be depressed as the bellies of the sterno-hyoidei and of the other lower muscles are by much the longest; but, on the contrary, we find that the os hyoides, with the thyroid cartilage, is a little raised in the depression of the jaw, which we may suppose to be done by the anterior belly of the digastricus; and, secondly, if these muscles were to act to bring about this motion of the jaw, these parts would be brought forwards, nearer to the straight line between the chin and sternum, which is not the case in this action; whereas we find it to be the case in deglutition, in which these evidently act. By applying our fingers upon the genio-hyoideus and mylo-hyoideus, near the os hyoides, between the two anterior bellies of the digastricus, (not near the chin, where the action of these two bellies may occasion a mistake,) we find these muscles quite flaccid, which is not the case in deglutition nor in speak-ing, in which they certainly do act; nor do we find the muscles under the os hyoides at all affected, as they are in the motion of the larynx.

It has been observed that when we open the mouth, while we keep the lower jaw fixed, the fore part of the head or face is necessarily raised. Authors have been at a good deal of pains to explain this. Some of them considered the condyles of the jaw as the centre of motion. But if this were the case, that part of the head where it articulates with the spine, and consequently the whole body, must be depressed in pro-portion as the upper jaw is raised, which is not true in fact. Others have considered the condyles of the occiput as the centre of motion; and they have conceived the extensor muscles of the head to be the moving powers. The muscles which move the head in this case are pointed out by two circumstances which attend all muscular mo-tion: in the first place, all actions of our body have muscles imme-diately adapted to them; and, secondly, when the mind wills any par-ticular action, its power is applied by instinct to those muscles only which are naturally adapted to that motion; and further, the mind being accustomed to see the part move which is naturally the most moveable, attends to its motion in the volition, although it be in that instance

fixed, and the other parts of the body move towards it; and although
the other parts of the body might be brought towards it by other muscles,
and would be so if the mind intended they should come towards it, yet
these muscles are not brought into action. Thus, the flexors of the arm
commonly move the hand to the body; but if the hand be fixed, the
body is moved by the same muscles to the hand. In this case, however, the mind wills the motion of the hand towards the body, and
brings the flexors into action; whereas if it wished to bring the body
towards the hand, the muscles of the fore part of the body would be
put into action, and this would produce the same effect.

To apply this to the lower jaw: when we attempt to open the mouth
while the lower jaw is immoveable, we fix our attention upon the very
same muscles (whatever they are) which we call into action when we
depress the lower jaw; and we find that we act with the·very same
muscles; for our mind attends to the depressing of the jaw, and not the
raising of the face, and under such circumstances the mouth is actually
opened. We find then by these means the head is raised; and the idea
that we have of this motion is the same that we have in the common
depression of the jaw; and we should not know, except from circumstances, that the jaw was not really depressed; we find also at this time
that the extensors of the head are not in action. On the contrary,
when the jaw is fixed in the same situation, if we have a mind to raise
the head or upper jaw, which of course must open the mouth, we fix
our attention to the muscles that move the head backwards, without
having the idea of opening our mouth; and at this time the extensors
of the head act. This plainly shows that the same muscles which depress the jaw when moveable, must raise the head when the jaw is kept
fixed.

This is a proof too that there are no other muscles employed in depressing the lower jaw than what will raise the head under the circumstances mentioned. This will further appear from the structure of the
parts; wherein four things are to be considered, viz. the articulation of
the jaw; the articulation of the head with the neck; the origin and the
insertion of digastric muscle.

Suppose i*, the upper jaw, to be fixed, and the lower jaw b, to be
moveable on the condyle a: if the digastric contracts, its origin g, and
insertion j, will approach towards one another; in which case it is
evident that the lower jaw will move downwards and backwards. But
if the lower jaw be fixed, as in the case supposed, and the vertebra h
also, the condyle will move upwards and forwards upon the eminence

* Pl. I. f. 3.

in the joint, the fore part of the head will be pushed upwards and backwards by the condyle, and the hind part of the head will be drawn down; so that the whole shall make a kind of circular motion upon the upper vertebræ; and the digastric muscle, pulling the hind part of the head towards the lower jaw, and at the same time pushing up the condyles against the fore part of the head, acquires by this mechanism a very considerable additional power.

Of the Structure of a Tooth; and, first, of the Enamel.

A tooth is composed of two substances, viz. enamel and bone. The enamel, called likewise the vitreous or cortical part, is found only upon the body of the tooth, and is there laid all around on the outside of the bony or internal substance*. It is by far the hardest part of our body; insomuch that the hardest and sharpest saw will scarce make an impression upon it, and we are obliged to use a file in dividing or cutting it. When it is broken it appears fibrous or striated, and all the fibres or striæ are directed from the circumference to the centre of the tooth†.

This in some measure prevents it from breaking in mastication, as the fibres are disposed in arches, and also keeps the tooth from wearing down, as the ends of the fibres are always acting on the food.

The enamel is thickest on the grinding surface and on the cutting edges or points of the teeth, and becomes gradually thinner on the sides as it approaches the neck, where it terminates insensibly, though not equally low, on all sides of the teeth‡. On the base or grinding surface it is of a pretty equal thickness, and therefore is of the same form with the bony substance which it covers§.

It would seem to be an earth united with a portion of animal substance, as it is not reducible to quick-lime by fire till it has first been dissolved in an acid. When a tooth is put into a weak acid, the enamel to appearance is not hurt; but on touching it with the fingers it crumbles down into a white pulp. The enamel of teeth, exposed to any degree of heat, does not turn to lime : it contains animal mucilaginous matter; for when exposed to the fire it becomes very brittle, cracks, grows black, and separates from the inclosed bony part of the tooth. It is capable, however, of bearing a greater degree of heat than the bony part, without becoming brittle and black‖. This substance has no

---

* Pl. V. f. 15, 16, 18.   † Pl. V. f. 22, 23, 24.   ‡ Ibid.   § Ibid.

‖ From this circumstance we can show the enamel better by burning a tooth, as the bony part becomes black sooner than the enamel. The method of burning, and showing them after they are burnt, is as follows: Let one half of a tooth be filed

marks of being vascular and of having a circulation of fluids : the most
subtile injections we can make never reach it; it takes no tinge from
feeding with madder, even in the youngest animals; and, as was observed above, when soaked in a gentle acid there appears no gristly or
fleshy part with which the earthy part had been incorporated*.

We shall speak of the use and formation of the enamel hereafter,
when they will be better understood[a].

Of the Bony Part of a Tooth.

The other substance of which a tooth is composed is bony, but much
harder than the most compact part of bones in general.   This substance
makes the interior part of the body, the neck, and the whole of the root
of a tooth.   It is a mixture of two substances, viz. calcareous earth and
an animal substance, which we might suppose to be organized and vascular.   The earth is in very considerable quantity : it remains of the
same shape after calcination, so that it is in some measure kept together
by cohesion; and it is capable of being extracted by steeping in the
muriatic and some other acids.   The animal substance, when deprived

away, from one end to the other, then burn it gently in the fire ; after this is done, wash
the filed surface with an acid, or scrape it with a knife.   By this method you will clean
the edge of the enamel, which will remain white, and the bony part will be found black.

* In all these experiments I never could observe that the enamel was in the least
tinged, either in the growing or formed tooth.   This looks as if the enamel were the
earth more fully depurated, or strained off, from the common juices in such a manner
as not to allow the gross particles of madder to pass.   Here it may not be amiss to
remark, that the names given to animal substance, such as gluten, &c., are not in the
least expressive of the thing meant, for there is no such thing as glue in an animal till
it has either undergone a putrefactive process or been changed by heat.   And here, too,
I wish it to be understood that I do not consider earth as any part of an animal, or that
it makes up any part of an animal substance.

[a] [The structure of the enamel is perfectly crystalline.   The crystals are fibrous in
appearance, and placed parallel to each other, at right angles with the surface of the
bony portion of the tooth with which their inner terminations are placed in contact.   It
is true that there is a trace of animal matter in this substance, according to the following analysis by Berzelius:

Phosphate of lime	85·3
Fluate of lime	3·2
Carbonate of lime	8·
Phosphate of magnesia	1·5
Soda and muriate of soda ...	1·
Animal matter and water ...	1·

100·]

of the earthy part by steeping in an acid, is more compact than the same substance in other bones, but still is soft and flexible.

That part of a tooth which is bony has nearly the same form as a complete tooth; and hence, when the enamel is removed, it has the same sort of edge or points as the enamel itself. We cannot by injection prove that the bony part of a tooth is vascular; but from some circumstances it would appear that it is so: for the fangs of teeth are liable to swellings, seemingly of the spina ventosa kind, like other bones, and they sometimes anchylose with the socket by bony and inflexible continuity, as all other contiguous bones are apt to do. But there may be a deception here, for the swelling may be an original formation, and the anchylosis may arise from the pulp, upon which the tooth is formed, being united with the socket. The following considerations would seem to show that the teeth are not vascular: first, I never saw them injected in any preparation, nor could I ever succeed in any attempt to inject them, either in young or old subjects, and therefore believe that there must have been some fallacy in the cases where they have been said to be injected. Secondly, we are not able to trace any vessels going from the pulp into the substance of the new-formed tooth; and whatever part of a tooth is formed, it is always completely formed, which is not the case with other bones. But, reasoning from analogy, we have a still more convincing proof in the effect of madder. Take, for example, any young animal, as a pig, and feed it with madder for three or four weeks; then kill the animal, and upon examination you will find the following appearances: first, if this animal had some parts of its teeth formed before the feeding with madder, those parts will be known by their remaining of the natural colour; but such parts of the teeth as were formed while the animal was taking the madder will be found to be of a red colour. This shows that it is only those parts that were formed while the animal was taking the madder that are dyed; for what were already formed will not be found in the least tinged. This is different in all other bones, for we know that any part of a bone which is already formed is capable of being dyed with madder, though not so fast as the part that is forming; therefore, as we know that all other bones when formed are vascular, and are thence susceptible of the dye, we may readily suppose that the teeth are not vascular, because they are not susceptible of it after being once formed. But we shall carry this still further: if you feed a pig with madder for some time, and then leave it off for a considerable time before you kill the animal, you will find the above appearances still subsisting, with this addition, that all the parts of the teeth which were formed after leaving off feeding with the madder will be white. Here thèn in some teeth we shall have white, then red, and then white again; and so we shall have the red and the white colour alternately through the whole tooth.

This experiment shows that the tooth, once tinged, does not lose its colour: now as all other bones that have not been tinged lose their colour in time, when the animal leaves off feeding with madder (though very slowly), and as that dye must be taken into the constitution by the absorbents, it would seem that the teeth are without absorbents as well as other vessels.

This shows that the growth of the teeth is very different from that of other bones. Bones begin at a point, and shoot out at their surface, and the part that seems already formed is not in reality so, for it is forming every day by having new matter thrown into it, till the whole substance is complete; and even then it is constantly changing its matter.

Another circumstance in which teeth seem different from bone, and a strong circumstance in support of their having no circulation in them, is, that they never change by age, and seem never to undergo any alteration when completely formed but by abrasion: they do not grow softer, like the other bones, as we find in some cases, where the whole earthy matter of the bones has been taken into the constitution.

From these experiments it would appear that the teeth are to be considered as extraneous bodies, with respect to a circulation through their substance; but they have most certainly a living principle, by which means they make part of the body, and are capable of uniting with any part of a living body, as will be explained hereafter. It is to be observed, that affections of the whole body have less influence upon the teeth than any other part of the body. Thus, in children affected with the rickets, the teeth grow equally well as in health, though all the other bones are much affected; and hence their teeth being of a larger size in proportion to the other parts, their mouths are protuberant[a].

---

[a] [As the arguments which are here adduced against the vascularity of the teeth are wholly insufficient, and in many respects inconsistent with each other, it will be useful to examine into the true bearing of the observations on which they are founded.

The failure of all attempts to inject the substance of the teeth, with even the finest of the matters usually employed for filling the minute branches of arteries in other structures of the body, can scarcely be considered as conclusive, since the colouring matter is, in all of them, too dense and coarse to pass into the vessels of many other parts, which, though in the healthy condition they do not convey red blood, yet, in a state of inflammation, become evidently injected with red particles. I have, however, on another occasion, alluded to two very conclusive facts, which appear unanswerably to prove the vascularity of the teeth. One is the occasional occurrence of red patches in

Of the Cavity of the Teeth.

Every tooth has an internal cavity, which extends nearly the whole length of its bony part*. It opens or begins at the point of the fang, where it is small; but in its passage it becomes larger, and ends in the body of the tooth†; the cavity at this end is exactly of the shape of the body of the tooth to which it belongs; and in general it may be said that the whole of the cavity is nearly of the shape of the tooth itself, larger, that is, in the body of the tooth, and thence gradually smaller to the extremity of the fang; simple where the tooth has but one root‡, and in the same manner compounded when the tooth has two or more fangs§.

This cavity is not cellular, but smooth in its surface: it contains no marrow, but appears to be filled with blood-vessels‖, and, I suppose,

* Pl. V. f. 1, 2, 3, &c.	† Ibid.	‡ Pl. V. f. 4, 5, 6, 7.
§ Pl. V. f. 1, 2.	‖ Pl. VIII. f. 7, 8.	

the otherwise healthy bony structure of a tooth when much inflamed, discoverable by breaking or sawing asunder the body of the tooth immediately after extraction. The other, the injection of a tooth with bile in cases of jaundice, of which I have seen more than one example. In the former instance, the red patches are of rather a bright colour, until they become dull and obscure by time; and in the latter the whole substance of the tooth is imbued with a bright yellow colour.

The experiments on madder would be far from conclusive on the point at issue, even were the details more complete. In the absence, however, of all information respecting the duration of each experiment, and especially the period which elapsed after the madder had been discontinued before the animal was killed, it would be futile to combat the conclusions which Hunter has deduced from them. Thus deficient, they only prove that the more highly organized bones, as might be expected, lose the colouring matter of the madder by absorption sooner than the teeth. The paragraph in which the results are summed up is perhaps as characteristic of the peculiar tendencies of Hunter's mind as any that can be found in his works. Concluding, from the failure of his experiments with madder, and from other peculiarities, that the teeth are devoid of a circulation through their substance, and therefore to be so far considered as extraneous bodies, his intense love of truth, which never suffered him even to escape from a dilemma by its slightest sacrifice, forces him to confess the existence of a living principle, because he found, from the result of other experiments, that they " were capable of uniting with any part of a living body." Instead, therefore, of endeavouring to render his theory consistent with itself, by disguising or perverting one of the two incompatible conclusions to which his observations had forced him, he adopts them both, and is thus driven to the inference, that an organ can, at the same time, be "an extraneous body," and yet possess "a living principle," and be " capable of uniting with any part of a living body."

The truth appears to be, that the teeth are truly organized bodies, having nerves and absorbent and circulating vessels, but possessing so low a degree of living power, and so dense a structure, as to exhibit phenomena, both in their healthy and diseased condition, which are very dissimilar from those which are observed in true osseous structures.]

nerves, united by a pulpy or cellular substance. The vessels are branches of the superior and inferior maxillaries, and the nerves must come from the second and third branches of the fifth pair.

By injections we can trace the blood-vessels distinctly through the whole cavity of the tooth; but I could never trace the nerves distinctly even to the beginning of the cavity.

Of the Periosteum of the Teeth.

The teeth, as we have observed, are covered by an enamel only at their bodies; but at their fangs they have a periosteum, which, though very thin, is vascular, and appears to be common to the tooth which it incloses, and the socket, which it lines as an investing internal membrane. It covers the tooth a little beyond the bony socket, and is there attached to the gum[a].

Of the Situation of the Teeth.

The general shape and situation of the teeth are obvious. The opposition of those of the two jaws, and the circle which each row describes, need not be particularly explained, as they may be very well seen in the living body, and may be supposed to be already understood from what has been said of the alveolar processes.

We may just observe, with regard to the situation of the two rows, that when they are in the most natural state of contact, the teeth of the upper jaw project a little beyond the lower teeth, even at the sides of the jaws, but still more remarkably at the fore part, where, in most people, the upper teeth lie before those of the lower jaw[*]; and at the lateral part of each row the line or surface of contact is hollow from behind forwards in the lower jaw, and in the same proportion it is convex in the upper jaw[†].

The edge of each row is single at the fore part of the jaws; but as the teeth grow thicker backwards, it there splits into an internal and ex-

---

* Pl. II. f. 1, 2.   † Ibid.

[a] [The periosteum can hardly be said to be common to the tooth and the socket. It is, in fact, continued from the external surface of the alveolar process into the socket, and then reflected over the surface of the root. Thus, if a healthy tooth be removed from a dead body, it will be found covered with an extremely thin periosteum, and the alveolar cavity will also often remain lined by a similar structure. Probably when inflammation has once existed to a considerable degree in this membrane, the two layers become permanently united.]

ternal edge. The canine tooth, which we shall call cuspidatus, is the point from which the two edges go off, so that the first grinder, or what we shall call the first bicuspis, is the first tooth that has a double edge*.

Of the Number of the Teeth.

Their number in the whole, at full maturity, is from twenty-eight to thirty-two : I once saw twenty-seven only ; never more than thirty-two. Fourteen of them are placed in each jaw when the whole number is no more than twenty-eight, and sixteen when there are thirty-two. If the whole be twenty-nine or thirty-one in number, the upper jaw sometimes, and sometimes the lower, has one more than the other; and when the number is thirty, I find them sometimes divided equally between the two jaws; and in other subjects sixteen of them are in one jaw and fourteen in the other. In speaking of the number of teeth, I am supposing that none of them have been pulled out, or otherwise lost; but that there are from eight to twelve of those large posterior teeth, which I call grinders, and that they are so closely planted as to make a continuity in the circle ; and in this case, when the number is less than thirty-two, the deficiency is in the last grinder.

The teeth differ very much in figure from one another, but those on the right side in each jaw resemble exactly those on the left, so as to be in pairs ; and the pairs belonging to the upper jaw nearly resemble the corresponding teeth of the lower jaw in situation, figure, and use†.

Each tooth is divided into two parts, viz. first, the body, or that part of it which is the thickest, and stands bare beyond the alveoli and gums ; secondly, the fang, or root, which is lodged within the gum and alveolar process : and the boundary between these two parts, which is grasped by the edge of the gum, is called the neck of a tooth. The bodies of the different teeth differ very much in shape and size, and so do their roots. The difference must be considered hereafter.

The teeth of each jaw are commonly divided into *three* classes, viz. Incisors, Canine, and Grinders ; but from considering some circumstances of their form, growth, and use, I choose to divide them into the *four* following classes, viz. Incisores, commonly called fore teeth ; Cuspidati, vulgarly called canine ; Bicuspides, or the first two grinders ; and Molares, or the last three teeth. The number of each class in each jaw, for the most part is four incisores, two cuspidati, four bicuspides, and four, five, or six molares.

* Pl. III. f. 1, 2.   † Pl. II. & III. and Pl. V. row 1, 2, 3, 4.

There is a regular gradation, both in growth and form, through these classes, from the incisores to the molares ; in which respect the cuspidati are of a middle nature between the incisores and bicuspides, just as the last-mentioned are intermediate between the cuspidati and molares : consequently the incisores and molares are the most unlike in every circumstance*.

Of the Incisores.

The incisores are situated in the anterior part of the jaw ; the others more backwards on each side, in the order in which we have named them. The bodies of the incisores are broad, having two flat surfaces, one anterior, the other posterior. These surfaces meet in a sharp cutting edge. The anterior surface is convex in every direction, and placed almost perpendicularly ; and the posterior is concave and sloping, so that the cutting edge is almost directly over the anterior surface†.

These surfaces are broadest and the tooth is thinnest at the cutting edge or end of the tooth, and thence they become gradually narrower and the tooth thicker towards the neck, where the surfaces are continued to the narrowest side or edge of the fang. The body of an incisor, in a side view, grows gradually thicker or broader from the edge of the tooth to its neck ; and these coincide with the flat or broad side of the fang : so that when we look on the fore or back part of an incisor, we observe it grows constantly narrower from its cutting edge to the extremity of its fang. But in a side view it is thickest or broadest at its neck, and thence becomes gradually more narrow, both to its cutting edge and to the point of its fang‡.

The enamel is continued further down and is thicker on the anterior and back part of the incisores than on their sides, and is even a little thicker on the fore part than upon the back part of the tooth. If we view them laterally, either when entire or when cut down through the middle, but especially in the latter case, it would seem as if the fang was driven like a wedge into and had split the body or enamel of the tooth§. They stand almost perpendicularly, their bodies being turned a little forwards. Their fangs are much shorter than those of the cuspidati, but pretty much of the same length with all the other teeth of this jaw‖.

---

* Pl. II. and Pl. V. f. 1.   It is here to be understood that the teeth from which we take our description are such as are just completely formed, and not therefore in the least worn down by mastication. Our description of each class is taken from the lower jaw ; and the difference between them and their corresponding classes in the upper jaw immediately follows that description.

† Pl. V.   ‡ Ibid.   § Ibid. f. 18.   ‖ Pl. III. f.4.

In the upper jaw they are broader and thicker, especially the two first : their length is nearly the same with those of the lower jaw. They stand a little obliquely, with their bodies turned much more forwards (the first especially), and they generally fall over those of the under jaw.

The two first incisores cover the two first and half of the second of the lower jaw, so that the second incisor of the upper jaw covers half of the second incisor and more than half of the cuspidatus of the under jaw *.

The edges of the incisores, by use and friction, in some people become blunt and thicker; and in others they sharpen one another, and become thinner.

Of the Cuspidatus.

The cuspidatus is the next after the incisores in each jaw, so that there are four of them in all. They are in general thicker than the incisores, and considerably the longest of all the teeth †.

The shape of the body of the cuspidatus may be very well conceived by supposing an incisor with its corners rubbed off, so as to end in a narrow point instead of a thin edge‡; and the fang differs from that of an incisor only in being much larger§.

The outside of the body of a cuspidatus projects most at the side next the incisores, being there more angular than anywhere else.

The enamel covers more of the lateral parts of these teeth than of the incisores. They stand perpendicularly, or nearly so, projecting further out in the circle than the others, so that the two cuspidati and the four incisores often stand almost in a straight line, especially in the lower jaw.

This takes place only in adults, and in them only when the second teeth are rather too large for the arch of the jaw; for we never find this when the teeth are at any distance from one another, or in young subjects. Their points commonly project beyond the horizontal plane formed by the row of teeth, and their fangs run deeper into the jaws, and are oftener a little bent.

In the upper jaw they are rather longer, and do not project much beyond the circle of the adjacent teeth; and in this jaw they are not placed vertically, their bodies being turned a little forwards and outwards.

When the jaws are closed, the cuspidatus of the upper jaw falls between and projects a little over the cuspidatus and first bicuspis of

* Pl. II. f. 1.   † Pl. III. f. 4.; Plate V. row 1, b.
‡ Pl. III. f. 1, at bb.   § Pl. III. f. 4.

the lower jaw. When they are a little worn down by use, they commonly first take an edge somewhat like a worn incisor, and afterwards become rounder.

The use of the cuspidati would seem to be to lay hold of substances, perhaps even living animals : they are not formed for dividing, as the incisores are, nor are they fit for grinding. We may trace in these teeth a similarity in shape, situation, and use, from the most imperfectly carnivorous animal, which we believe to be the human species, to the most perfectly carnivorous, viz. the lion[a].

Of the Bicuspides.

Immediately behind the cuspidati, in each jaw, stand two teeth, commonly called the first and second grinders, but which, for reasons hinted at above, I shall suppose to constitute a particular class, and call them bicuspides.

These (viz. the fourth and fifth tooth from the symphysis of the jaw) resemble each other so nearly that a description of the first will serve for both. The first indeed is frequently the smallest, and has rather the longest fang, having somewhat more of the shape of the cuspidatus than the second.

The body of this tooth is flattened laterally, answering to the flat side of the fang. It terminates in two points, viz. one external and one internal. The external is the longest and thickest; so that on looking into the mouth from without, this point only can be seen, and the tooth has very much the appearance of a cuspidatus, especially the first of these teeth. The internal point is the least, and indeed sometimes so very small that the tooth has the greatest resemblance to a cuspidatus in any view*. At the union of the points the tooth is thickest, and

* Pl. III. f. 1, 2, c c.

---

[a] [That our conclusions as to the functions of an organ as it exists in man, when drawn exclusively from analogous structures in the lower animals, will frequently prove erroneous, is strikingly shown in these observations on the use of the cuspidatus. The simple and obvious use of this tooth, in the human species, is to tear such portions of food as are too hard or tough to be divided by the incisores; and we frequently find it even far more developed in animals which are known to be exclusively frugivorous. Not only is its structure wholly unadapted for such an object as that assigned to it in the text, but there is no analogous or other ground for supposing that man was originally constructed for the pursuit and capture of living prey. His naturally erect position and the structure of the mouth would render this impossible by the means inferred by Hunter, and the possession of so perfect an instrument as the hand obviates the necessity of his ever employing any other organ for the purpose of seizing or holding food of whatever description.]

thence it loses in thickness, from side to side, to the extremity of the fang, so that the fang continues pretty broad to the point, and is often forked there. All the teeth hitherto described often have their points bent, and more particularly the cuspidati.

The enamel passes somewhat further down externally and upon the inside, than laterally : but this difference is not so considerable as in the incisores and cuspidati; in some, indeed, it terminates equally all round the tooth. They stand almost perpendicularly, but seem to be a little turned inwards, especially the last of them.

In the upper jaw they are rather thicker than in the lower, and are turned a very little forwards and outwards. The first in the upper jaw falls between the two in the lower, the second falls between the second and the first grinder; and both project over those of the lower jaw, but less than the incisores and cuspidati.

The bicuspides, and especially the second of them, in both jaws, are oftener naturally wanting than any of the teeth, except the dentes sapientiæ; hence we might conjecture that they are less useful; and this conjecture appears less improbable when we consider that in their use they are of a middle nature between cutters and grinders, and that in most animals, so far as I have observed, there is a vacant space between the cutters and grinders. I have also seen a jaw in which the first bicuspis was of the same shape and size as a grinder, and projected, for want of room, between the cuspidatus and second bicuspis. These and the grinders alter very little in shape on their grinding surfaces by use; their points only wear down and become obtuse.

Of the Grinders.

In describing the grinders we shall first consider the first and second conjointly, because they are nearly the same in every particular, and then give an account of the third or last grinder, which differs from the former in some circumstances.

The two first grinders differ from the bicuspides principally in being much larger, and in having more points upon their body and more fangs*.

The body forms almost a square, with rounded angles. The grinding surface has commonly five points, or protuberances, two of which are on the inner, and three on the outer part of the tooth; and generally some smaller points at the roots of these larger protuberances. These protuberances make an irregular cavity in the middle of the tooth. The three outer points do not stand so near the outer edge of the tooth as

* Pl. III. f. 1, 2, *d d*.

the inner do on the inside; so that the body of the tooth swells out more from the points, or is more convex, on the outside. The body towards its neck becomes but very little smaller, and there divides into two flat fangs, one forwards the other backwards, with their edges turned outwards and inwards, and their sides consequently forwards and backwards: the fangs are but very little narrower at their ends, which are pretty broad and often bifurcated. There are two cavities in each fang, one towards each edge leading to the general cavity in the body of the tooth. These two cavities are formed by the meeting of the sides of the fang in the middle, thereby dividing the broad and flat cavity into two*; and all along the outside of these (and all the other flat fangs) there is a corresponding longitudinal groove. These fangs at their middle are generally bent a little backwards†.

The enamel covers the bodies of these teeth pretty equally all round.

The first grinder is somewhat larger and stronger than the second; it is turned a little more inwards than the adjacent bicuspides, but not so much as the second grinder. Both of them have generally shorter fangs than the bicuspides.

There is a greater difference between these grinders in the upper and lower jaw than between any of the other teeth. In the upper jaw they are rather rhomboidal than square in their body, with one sharp angle turned forwards and outwards, the other backwards and inwards; besides, they have three fangs, which diverge, and terminate each in a point: these are almost round, and have but one cavity. Two of them are placed near each other perpendicularly over the outside of the tooth; and the other, which generally is the largest, stands at a greater distance on the inside of the tooth, slanting inwards. In this jaw these two grinders are inclined outwards, and a little forwards; they project a little over the corresponding teeth of the lower jaw, and are placed further back in the mouth, so that each is partly opposed to two of the lower jaw. The second in the upper jaw is smaller than the others; and the first and second are placed directly under the maxillary sinus. I once saw the second grinder naturally wanting on one side of the lower jaw.

The third grinder is commonly called dens sapientiæ: it is a little shorter and smaller than the others, and inclined a little more inwards and forwards. Its body is nearly of the same figure, but rather rounder, and its fangs are generally not so regular and distinct, for they often appear squeezed together; and sometimes there is only one fang, which makes the tooth conical: it is much smaller than the rest of the grinders. In the upper jaw this tooth has more variety than in the lower,

* Pl. V. f. 8, where four dark spots are observed.   † Pl. III. f. 4.

and is even smaller than the corresponding tooth of the lower, and consequently stands directly opposed to it: but for this circumstance the grinders would reach further back in the upper jaw than in the lower, which is not commonly the case.

In the upper jaw this third grinder is turned but a very little outwards, is frequently inclined somewhat backwards, and projects over that of the under jaw. It oftener becomes loose than any of the other teeth.

It is placed under the posterior part of the maxillary sinus, where the parts which compose the sinus are thicker than in the middle. The variations as to the natural number of the teeth depend commonly upon the dentes sapientiæ.

Thus, from the incisores to the first grinder, the teeth become gradually thicker at the extremity of their bodies, and smaller from the first grinder to the dens sapientiæ. From the cuspidatus to the dens sapientiæ the fangs become much shorter: the incisores are nearly of the same length with the bicuspides. From the first incisor to the last grinder the teeth stand less out from the sockets and gums.

The bodies of the teeth in the lower jaw are turned a little outwards at the anterior part of the jaw, and thence, to the third grinder, they are inclined gradually more inwards. The teeth in the upper jaw project over those of the under, especially at the fore part, which is owing to the greater obliquity of the teeth in the upper jaw; for the circle of the sockets is nearly the same in both jaws. This oblique situation, however, becomes gradually less, from the incisores backwards to the last grinder, which makes them gradually project less in the same proportion.

The teeth in the upper jaw are placed further back in the circle than the corresponding teeth of the lower; this is owing to the two first incisores above being broader than the corresponding incisores below. All the teeth have only one fang, except the grinders, each of which has two in the lower jaw and three in the upper*

The fangs bear a proportion to the bodies of the teeth; and the reason is evident, for otherwise they would be easily broken, or pushed out of their sockets. The force commonly applied to them is oblique, not perpendicular; and they are not so firmly fixed in the upper jaw, that is, the alveolar process in that is not so strong, as in the under jaw: it is perhaps on this account that the grinders in that jaw have three fangs.

This particular structure in the alveolar process of the upper jaw is

---

* Those anatomists who allow the teeth to have more fangs have been led into a mistake; I suppose, by often observing two canals in one fang, and thence concluding that such a fang was originally two, and that these were now grown together.

perhaps to give more room for the antrum Highmorianum. On this supposition the fangs must be made accordingly, *i. e.* so that they shall not
be pushed into that cavity : now, by their diverging they inclose, as it
were, the bottom of the antrum, and do not push against its middle,
which is the weakest part ; and the points of three diverging fangs will
make a greater resistance (or not be so easily pushed in) than if they
were placed parallel. If there had been only two, as in the lower jaw,
they must have been placed opposite to the thinnest part of the antrum ;
and three points placed in any direction but a diverging one would have
had here much the same effect as two ; and as the force applied is endeavouring to depress the tooth, and push it inwards, the innermost fang
diverges most, and is supported by the inner wall of the antrum. That
all this weakness in the upper jaw is for the increase of the antrum is
probable, because all the teeth in the upper jaw are a good deal similar
to those in the lower, excepting those that are opposite to the maxillary
sinus ; and here they differ principally in the fangs, without any other
apparent reason : and what confirms this is, that the dentes sapientiæ in
both jaws are more alike than the other grinders,—for this reason, as I
apprehend, because the dens sapientiæ in the upper jaw does not interfere
so much with the maxillary sinus.

What makes it still more probable that the two first superior grinders
have three fangs on account of the maxillary sinus is, that the two
grinders on each side of the upper jaw, in the child, have three fangs, and
we find them underneath the antrum ; but those that succeed them
have only one fang, as in the lower jaw : but by that time the antrum
has passed further back, or rather the arch of the jaw has projected, or
shot forwards, as it were, from under the antrum, so that the alveolar
processes that were under it at one age are got before it in another.

That the edge of every fang is turned towards the circumference of the
jaw, in order to counteract the acting power, we shall see when we consider the motion of the jaw and the use of the teeth.

Of the Articulation of the Teeth.

The fangs of the teeth are fixed in the gum and alveolar processes by
that species of articulation called gomphosis, which in some measure
resembles a nail driven into a piece of wood*.

They are not, however, firmly united with the processes, for every
tooth has some degree of motion ; and in heads which have been boiled

* See Plate I. for the sockets; and Pl. III. f. 4, for the teeth themselves in their
sockets.

or macerated in water, so as to destroy the periosteum and adhesion of the teeth, we find the teeth so loosely connected with their sockets that all of them are ready to drop out, except the grinders, which remain, as it were, hooked from the number and shape of their fangs.

Of the Gums.

The alveolar processes are covered by a red vascular substance, call d the gums, which has as many perforations as there are teeth, and the neck of a tooth is covered by and fixed to this gum. Hence there are fleshy partitions between the teeth, passing between the external and internal gum, and, as it were, uniting them : these partitions are higher than the other parts of the gum, and form an arch between every two adjacent teeth. The thickness of that part of the gum which projects beyond the sockets is considerable, so that when the gum is corroded by disease, by boiling, or otherwise, the teeth appear longer, or less sunk into the jaw. The gum adheres very firmly in a healthful state both to the alveolar process and to the teeth, but its extreme border is naturally loose all around the teeth. The gum, in substance, has something of a cartilaginous hardness and elasticity, and is very vascular, but seems not to have any great degree of sensibility; for though we often wound it in eating, and in picking our teeth, yet we do not feel much pain upon these occasions; and both in infants and old people, where there are no teeth, the gums bear a very considerable pressure without pain.

The advantage arising from this degree of insensibility in the gums is obvious, for till the child cuts its teeth the gums are to do the business of teeth, and are therefore formed for this purpose, having a hard ridge running through their whole length. Old people who have lost their teeth have not this ridge. When in a sound state, the gums are not easily irritated by being wounded, and therefore are not so liable to inflammation as other parts, and soon heal.

The teeth being united to the jaw by the periosteum and gum, have some degree of a yielding motion in the living body. This circumstance renders them more secure ; it breaks the jar of bony contact, and prevents fractures both of the sockets and of the teeth themselves.

Of the Action of the Teeth, arising from the Motion of the Lower Jaw.

The lower jaw may be said to be the only one that has any motion in mastication, for the upper jaw can only move with the other parts of the head. That the upper jaw and head should be raised in the common act of opening the mouth or chewing, would seem, at first sight, improbable; and from an attentive view of the mechanism of the joints and muscles of those parts, from experiment and observation, we find that they do not sensibly move. We shall only mention one experiment in proof of this, which seems conclusive. Let a man place himself near some fixed point, and look over it, to another distant and immoveable object, when he is eating. If his head should rise in the least degree he would see more of the distant object over the nearest fixed point, which in fact he does not. The nearer the fixed point is, and the more distant the object, the experiment will be more accurate and convincing. The result of the experiment will be the same if the nearest point has the same motion with the head, as when he looks from under the edge of a hat, or anything else put upon his head, at some distant fixed object. We may conclude, then, that the motion is entirely in the lower jaw; and, as we have already described both the articulation and the motion of the bone, we shall now explain the action of mastication, and at the same time consider the use of each class of teeth.

With regard to the action of the teeth of both jaws in mastication, we may observe once for all that their action and reaction must be always equal, and that the teeth of the upper and lower jaws are complete and equal antagonists both in cutting and grinding.

When the lower jaw is depressed, the condyles slide forwards on the eminences, and they return back again into the cavities when the jaw is completely raised. This simple action produces a grinding motion of the lower jaw, backwards on the upper, and is used when we divide anything with our fore teeth, or incisores. For this purpose the incisores are well formed: for as they are higher than the others, their edges must come in contact sooner; and as the upper project over the under, we find, in dividing any substance with them, that we first bring them opposite to one another, and as they pass through the part to be divided, the lower jaw is brought back, while the incisores of that jaw slide up behind those of the upper jaw, and of course pass by one another. In this way they complete the division, like a pair of scissors, and at the same time they sharpen one another. There are exceptions to this, for these teeth in some people meet equally, viz. in those people whose fore teeth do not project further from the gum, or socket, than the back teeth; and such teeth are not so fit for dividing: and in some people the teeth of the lower jaw are so placed as to come before those of the upper jaw. This last situation is as favourable for cutting as when the overlapping of the teeth is the reverse, except for this circumstance, that the lower jaw must be longer, and therefore its action weaker.

The other motion of the lower jaw, viz. when the lateral teeth are used, is somewhat different from the former. In opening the mouth one condyle slides a little forwards, and the other slides a little further back into its cavity; this throws the jaw a little to that side, just enough to bring the lower teeth directly under their corresponding teeth in the upper jaw: this is done either in dividing or holding of substances, and these are the teeth that are generally used in the last-mentioned action. When the true grinding motion is to be performed, a greater degree of this last motion takes place; that is, the condyle of the opposite side is brought further forwards, and the condyle of the same side is drawn further back into the cavity of the temporal bone, and the jaw is a little depressed. This is only preparatory for the effect to be produced, for the moving back of the first-mentioned condyle into the socket is what produces the effect in mastication.

The lateral teeth in both jaws are adapted to this oblique motion. In the lower they are turned a little inwards, that they may act more in the direction of their axis; and here the alveolar process is strongest upon the outside, being there supported by the ridge at the root of the coronoid process. In the upper jaw the obliquity of the teeth is the reverse, that is, they are turned outwards, for the same reason; and the longest fang of the grinders is upon the inside, where the socket is strengthened by the bony partition between the antrum and nose. Hence it is that the teeth of the lower jaw have their outer edges worn down first, and *vice versâ* in the upper jaw.

General Comparisons between the Motion of the Jaw in young and in old People.

In children who have not yet teeth there does not seem to be a sliding motion in the lower jaw. The articular eminence of the temporal bone is not yet formed, and the cavity is not larger than the condyle; therefore the centre of motion in such must be in the condyle. In old people who have lost their teeth the centre of motion appears to be in the condyles, and the motion of their jaw to be only depression and elevation. They never depress the jaw sufficiently to bring the condyle forwards on the eminence, because in them the mouth is sufficiently opened when the jaw is in its natural position.

Hence it is that in old people the gums of the two jaws do not meet in the fore part of the mouth*, and they cannot bite at that part so well as at the side of the jaw; and, instead of the grinding motion, which would be useless where there are no grinders, they bruise their food rather by a simple motion of the jaw upwards and downwards.

It is from the want of teeth in both these ages that the face is shorter in proportion to its breadth. In an old person, after the teeth are gone the face is shorter while the mouth is shut by almost the whole lengths of the teeth in both jaws; that is, about an inch and a half.

From the want of teeth, too, at both those ages, the cavity of the mouth is then smaller, and the tongue seems too large and unmanageable, more especially in old people. In these last we observe also that the chin projects forwards in proportion as the mouth is shut, because the basis of the lower jaw (which is all that now remains,) describes a wider circle than the alveolar process in younger people. The jaws do not project so much forwards in a child as in an adult; hence the face is flatter, especially at the lower part. In proportion as the last grinders are produced, the sides of the curve formed by the jaws become longer, and push forward the fore part, none of the additional part passing backwards. The fore part also continues nearly of the same size, so that the whole jaw is longer in proportion to its breadth, and projects further forwards.

Of the Formation of the Alveolar Processes.

Having considered the alveolar processes in their adult, or perfect state, we shall next examine and trace them from their beginning.

We may observe the beginning of the alveolar process at a very early period. In a fœtus of three or four months it is only a longitudinal groove, deeper and narrower forwards, and becoming gradually more shallow and wider backwards : instead of bony partitions, dividing that groove into a number of sockets, there are only slight ridges across the bottom and sides, with intermediate depressions, which mark the situation of the future alveoli†.

In the lower jaw the vessels and nerves run along the bottom of this alveolar cavity in a slight groove, which afterwards becomes a complete and distinct bony canal.

---

* Pl. IV., where the symphysis of the lower jaw, when the mouth is shut, projects considerably further forwards than that of the upper.

† Pl. VI. f. 1, 2.

The alveolar process grows with the teeth, and for some time keeps the start of them. The ridges which are to make the partitions shoot from the sides across the canal, at the mouth of the cell, forming hollow arches : this change happens first at the anterior part of the jaws*. As each cell becomes deeper, its mouth also grows narrower, and at length is almost, but not quite, closed over the contained tooth.

The disposition for contracting the mouth of the cell is chiefly in the outer plate of the bone, which occasions the contracted orifices of the cells to be nearer the inner edge of the jaw†. The reason, perhaps, why the bone shoots over, and almost covers the tooth, is that the gum may be firmly supported before the teeth have come through.

The alveoli which belong to the adult grinders are formed in another manner : in the lower jaw they would seem to be the remains of the root of the coronoid process‡, for the cells are formed for those teeth in the root of that process ; and in proportion as the body of the bone, and the cells already formed, push forwards from under that process, the succeeding cells and their teeth are formed, and pushed forward in the same manner.

In the upper jaw there are cells formed in the tubercles for the young grinders, which at first are very shallow, and become deeper and deeper as the teeth grow ; and they grow somewhat faster, so as almost to inclose the whole tooth before it is ready to push its way through that inclosure and gum§. There is a succession of these till the whole three grinders are formed.

Of the Formation of the Teeth in the Fœtus.

The depressions or first rudiments of the alveoli observable in a fœtus of three or four months, are filled with four or five little pulpy substances, which are not very distinct at this age. About the fifth month both the processes themselves and the pulpy substances become more distinct, the anterior of which are the most complete. About this age, too, the ossifications begin on the edge of the first incisores. The cuspidati are not in the same circular line with the rest, but somewhat on the outside, making a projection there at this age, there not being sufficient room for them.

About the sixth or seventh month the edges or tips of all these five sub-

* Pl. VI. f. 1, 2, 3, 4, 5, 6.
† Pl. VI., which is most remarkable in those of the grinders, as the alveoli of these are not opened for the exit of the teeth.
‡ Pl. VI. f. 7. § Pl. VI. f. 11.

stances have begun to ossify, and the first of them is a little advanced*;
and besides these, the pulp of the sixth tooth has begun to be formed:
it is situated in the tubercle of the upper jaw, and under and on the inside of the coronoid process in the lower jaw. So that at this age, in
both jaws, there are in all twenty teeth which have begun to ossify, and
the stamina of twenty-four. They may be divided into the incisores,
cuspidati, and molares, for at this age there are no bicuspides, the two
last teeth on each side of both jaws having all the characteristics and
answering all the purposes of the true molares in the adult, though when
these first molares fall out their places are taken by the bicuspides.

The teeth gradually advance in their ossification, and about the seventh, eighth, or ninth month after birth, the incisores begin to cut or
pass through the gums, first, generally, in the lower jaw. Before this
time the ossifications in the third grinder, or that which makes the first
in the adult, have begun†.

The cuspidati and molares of the fœtus are not formed so fast as the
incisores; they generally all appear nearly about the same time, viz.
about the twentieth or twenty-fourth month; however, the first grinder
is often more advanced within the socket than the cuspidatus, and most
commonly appears before it.

These twenty are the only teeth that are of use to the child from the
seventh, eighth, or ninth month, till the twelfth or fourteenth year.
These are called the temporary, or milk teeth, because they are all shed
between the years of seven and fourteen, and are supplied by others.

Of the Cause of Pain in Dentition.

These twenty teeth in cutting the gum give pain, and produce many
other symptoms which often prove fatal to children in dentition. It
has been generally supposed that these symptoms arise from the tooth's
pressing upon the inside of the gum, and working its way mechanically;
but the following observations seem to be nearer the truth.

The teeth, when they begin to press against the gum, irritate it, and
commonly give pain. The gums are then affected with heat, swelling,
redness, and the other symptoms of inflammation. The gum is not cut
through by simple or mechanical pressure, but the irritation and consequent inflammation produces a thinning or wasting of the gum at
this part; for it often happens, that when an extraneous or a dead sub-

---

* Pl. VII. f. 1 & 2, where these ossifications are represented.

† Pl. VII. f. 3, where the first incisors had cut the gum, and where the third grinder
in the child, or first in the adult, had begun to ossify.

stance is contained in the body, it produces a destruction of the part between it and that part of the skin which is nearest it, and seldom of the other parts, excepting those between it and the surface of a cavity opening externally, and that by no means so frequently; and in those cases there is an absorption of the solids, or of the part destroyed, not a melting down or solution of them into pus. The teeth are to be looked upon as extraneous bodies with respect to the gum, and as such they irritate the inside of that part in the same manner as the pus of an abscess, an exfoliation of a bone, or any other extraneous body, and therefore produce the same symptoms, excepting only the formation of matter. If, therefore, these symptoms attend the cutting of the teeth, there can be no doubt of the propriety of opening the way for them; nor is it ever, as far as I have observed, attended with any dangerous consequence[a].

Of the Formation and Progress of the Adult Teeth.

Having now considered the first formation and the progress of the temporary teeth, we shall next describe the formation of those teeth which are to serve through life.

In this inquiry, to avoid confusion, I shall confine the description to the teeth in the lower jaw, for the only difference between those in the two jaws is in the time of their appearance, and generally it is later in the upper jaw. Their formation and appearance proceed not regularly from the first incisor backwards to the dens sapientiæ, but begin at two points on each side of both jaws, viz. at the first incisor and at the first molaris. The teeth between these two points make a quicker progress than those behind.

The pulps of the first adult incisor and of the first adult molaris begin to appear in a fœtus of seven or eight months; and five or six months after birth the ossification begins in them. Soon after birth the

---

a [There can indeed be no doubt that the emancipation of the rising tooth is occasioned by absorption of the gum, but it is also probable that this absorption is increased, if not wholly produced, by the pressure of its edge on the horizontal surface of the tooth. It appears probable, therefore, that when, in consequence of the rapid elongation of the root, the crown of the tooth rises faster than this process for the removal of the containing parts goes on, an undue pressure takes place on the inside of the gum, and local inflammation, accompanied by much constitutional disturbance, is the result. The mere existence of the tooth in contact with the gum "as an extraneous body," would not account for all this disturbance, for after the gums are lanced the tooth is still in contact with the soft parts; but because the pressure is thus taken off, the irritation immediately subsides.]

pulps of the second incisor and cuspidatus begin to be formed, and about eight or nine months afterwards they begin to ossify. About the fifth or sixth year the first bicuspis appears ; about the sixth or seventh, the second bicuspis and the second molaris ; and about the twelfth, the third molaris, or dens sapientiæ.

The first five may be called the permanent teeth : they differ from the temporary in having larger fangs. The permanent incisores and cuspidati are much thicker and broader; and the molares are succeeded by bicuspides, which are smaller, and have but one fang.

All these permanent or succeeding teeth are formed in distinct alveoli of their own, so that they do not fill up the old sockets of the temporary teeth, but have their new alveoli formed as the old ones decay*.

The first incisor is placed on the inside of the root of the corresponding temporary tooth, and deeper in the jaw. The second incisor and the cuspidatus begin to be formed on the inside, and somewhat under the temporary second incisor and cuspidatus. These three are all situated much in the same manner with respect to the first set, but as they are larger they are placed somewhat further back in the circle of the jaw.

The first bicuspis is placed under, and somewhat further back than the first temporary grinder, or fourth tooth of the child.

The second bicuspis is placed immediately under the second temporary grinder.

The second molaris is situated in the lengthening tubercle in the upper jaw, and directly under the coronoid process in the lower.

The third molaris, or dens sapientiæ, begins to form immediately under the coronoid process.

The first adult molaris comes to perfection and cuts the gum about the twelfth year of age, the second about the eighteenth, and the third, or dens sapientiæ, from the twentieth to the thirtieth ; so that the incisores and cuspidati require about six or seven years from their first appearance to come to perfection, the bicuspides about seven or eight, and the molares about twelve.

It sometimes happens that a third set of teeth appears in very old people; when this does happen it is in a very irregular manner, sometimes only one, at other times more, and now and then a complete set comes in both jaws. I never saw an instance of this kind but once, and there two fore teeth shot up in the lower jaw.

I should suppose that a new alveolar process must be also formed in such cases, in the same manner as in the production of the first and

* Pl. VI. f. 11, 12, 13.

second sets of teeth. From what I can learn, the age at which this happens is generally about seventy. From this circumstance, and another that sometimes happens to women at this age, it would appear that there is some effort in nature to renew the body at that period. When this set of teeth which happens so late in life is not complete, especially where they come in one jaw and not in the other, they are rather hurtful than useful, for in that case we are obliged to pull them out, as they only wound the opposite gum[a].

---

[a] [This account of the manner in which the permanent teeth are formed is exceedingly imperfect. The observations of Dr. Blake, (recorded first in his inaugural thesis, and afterwards published in English in an enlarged form,) first made known the process by which this extraordinary formation is produced. Subsequent investigations have confirmed the general views given by Blake, and I make no apology for offering the following account of the process, which is substantially the same as I have already given in another work.

The formation of the permanent teeth, although essentially proceeding upon the same general principle, and produced by means of similar structures as those by which the temporary ones are formed, differs in some very remarkable points from that process. The rudiments of the permanent teeth, instead of being original and independent, like those of the temporary, are, in fact, derived from them, and remain for a considerable time attached to and intimately connected with them. (See Pl. VIII. f. 9, 10, 11, 12.)

At an early period in the formation of the temporary teeth, by a process which reminds us of the gemmiparous reproduction in the lower grades, both of animal and vegetable life, the investing sac, or capsule, gives off a small process, a bud containing a portion of the essential rudiments, namely, the pulp, covered by its proper membrane. This constitutes the rudiment of the permanent tooth. It commences in a small thickening on one side of the parent sac, which gradually becomes more and more circumscribed, and at length assumes a distinct form, though still connected with it by a peduncle, which is nothing more than a process of the investing sac. For a time the new rudiment is contained within the same alveolus with its parent, which is excavated by the absorbents for its reception, by a process almost unparalleled in the phenomena of physiology. It is not produced by the pressure of the new rudiment, as has been erroneously believed, but commences in the cancelli of the bone immediately within its smooth surface, thus constituting what may be termed a process of anticipation. The new cell, after being sufficiently excavated, and as the rudiment continues to increase, is gradually separated from the former one, by being more and more deeply excavated in the substance of the bone, and also by the deposition of a bony partition between them; and at length the new rudiment is shut up in its proper socket, though still connected with the temporary tooth by the cord or process of the capsule already described, which has in the mean time been gradually attenuated and elongated.

The situation of each permanent rudiment when its corresponding temporary tooth has made its appearance through the gum, is beneath and a little behind the latter, and rather further from the centre of the jaw. From the preceding statement, then, it will be readily understood that the upper part of the new sac being, by means of the cord, connected with the gum, assumes, by and by, the same relation to that substance as that which the temporary rudiment, as before described, had originally sustained; whilst, from its substance being deeply imbedded in the jaw, the vessels and nerves which had entered into the composition of the new process of pulp in its first production, probably became so enlarged and modified in their structure as ultimately to form the true dental

The Manner in which a Tooth is formed.

The body of the tooth is formed first, afterwards the enamel and fangs are added to it. All the teeth are produced from a kind of pulpy substance, which is pretty firm in its texture, transparent, excepting at the surface, where it adheres to the jaw, and has at first the shape of the bodies of the teeth which are to be formed from it*. These pulpy substances are very vascular: they adhere only at one part to the jaw, viz. at the bottom of the cavity which is to form the socket, and at that place their vessels enter, so that they are prominent and somewhat loose in the bony cavity which lodges them.

They grow nearly as large as the body of the tooth before the ossification begins, and increase a little for some time after the ossification has begun. They are surrounded by a membrane, which is not connected with them, excepting at their root or surface of adhesion. This membrane adheres by its outer surface all around the bony cavity in the jaw, and also to the gum where it covers the alveoli.

When the pulp is very young, as in the foetus of six or seven months, this membrane itself is pretty thick and gelatinous†. We can examine it best in a new-born child, and we find it made up of two lamellæ, an external and internal: the external is soft and spongy, without any vessels; the other is much firmer and extremely vascular, its vessels coming from those that are going to the pulp of the tooth: it makes a kind of capsule for the pulp and body of the tooth. While the tooth is within the gum there is always a mucilaginous fluid, like the synovia in the joints, between this membrane and the pulp of the tooth.

When the tooth cuts the gum, this membrane likewise is perforated, after which it begins to waste, and is entirely gone by the time the tooth is fully formed, for the lower part of the membrane continues to adhere to the neck of the tooth, which has now risen as high as the edge of the gum[a].

* Pl. VIII. f. 4, 5, 6.   † Pl. VIII. f. 1, 2.

---

branches. This is much more probable than to suppose that a new set of nerves and vessels is given off from the maxillary branches to join the pulps at a distance, through an intervening layer of bone of an indefinite thickness, to supply every new tooth.

We now, therefore, find the new rudiment in a state nearly analogous to that in which the parent tooth was originally placed, and with similar relations to the surrounding parts; the sac above, attached to the gum, and the pulp beneath, (covered with its proper membrane,) connected by its vessels &c. with the jaws.]

[a] [The statement that the bone of a tooth is produced from the pulp is erroneous. This substance constitutes only the mould upon which the ossification is formed, be-

Of the Ossification of a Tooth upon the Pulp.

The beginning of the ossification upon the pulp is by one point, or more, according to the kind of tooth. In the incisores it is generally by three points, the middle one being the highest, and the first that begins to ossify. The cuspidatus begins by one point only ; the bicuspis by two, one external, which is the first and the highest, and the other internal. The molares, either in a child or an adult, begin by four or five ossifications, one on each point, the external always the first*. Where the teeth begin to ossify at one point only, that ossification gradually advances till the tooth is entirely completed† ; but if there is more than one point of ossification, each ossification increases till their bases come in contact with one another, and there all unite into one‡, after which they advance in growth as one ossification.

The ossifications in their progress become thicker and thicker where they first began, but increase faster on the edges of the teeth; so as thence to become more and more hollow, and the cavity becomes deeper§. As the ossification advances, it gradually surrounds the pulp till the whole is covered by bone, excepting the under surface ; and while the ossifications advance, that part of the pulp which is covered by bone is always more vascular than the part which is not yet covered‖.

The adhesion of the pulp to the new-formed tooth or bone is very

---

* Pl. VII. f. 1, where some of the distinct ossifications may be observed.

† Pl. VII. f. 1, 2, 3.   ‡ Pl. VII. f. 2.

§ Pl. VIII. f. 14, *a, b, c, d,* two rows of incisors sawed down the middle, the highest of the child, the other of the adult: *e, f, g,* two rows of grinders showing the same circumstances.   ‖ Pl. VIII. f. 5, 6.

---

tween which and the pulp is placed a membrane of extreme tenuity, which I have termed the proper membrane of the pulp. It is slightly attached to the surface of the pulp, which it completely covers, and it is from the outer surface of this membrane that the bone is secreted. As the pulp recedes on the deposit of the successive laminæ of bone, the ossific membrane continues to cover it, and ultimately forms the well-known membrane lining the internal cavity of the perfect tooth.

The double investing membrane or sac which surrounds the whole rudiment as far as the neck of the tooth, and no further, has been proved, by repeated injections, to be vascular throughout, though Hunter states the internal, and Blake the external layer to be exclusively so. It is from the inner surface of this capsule that the enamel is secreted, as will be more particularly noticed hereafter. As soon as the enamel is secreted the capsule becomes absorbed, beginning at the edge or horizontal surface of the tooth, where the enamel is first deposited. It is, therefore, not perforated by the rising of the tooth, as inferred in the text, but absorbed as soon as it has performed its single function.]

slight, for it can always be separated from it without any apparent violence, nor are there any vessels going from the one to the other; the
place, however, where it is most strongly attached is round the edge of
the bony part, which is the last part formed. When the bone has covered all the pulp, it begins to contract a little and becomes somewhat
rounded, making that part of the tooth which is called the neck; and
from this place the fangs begin*. When the fangs form, they push up
the bodies of the teeth through the sockets, which waste, and afterwards through the gum, which also wastes, as has been explained upon
the cutting of the teeth; for before this time the rising of the teeth is
scarce observable, as the pulp was at first nearly of the size of the body
of the tooth itself, and wasted nearly in proportion to the increase of
the whole ossification.

The pulp has originally no process answering to the fang† ; but as
the cavity in the body of the tooth is filled up by the ossification, the
pulp is lengthened into a fang. The fang grows in length and rises
higher and higher in the socket till the whole body of the tooth is
pushed out. The socket at the same time contracts at its bottom and
grasping the neck or beginning fang, adheres to it and rises with it, which
contraction is continued through the whole length of the socket as the
fang rises ; or the socket which contained the body of the tooth, being
too large for the fang, is wasted or absorbed into the constitution, and
a new alveolar portion is raised with the fang ; whence in reality the
fang does not sink or descend into the jaw. Both in the body and in
the fang of a growing tooth, the extreme edge of the ossification is so
thin, transparent, and flexible, that it would appear rather to be horny
than bony, very much like the mouth or edge of the shell of a snail
when it is growing ; and indeed it would seem to grow much in the
same manner‡, and the ossified part of a tooth would seem to have
much the same connexion with the pulp as a snail has with its shell.

As the tooth grows, its cavity becomes gradually smaller, especially
towards the point of the fang. In tracing the formation of the fang of
a tooth we hitherto have been supposing it to be single, but where
there are two or more it is somewhat different and more complicated.

When the body of a molaris is formed, there is but one general cavity in the body of the tooth, from the brim of which the ossification
is to shoot, so as to form two or three fangs§. If two only, then the
opposite parts of the brim of the cavity of the tooth shoot across where
the pulp adheres to the jaw, meet in the middle, and thereby divide

---

* Pl. VIII. f. 13, 14, 15.　　　　　　　† Pl. VIII. f. 1, 4, 5, 6.
‡ Pl. VIII. f. 13, 14, 15.　　　　　　　§ Pl. VIII. f. 13, A, A.

the mouth of the cavity into two openings *; and from the edges of these two openings the two fangs grow †.

We often find that a distinct ossification begins in the middle of the general cavity upon the root of the pulp, and two processes coming from the opposite edges of the bony shell join it; which answers the same purpose.

When there are three fangs, we see three processes coming from so many points of the brim of the cavity, which meet in the centre and divide the whole into three openings‡; and from these are formed the three fangs §. We often find the fangs forked at their points, especially in the bicuspides. In this case the sides of the fang as it grows come close together in the middle, making a longitudinal groove on the outside; and this union of the opposite sides divides the mouth of the growing fang into two orifices, from which the two points are formed.

By the observations which I have made in unravelling the texture of the teeth when softened by an acid, and from observing the disposition of the red parts in the tooth of growing animals interruptedly fed with madder, I find that the bony part of a tooth is formed of lamellæ placed one within another. The outer lamella is the first formed and is the shortest; the more internal lamellæ lengthen gradually towards the fang, by which means, in proportion as the tooth grows longer, its cavity grows smaller, and its sides grow thicker ‖.

How the earthy and animal substance of the tooth is deposited on the surface of the pulp is not perhaps to be explained [a].

Of the Formation of the Enamel.

In speaking of the enamel we postponed treating of its formation till it could be more clearly understood; and now we shall previously describe some parts which we apprehend to be subservient to its formation, much in the same manner as the pulp is to the body of the tooth.

From its situation and from the manner in which the teeth grow, one would imagine that the enamel is first formed; but the bony part begins first, and very soon after the enamel is formed upon it. There is an-

* Pl. VIII. f. 13, B.　　　　　　　　 † Pl. VIII. f. 13, C, D.
‡ Pl. VIII. f. 13, F, G.　　　　　　　§ Pl. VIII. f. 13, H, I, K.
‖ Pl. VIII. f. 7, 8.

[a] This is explained in the note to the preceding section.

other pulpy substance opposite to that which we have described : it adheres to the inside of the capsule, where the gum is joined to it, and
its opposite surface lies in contact with the basis of the above-described
pulp, and afterwards with the new-formed basis of the tooth. Whatever
eminences or cavities the one has, the other has the same, but reversed,
so that they are moulded exactly to each other.

In the incisores it lies in contact, not with the sharper cutting edge
of the pulp or tooth, but against the hollowed inside of the tooth ; and
in the molares it is placed directly against their base, like a tooth of the
opposite jaw. It is thinner than the other pulp, and decreases in
proportion as the teeth advance. It does not seem to be very vascular.
The best time for examining it is in a fœtus of seven or eight months
old.

In the graminivorous animal, such as the horse, cow, &c., whose
teeth have the enamel intermixed with the bony part*, and whose teeth,
when forming, have as many interstices as there are continuations of
the enamel, we find processes from the pulp passing down into those
interstices as far as the pulp which the tooth is formed from, and there
coming into contact with it.

After the points of the first-described pulp have begun to ossify, a thin
covering of enamel is spread over them, which increases in thickness
till some time before the tooth begins to cut the gum.

The enamel appears to be secreted from the pulp above described,
and perhaps from the capsule which incloses the body of the tooth.
That it is from the pulp and capsule seems evident in the horse, ass,
ox, sheep, &c., therefore we have little reason to doubt of it in the human species. It is a calcareous earth, probably dissolved in the juices
of our body, and thrown out from these parts, which act here as a gland.
After it is secreted, the earth is attracted by the bony part of the tooth
which is already formed, and upon that surface it crystallizes.

The operation is similar to the formation of the shell of the egg, the
stone in the kidneys and bladder, and the gall stone. This accounts
for the striated crystallized appearance which the enamel has when
broken, and also for the direction of these striæ †.

The enamel is thicker at the points and basis than at the neck of the
teeth, which may be easily accounted for from its manner of formation ;
for if we suppose it to be always secreting, and laid equally over the

* Pl. V. f. 20, 21.

† The author has made many experiments on the formation of different calculi, and
finds they are formed by crystallization, which were communicated to his brother, and
taught by him to his pupils in 1761, and which he proposes to give to the public as soon
as his time will permit.

whole surface, as the tooth grows, the first formed will be the thickest; and the neck of the tooth, which is the last-formed part inclosed in this capsule, must have the thinnest coat; and the fang, where the periosteum adheres, and leaves no vacant space, will have none of the enamel.

At its first formation it is not very hard; for by exposing a very young tooth to the air the enamel cracks and looks rough; but by the time that the teeth cut the gum, the enamel seems to be as hard as ever it is afterwards; so that the air seems to have no effect in hardening it [a].

Of the Manner of Shedding the Teeth.

An opinion has commonly prevailed that the first set of teeth is pushed out by the second; this, however, is very far from being the case: and were it so, it would be attended with a very obvious inconvenience; for, were a tooth pushed out by one underneath, that tooth must rise in proportion to the growth of the succeeding one, and stand in the same proportion above the rest. But this circumstance never happens, neither can it, for the succeeding teeth are formed in new and distinct sockets, and generally the incisores and the cuspidati of the second set are situated on the inside of the corresponding teeth of the first set [*]; and we find that in proportion to the growth of the succeeding teeth, the fangs of the first set decay, till the whole of the fang is so far destroyed that nothing remains but the neck, or that part of the fang to which the gum adheres [†], and then the least force pushes the tooth out. It would be very natural to suppose that this was owing

* Pl. VI. f. 12, 13.

† Pl. VIII. f. 16, 17, & 18, which show the gradual decay in the single and double teeth, and also in one grinder of a horse.

---

[a] [According to the most accurate observations which I have been able to make, and they are confirmed by those of others, the substance which Hunter terms "another pulpy substance," adhering to the inside of the capsule, is nothing more than a thickened and turgid state of the inner layer of the capsule itself, surcharged with blood and probably also with the earthy matter which it is about to deposit, constituting the future enamel-covering of the crown of the tooth. This thickening appears to be somewhat analogous to that extraordinary turgescence which is observable in the mantle of certain species of snail, as our own *Helix Pomatia* immediately before the calcareous winter operculum is poured out from every part of its surface.

The enamel when just deposited is not much more solid than thick cream. It soon sets, but is at first but little coherent, being easily pulverized; it gradually, however, assumes its crystalline form, becomes semitransparent, and extremely hard.]

to a constant pressure from the rising teeth against the fangs or sockets of the first set, but it is not so; for the new alveoli rise with the new teeth, and the old alveoli decay in proportion as the fangs of the old teeth decay, and when the first set falls out, the succeeding teeth are so far from having destroyed, by their pressure, the parts against which they might be supposed to push, that they are still inclosed and co-vered by a complete bony socket. From this we see that the change is not produced by a mechanical pressure, but is a particular process in the animal œconomy.

I have seen two or three jaws where the second temporary grinders were shedding in the common way, without any tooth underneath; and in one jaw, where both the grinders were shedding, I met with the same circumstance.

A remarkable instance of this sort occurred to me in a lady who de-sired me to look at a loose tooth, which I found was the last temporary tooth not yet shed. I desired that it might be drawn out, and told her it was of no use and could not by any art be fixed, as it was one of the teeth that is naturally shed, and that another might come in its place : however, she was disappointed.

These cases prove evidently, that in shedding, the first teeth are not pushed out by the second set, but that they grow loose and fall out of their own accord. That the succeeding teeth have some influence on the shedding of the temporary set is proved by those very cases ; since in one of the first mentioned the person was above twenty years of age, and in the other the lady was thirty; and it is reasonable to believe, that the shedding of these teeth was so late in those instances from the want of the influence, whatever it is, of the new teeth. When the in-cisores and cuspidati of the new set are a little advanced, but long be-fore they appear through their bony sockets, there are small holes leading to them on the inside, or behind the temporary sockets and teeth ; and these holes grow larger and larger, till at last the body of the tooth passes quite through them[a].

Of the Growth of the Two Jaws.

As a knowledge of the manner in which the two jaws grow will lead

---

[a] [In the last paragraph of the section is an additional instance of the total misunder-standing of the relation of the permanent to the temporary teeth during their formation. The holes which have been described in a former note, as the foramina through which the communicating cord passes from the permanent rudiment to the neck of the tempo-rary tooth are here erroneously stated to be the commencement of the openings through which the permanent teeth pass in their subsequent progress. See Pl. VIII. f. 9, 10, 11, 12.]

to the better understanding of the shedding of the teeth, and as the jaws seem to differ, in their manner of growing, from other bones, and also vary according to the age, it will be here proper to give some account of their growth.

In a fœtus three or four months old, we have described the marks of four or five teeth, which occupy the whole length of the upper jaw, and all that part of the lower which lies before the coronoid process, for the fifth tooth is somewhat under that process *.

These five marks become larger, and the jaw-bones of course increase in all directions, but more considerably backwards; for in a fœtus of seven or eight months the marks of six teeth in each side of both jaws are to be observed, and the sixth seems to be in the place where the fifth was; so that in these last four months the jaw has grown in all directions in proportion to the increased size of the teeth, and besides has lengthened itself at its posterior end as much as the whole breadth of the socket of that sixth tooth†.

The jaw still increases in all points till twelve months after birth, when the bodies of all the six teeth are pretty well formed; but it never after increases in length between the symphysis and the sixth tooth; and from this time, too, the alveolar process, which makes the anterior part of the arches of both jaws, never becomes a section of a larger circle, whence the lower part of a child's face is flatter, or not so projecting forwards as in the adult‡.

After this time the jaws lengthen only at their posterior ends; so that the sixth tooth, which was under the coronoid process in the lower jaw, and in the tubercles of the upper jaw of the fœtus, is at last, viz. in the eighth or ninth year, placed before these parts; and then the seventh tooth appears in the place which the sixth occupied, with respect to the coronoid process and tubercle; and about the twelfth or fourteenth year, the eighth tooth is situated where the seventh was placed. At the age of eighteen or twenty, the eighth tooth is found before the coronoid process in the lower jaw and under, or somewhat before the tubercle in the upper jaw, which tubercle is no more than a succession of sockets for the teeth till they are completely formed.

In a young child the cavity in the temporal bone for the articulation of the jaw is nearly in a line with the gums of the upper jaw; and for this reason the condyle of the lower jaw is nearly in the same line §; but afterwards, by the addition of the alveolar process and teeth, the

* Pl. VI. f. 1, 2.

† Pl. VI. f. 3, 4, 5, & 6, for the general increase of the jaws, but more particularly backwards.

‡ Pl. VI. f. 7. for these facts.   § Pl. VI. f. 10.

line of the gums in the upper jaw descends considerably below the articular cavity; and for that reason the condyloid process is then lengthened in the same proportion.

In old people who have lost all their teeth, the articulation comes again into the same line with the gums of the upper jaw *; but in the lower jaw, the condyles cannot be diminished again for accommodating it to the upper, so that it necessarily projects beyond the gums of the upper jaw at the fore part. When the mouth is shut, the projection of the jaw at the chin fits the two jaws to each other at that place where the grinders were situated, and where the strength of mastication lies; for if the chin was not further from the centre of motion than the gums of the upper jaw, at the fore part, the jaws, in such people as have lost all their teeth, would meet in a point at the fore part, like a pair of pincers, and be at a considerable distance behind †.

The Reason for the Shedding of the Teeth.

As the shedding of the teeth is a very singular process in the animal œconomy, many reasons have been assigned for it; but these reasons have not carried along with them that conviction which is desired. Authors have not fully considered the appearances; which naturally explain themselves; nor have they considered the advantages necessarily arising from the size and construction of only such a number as the first set; nor have they considered fully the disadvantages that such size and construction would have, if continued when it is necessary to have a great number, which is the case with the adult.

We shall consider these advantages in a child where the shedding-teeth are all completely formed, which will be setting them in the clearest point of light; and also the disadvantages that would occur if in the adult these were not changed for another set somewhat different.

If the child had been so contrived as not to have required teeth till the time of the second set appearing, there would have been no occasion for a new set; but the jaw-bones being considerably smaller in children than in adults, and it being necessary that they should have two grinders, there is not room for incisores and cuspidati of sufficient size to serve through life; and the first-formed grinders having necessarily too small fangs, and the jaw increasing at the back part only, these two grinders would have been protruded too far forwards, and at too great a distance from the centre of motion. This variation in the

* Pl. IV.   † Ibid.

size of the teeth is likewise a reason why the second set are not formed in the sockets of the first, and why the old sockets are destroyed.

These circumstances, with regard to the shedding of the teeth, contradict the notion of the second set being made broader and thicker by the resistance they meet with in pushing out the first. For were we, on a partial view of the subject, to admit the supposition, the bicuspides would effectually overturn our hypothesis, because here the second set are much smaller than the first, and yet the resistance would be greater to them than to the incisores.

From the manner in which the teeth are shed, it is evident that drawing a temporary tooth for the easier protrusion of the one underneath, will be of no great service; for in general it falls out before the other can touch it. But it is often of much more service to pull out the neighbouring or adjacent temporary tooth, for we must be convinced by what has been advanced with regard to the changes in size, that excepting the whole were to be shed at the same time, or the order of shedding, viz. from before backwards, were to be inverted, that the second set of incisores and cuspidati must be pinched in room till the grinders are also shed, and therefore we find it often of use to draw a temporary tooth that is placed further back; and it would, perhaps, be right upon the whole, always to draw at least the first grinder, and perhaps, some time after, the second grinder also[a].

Of the Cavity filling up as the Teeth wear down.

A tooth very often wears down so low that its cavity would be exposed if no other alteration were produced in it. To prevent this, Na-

---

a [The practice here recommended, "always to draw at least the first grinder" of the temporary set, has been but too much followed by the interested or ignorant, who have readily shielded their malpractice under the authority of Hunter's name. The early extraction of any of the temporary teeth to make room for the permanent ones is rarely necessary, and it is on all accounts to be deprecated, unless the peculiar circumstances of the case imperatively call for it. But the removal of the large molar teeth of the child, in *anticipation* of a future deficiency of room, is so obviously uncalled for, and such a wanton interference with the usual process of nature, that we cannot but wonder at its being proposed as a general rule, even were there no positive evils to be apprehended from it: but this is not all; not only does the premature removal of the temporary molares endanger the perfect formation of the bicuspides which succeed them, by the forcible laceration of the connecting cord before described, but, if it take place before the permanent teeth are ready to fall into their ultimate situation, the jaw will contract as the child grows, and the second set of teeth will be forced into an irregular position, from permanent want of room. These arguments hold good against the too early removal of any of the deciduous teeth.]

ture has taken care that the bottom part of the cavity should be filled up by new matter in proportion as the surface of the teeth is worn down. This new matter may be easily known from the old, for when a tooth has been worn down almost to the neck, a spot may always be seen in the middle, which is more transparent, and at the same time of a darker colour (occasioned in some measure by the dark cavity under it), and generally softer than the other*. Any person may be convinced of thetruth of these observations by taking two teeth of the same class, but of very different ages, one just completely formed, the other worn down almost to its neck. In the last he will observe the dark spot in the centre, and if as much is cut off from the complete tooth as has been worn off from the old one, the cavity of the young tooth will be found cut through; and on examining the other, its cavity will be found filled up below that surface. Now this observation contra-dicts the idea of the hole leading into the cavity of the tooth being closed up; and what is still a further proof of it, I have been able to inject vessels in the cavities of the teeth in very old people when the alveolar process has been gone, and the teeth very loose in the gum.

Old people are often found to have very good sets of teeth, only pretty much worn down. The reason of this is, that such people never had any disorder in their teeth, or alveolar processes, sufficient to occasion the falling of one tooth. For if by accident one tooth is lost, the rest will necessarily fail in some degree, even though they are sound, and likely to remain so, had not this accident happened; and this weakening cause is greater in proportion to the number that are lost. From this observation we see that the teeth support one another[a].

Of the Continual Growth of the Teeth.

It has been asserted that the teeth are continually growing, and that the abrasion is sufficient to keep them always of the same length; but

* Pl. V. f. 25, 26.

---

[a] [The filling up of the internal cavity of the teeth in old people here alluded to, appears to be consequent upon the loss of substance from the surface. As the superstratum of bone becomes thinner by abrasion, the membrane lining the internal cavity, from which, as I have before shown, *the bone of the tooth was originally produced,* now again resumes its ossific action, and produces a fresh layer of bony matter, which in some cases at length fills the socket, and obliterates the membrane from which it has been secreted. This is particularly the case in sailors who have lived much upon hard biscuits, a circumstance which tends greatly to accelerate this abrasion of the surface, a process perfectly and obviously analogous to that of the wearing of the teeth in graminivorous animals.]

we find that they grow at once to their full length, and that they gradually wear down afterwards, and that there is not even the appearance of their continuing to grow. The teeth would probably project a little further out of the gum if they were not opposed by those in the opposite jaw; for in young people who had lost a tooth before the rest had come to their full length, I have seen the opposite tooth project a little beyond the rest before they were at all worn down. It may be further observed, that when a tooth is lost, the opposite one may project from the disposition of the alveolar process to rise higher, and fill up at the bottom of the sockets; and the want of that natural pressure seems to give that disposition to these processes, which is best illustrated in those teeth which are formed deeper in their sockets than usual. As a proof that the teeth continue growing, it has been said that the space of a fallen tooth is almost filled up by the increased thickness of the two adjacent teeth, and the lengthening of that which is opposite. There is an evident fallacy in the case; either the observations have been made upon such jaws as above described, or the appearances have not been examined with sufficient accuracy; for when the space appears to have become narrow by the approximation of the two adjacent teeth, it is not owing to any increase of their breadth, but to their moving from that side where they are well supported to the other side, where they are not. For this reason they get an inclined direction; and I observe it extends to the several adjacent teeth in a proportionally less degree, and affects those which are behind more than those which are before the vacant space.

In the lower jaw the back teeth are not fixed perpendicularly, but all inclined forward, and the depression of the jaw increases this position; the action of the teeth, when thrown out of the perpendicular, has also a tendency to increase that oblique direction, as a pair of scissors, in cutting, pushes everything forward, or from the centre of motion; therefore this alteration, I think, is most commonly observable in the lower jaw.

And that teeth are not actually always growing in breadth, must be obvious to every person who considers, that in many people, through life, the teeth stand so wide from each other that there are considerable spaces between them, which could not be the case if they were always growing in thickness.

We might add, too, that according to the hypothesis the dens sapientiæ should grow to an enormous size backward, because there it has no check from pressure; and in people where the dens sapientiæ is wanting in one jaw, which is very common, it should grow to an uncommon length in the opposite jaw, for the same reason. But neither of these things happens.

I need hardly take notice, that when a tooth has lost its opposite it will in time become really so much longer than the rest, as the others grow shorter by abrasion; and I observe that the tooth which is opposite to the empty space becomes in time not only longer, for the above-mentioned reason, but more pointed. The apex falls into the void space, and the two sides are rubbed away against the sides of the two approaching teeth next to that space.

The manner of their formation likewise shows that teeth cannot grow beyond a certain limited size. To illustrate this I may observe, that I have often, in the dead body of adults, found the left cuspidatus of the upper jaw with its points scarcely protruding out of the alveolar process, though the tooth was completely formed, and longer than the other by the whole point, which in that other was worn away*. This tooth, at its first formation, had been deeper in the jaw than what is common; and after it had grown to the ordinary size it grew no longer, though it had not the resistance of the opposite teeth to set bounds to its increase; yet commonly in these cases the tooth continues to project further and further through the gum, though this is not owing to its growing longer, but to the socket filling up behind it, and thereby continuing to push it out by slow degrees.

Of the Sensibility of the Teeth.

The teeth would seem to be very sensible, for they appear to be subject to great pain, and are easily and quickly affected by either heat or cold.

We may presume that the bony substance itself is not capable of conveying sensations to the mind, because it is worn down in mastication, and occasionally worked upon by operators in living bodies, without giving any sensation of pain in the part itself.

In the cavity of a tooth it is well known that there is exquisite sensibility, and it is likewise believed that this is owing to the nerve in that cavity. This nerve would seem to be more sensible than nerves are in common, as we do not observe the same violent effects from any other nerve in the body being exposed either by wound or sore, as we do from the exposure of the nerve of a tooth. Perhaps the reason of the intenseness, as well as the quickness of the sense of heat and cold in the teeth, may be owing to their communicating these to the nerve sooner than any other part of the body[a].

* Pl. VI. f. 8.

---

[a] [That the bony substance of the teeth "is itself capable of conveying sensation to the mind" is, notwithstanding the author's presumption to the contrary, easily proved. Whence otherwise arises that acute sensation so commonly felt when the neck of a tooth

Of Supernumerary Teeth.

We often meet with supernumerary teeth, and this, as well as some other variations, happens oftener in the upper than in the lower jaw, and, I believe, always in the incisores and cuspidati. I have only met with one instance of this sort, and it was in the upper jaw of a child about nine months old : there were the bodies of two teeth, in shape like the cuspidati, placed directly behind the bodies of the two first permanent incisores, so that there were three teeth in a row, placed behind one another, viz. the temporary incisor, the body of the permanent incisor, and that supernumerary tooth. The most remarkable circumstance was, that these supernumerary teeth were inverted, their points being turned upwards, and bended by the bone which was above them not giving way to their growth, as the alveolar process does.

It often happens that the incisores and cuspidati, in the upper jaw especially, are so irregularly placed as to give the appearance of a double row. I once saw a remarkable instance of this in a boy ; the second incisor in each side was placed further back than what is common, and the cuspidatus and first incisor closer together than if the second incisor had been directly between them, so that the appearance gave an idea of a second row of teeth.

This happens only in the adult set of teeth, and is owing to there not being room in the jaw for this second set, the jaw-bone being formed with.the first set of teeth, and never increasing afterwards ; so that if the adult set does not pass further back, they must overlap each other, and give the appearance of a second row[a].

Of the Use of the Teeth, so far as they affect the Voice.

The teeth serve principally for mastication, and that use need not be further explained.

---

is touched with the nail or with any sharp hard instrument, or when a portion of the enamel only is broken from the surface of a tooth? In the latter case every other part of the tooth may be touched without any sensation being produced, but as soon as the instrument comes in contact with the denuded portion of the bone, a painful acute sensation is instantly perceived.]

[a] [The occurrence of supernumerary teeth is not at all uncommon, and they are found not as Hunter supposes, only amongst the incisores and cuspidati, but not unfrequently also near the posterior molares. When found near the front of the mouth they always resemble a small and ill-formed cuspidatus, and when near the molares the crown is broader and truncated, somewhat like the neighbouring teeth. It is almost unnecessary to add that the case of irregularity mentioned in the second paragraph is one of very frequent occurrence.]

They serve likewise a secondary or subordinate purpose, giving strength and clearness to the sound of the voice, as is evident from the alteration produced in speaking, when the teeth are lost.

This alteration, however, may not depend entirely upon the teeth, but, in some measure, on the other organs of the voice having been accustomed to them ; and therefore when they are gone those other organs may be put out of their common play, and may not be able to adapt themselves so well to this new instrument. Yet I believe that habit in this case has no great effect, for those people seldom or never get the better of the defect; and young children who are shedding their teeth, and are, perhaps, without any fore teeth for half a year or more, always have that defect in their voice till the new teeth come, and as these grow the voice becomes clear again.

This use seems to be entirely in the fore teeth, for the loss of one of these makes a great alteration, and the loss of two or three grinders seems to have no sensible effect. As an argument for the use of the teeth in modifying the sound of the voice, we may observe, that the fore teeth come at a time when the child begins to articulate sounds, and at that time they are so loose in the gums that they can be of very little service in mastication.

Every defect in speech, arising from this defect in the organ, is generally attended with what we call a lisp. People who have lost all their teeth, and most old people for that reason, lose, in a great measure, their voice. This arises partly from the loss of the fore teeth, but principally from the loss of all the teeth, and of the alveolar processes of both jaws, by which means the mouth becomes too small for the tongue, and the lips and cheeks become flaccid, insomuch that the nicer movements of these parts, in the articulation of sounds, are obstructed, and thence the words and syllables are indistinctly pronounced and slurred, or run into one another.

Under what Class do the Human Teeth come.

Natural historians have been at great pains to prove, from the teeth, that man is not a carnivorous animal; but in this, as in many other things, they have not been accurate in their definitions; nor have they determined what a carnivorous animal is.

If they mean an animal that catches and kills his prey with his teeth, and eats that flesh of the prey just as it is killed, they are in the right; man is not in this sense a carnivorous animal, and therefore he has not teeth like those of a lion ; and this, I presume, is what they mean.

But if their meaning were that the human teeth are not fitted for eating meat that has been caught, killed, and dressed by art, in all the various ways that the superiority of the human mind can invent, they are in the wrong. Indeed, from this confined way of thinking, it would be hard to say what the human teeth are fitted for, because, by the same reasoning, man is not a graminivorous animal, as his teeth are not fitted for pulling vegetable food, &c. They are not made like those of cows or horses, for example.

The light in which we ought to view this subject is, that man is a more perfect or complicated animal than any other, and is not made, like others, to come at his food by his teeth, but by his hands, directed by his superior ingenuity, the teeth being given only for the purpose of chewing the food, in order to its more easy digestion ; and they, as well as his other organs of digestion, are fitted for the conversion of both animal and vegetable substances into blood, and thence he is able to live in a much greater variety of circumstances than any other animal, and has more opportunities of exercising the faculties of his mind. He ought, therefore, to be considered as a compound, fitted equally to live upon flesh and upon vegetables.

Of the Diseases of the Teeth.

The teeth are subject to diseases as well as other parts of the body. Whatever the disorder is that affects them, it is generally attended with pain; and from this, indeed, we commonly first know that they are affected.

Pain in the teeth proceeds, I believe, in a great measure from the air coming into contact with the nerve in the cavity of the tooth, for we seldom see people affected with the tooth-ache but when the cavity is exposed to the air.

It is not easy to say by what means the cavity comes to be exposed.

The most common disease to which the teeth are subject begins with a small dark-coloured speck, generally on the side of the tooth where it is not exposed to pressure ; from what cause this arises is hitherto unknown. The substance of the tooth thus discoloured gradually decays, and an opening is made into the cavity. As soon as the air is thereby admitted a considerable degree of pain arises, which is probably owing to the admission of the air, as it may be prevented by filling the cavity with lead, wax, &c. This pain is not always present; the food and other substances perhaps fill up the hole occasionally, and prevent the access of the air, and of consequence the pain, during the time they remain in it.   When an opening is made into the cavity of the tooth the inside begins to decay, the cavity becomes larger, the breath at the same time often acquires a putrid *fœtor*, the bone continues to decay till it is no longer able to support the pressure of the opposite tooth; it breaks and lays the cavity open.   We have not as yet found any means of preventing this disease, or of curing it; all that can be done is to fill the hole with lead, which prevents the pain and retards the decay; but after the tooth is broken this is not practicable, and for that reason it is then best to extract it.

It would be best of all to attempt the extraction of a tooth by drawing it in the direction of its axis, but that not being practicable by the instruments at present in use, which pull laterally, it is the next best to draw a tooth to that side where the alveolar process is weakest, which is the inside in the two last grinders on each side of the lower jaw, and the outside in all the others.

It generally happens in drawing a tooth that the alveolar process is broken, particularly when the grinders are extracted; but this is attended with no bad consequences, as that part of the alveolar process from which the tooth was extracted always decays.

In drawing a tooth the patient complains of a disagreeable jarring noise, which always happens when anything grates against the bones of the head[a].

Of Cleaning the Teeth.

From what was said of the nature and use of the enamel, it is evident that whatever is capable of destroying it must be hurtful; therefore all acids, gritty powders, and injudicious methods of scaling the teeth are prejudicial; but simply scaling the teeth, that is, clearing them of the stony concretions which frequently collect about their necks, while nothing is scraped off but that adventitious substance, is proper and useful.   If not removed by art, the quantity of the stony matter is apt to increase and to affect the gum.   This matter first begins to form on the tooth near to the gum; but not in the very angle, because the motion of the gum commonly prevents the accumulation of it at this part.   I have seen it cover not only the whole tooth, but a great part of the gum: in this case there is always an accumulation of

---

[a] [The introduction of forceps of various forms, and of simple elevators, has greatly facilitated the extraction of single-rooted teeth and of stumps; but the key instrument must still be acknowledged to be the most certain instrument in many, perhaps in most, cases.]

a very putrid matter, frequently considerable tenderness and ulceration of the gum, and scaling becomes absolutely necessary*.

Of Transplanting the Teeth.

From considering the almost constant variety of the size and shape of the same class of teeth in different people it would appear almost impossible to find the tooth of one person that should fit, with any degree of exactness, the socket of another; and this observation is supported, and indeed would seem to be proved, by observing the teeth in skeletons. Yet we can actually transplant a tooth from one person to another without great difficulty, Nature assisting the operation if it is done in such a way that she can assist; and the only way in which Nature can assist, with respect either to size or shape, is by having the fang of the transplanted tooth rather smaller than the socket. The socket in this case grows to the tooth. If the fang is too large, it is impossible indeed to insert it at all in that state; however, if the fang should be originally too large, it may be made less, and this seems to answer the purpose as well.

The success of this operation is founded on a disposition in all living substances to unite when brought into contact with one another, al-

---

* The animal fluids, when out of the course of the general circulation, especially when they stagnate in cavities, are apt to deposit an absorbent earth, and form concretions. This earth is sometimes contained in the fluids, and is only deposited, as in the formation of the stone in the urinary passages; in some cases, perhaps, the fluids undergo a change, by which the earth is first formed, and afterwards deposited. This deposition takes place particularly in weakened parts, or where the circulation is languid, or where there are few arteries, such as about joints and tendons, as if it were intended to strengthen these parts if they should at any time give way; for if an artery, for instance, is overcome by the action of the heart, and unnaturally dilated, its coats have commonly these concretions formed everywhere in their interstices. The same thing happens also in the coats of encysted tumours, which are constantly distended, in cases of distentions of the tunica vaginalis testis, &c. It is also apt to take place in parts which have lost their natural functions, as in the coats of the eye in cases of blindness, and in diseased lymphatic glands, &c., and where the living power is diminished in the system, as in the arteries, membranes, &c. of old people; and in some particular habits, as in those who are affected by the gout[a].

The same sort of deposition takes place likewise where there is any substance with such properties as render it a fit basis for crystallization, as when extraneous bodies are lodged in the bladder; whence such bodies are so often found to form the nucleus of a stone. The same thing happens in the bowels of many animals, whence the nucleus of intestinal concretions, or bezoars, is commonly a nail, or some indigestible substance which had been swallowed. The crust which collects upon the teeth seems to be a crystallization of the same nature.

---

[a] [This substance consists, in a very large proportion, of earthy phosphates, combined with mucus.]

though they are of a different structure, and even although the circulation is only carried on in one of them.

This disposition is not so considerable in the more perfect or complex animals, such as quadrupeds, as it is in the more simple or imperfect, nor in old animals, as in young; for the living principle in young animals, and those of simple construction, is not so much confined to, or derived from, one part of the body; so that it continues longer in a part separated from their bodies, and even would appear to be generated in it for some time; while a part, separated from an older or more perfect animal, dies sooner, and would appear to have its life entirely dependent on the body from which it was taken.

Taking off the young spur of a cock and fixing it to his comb is an old and well-known experiment.

I have also frequently taken out the testis of a cock and replaced it in his belly, where it has adhered and has been nourished; nay, I have put the testis of a cock into the belly of a hen with the same effect[a].

In like manner a fresh tooth, when transplanted from one socket to another, becomes, to all appearance, a part of that body to which it is now attached as much as it was of the one from which it was taken; while a tooth which has been extracted for some time, so as to lose the whole of its life, will never become firm or fixed; the sockets will also in this case acquire the disposition to fill up, which they do not in the case of the insertion of a fresh tooth.

These appearances show that the living principle exists in the several parts of the body, independent of the influence of the brain or circulation, and that it subsists by these, or is indebted to them for its continuance; and in proportion as animals have less of brain and circulation the living power has less dependence on them, and becomes a more active principle in itself; and in many animals there is no brain nor circulation, so that this power is capable of being continued equally by all the parts themselves, such animals being nearly similar in this respect to vegetables[b].

---

a [These experiments are related in the Animal Œconomy, see Vol. IV.]

b [The practice of transplanting teeth from one person to another originated, I believe, with Hunter, under whose superintendence it was frequently performed. Had the results of all these cases been known to him, it is probable that this recommendation would not have been written; there is not, I believe, a single instance of its perfect success, and there are many in which it has been followed by even fatal results. Fox, in his excellent practical work on the teeth, strongly reprobates this practice, and has probably prevented much pain and disease by exposing its continual failure, its occasional injurious results, and the want of correct feeling which seems to be necessarily involved in its performance. The tooth figured by Fox as having been the subject of this operation is now in the collection of Guy's Hospital; its root is deeply eroded by absorption.]

THE NATURAL HISTORY

OF

THE HUMAN TEETH.

PART II.

INTRODUCTION.

THE importance of the teeth is such that they deserve our utmost attention, as well with respect to the preservation of them when in a healthy state, as to the methods of curing them when diseased. They require this attention not only for the preservation of themselves, as instruments useful to the body, but also on account of other parts with which they are connected, for diseases in the teeth are apt to produce diseases in the neighbouring parts, frequently of very serious consequences, as will evidently appear in the following treatise.

One might at first imagine that the diseases of the teeth must be very simple, and like those which take place everywhere else in the bony parts of our body; but experience shows the contrary. The teeth, being singular in their structure and some other circumstances, have diseases peculiar to themselves. These diseases, considered abstractedly, are indeed very simple; but by the relations which the teeth bear to the body in general, and to the parts with which they are immediately connected, they become extremely complicated. The diseases which may arise in consequence of those of the teeth are various, such as abscesses, carious bones, &c., many of which, although proceeding originally from the teeth, are more the object of the surgeon than of the dentist, who will find himself as much at a loss in such cases as if the abscess or carious bone were in the leg or any other distant part. All the diseases of the teeth which are common to them with the other parts of the body, should be put under the management of the physician or surgeon, but those which are peculiar to the teeth and their connexions belong properly to the dentist.

It is not my present purpose to enumerate every disease capable of producing such symptoms as may lead us to suspect the teeth, for the jaws may be affected by almost every kind of disorder. I shall therefore confine myself to the diseases of the teeth, gums, and alveolar processes; which parts, having a peculiar connexion, their diseases fall properly within the province of the dentist. I shall also purposely avoid entering into common surgery, so as not to lead the dentist beyond his depth, into matters of which (it is to be supposed) he has not acquired a competent knowledge.

In order that the reader may perfectly understand what follows, it will be necessary for him previously to consider and comprehend the anatomy and uses of every part of a tooth, as explained in my *Natural History of the Human Teeth*, to which I shall be obliged frequently to refer. Without such previous study the dentist will often be at a loss to account for many of the diseases and symptoms mentioned here, and will retain many vulgar errors imbibed by conversing with ignorant people, or by reading books in which the anatomy and physiology of the teeth are treated without a sufficient knowledge of the subject.

Whichever of the connected parts be originally diseased, the teeth are commonly the greatest sufferers. None of those parts can be distempered without communicating to the teeth such morbid effects as tend to the destruction of them[a].

---

[a] [The object of the author in writing this work, as given in the introduction to the second part, was indeed worthy of himself. That the dentists of his day required such information as he professes to give them, nearly as much as those of the present, may be fairly inferred; but it also may be reasonably asked, how the unfortunate dentist who is supposed by our author not to have acquired a knowledge of common surgery, as "a matter beyond his depth", is to understand the diseases "which are peculiar to the teeth *and their connexions*"; as if abscess, ulceration, tumours, caries, necrosis, &c., are to be readily understood by the charlatan who knows nothing of the principles of common surgery, when they occur in the gums and alveolar processes; whilst, if they take place in other parts of the body, they fall within the province of the surgeon. Had Hunter endeavoured to rescue the surgical treatment of the teeth altogether from the hands of the mere mechanic, and urged the study of this not uninteresting portion of professional knowledge upon the notice of the scientific practitioner, he would have done more to raise it from its present degradation than it can ever be in the power of a less influential author to effect; and we should not now have had to deplore, in his own quaint but expressive words, that the dentist should be "at a loss to account for many of these diseases and symptoms," and "retain many vulgar errors imbibed by conversing with ignorant people."]

CHAPTER I.

OF THE DISEASES OF THE TEETH, AND THE CONSE-
QUENCES OF THEM.

---

§. 1. *The Decay of the Teeth, arising from Rottenness.*

THE most common disease to which the teeth are exposed is such a decay as would appear to deserve the name of mortification. But there is something more; for the simple death of the part would produce but little effect, as we find that teeth are not subject to putrefaction after death, and therefore I am apt to suspect, that during life there is some operation going on which produces a change in the diseased part. It almost always begins externally in a small part of the body of the tooth, and commonly appears at first as an opake white spot. This is owing to the enamel's losing its regular and crystallized texture, and being reduced to a state of powder, from the attraction of cohesion being destroyed, which produces similar effects to those of powdered crystal. When this has crumbled away, the bony part of the tooth is exposed; and when the disease has attacked this part, it generally appears like a dark brown speck. Sometimes, however, there is no change of colour, and therefore the disease is not observable till it has made a considerable hole in the tooth. The dead part is generally at first round, but not always, its particular figure depending more on the place where it begins than on any other circumstance. It is often observed on the hollow parts of the grinding surface of the molares, and there looks like a crack filled with a very black substance. In the incisores the disease usually begins pretty near the neck of the tooth, and the scooping process goes on enlarging the cavity, commonly across the same part of the tooth, which almost divides it into two. When such a diseased tooth gives way, the mischief is occasioned by its body breaking off.

When it attacks the bony part it appears first to destroy the earth; for the bone becomes softer and softer, and is at last so soft on the exterior exposed surface that it can be picked away with a pin, and when allowed to dry it cracks like dried clay.

It begins sometimes in the inside of the tooth, although but rarely. In this case the tooth becomes of a shining black, from the dark colour being seen through the remaining shell of the tooth, and no hole is found leading into the cavity.

This blackness is seldom more than a portion of the bony part de-cayed or mortified. However, it often happens that the remaining part of the tooth becomes simply dead, in which state it is capable of taking on a dye. As it is generally on the external surface, one might expect no great mischief would ensue; but the tendency to mortification goes deeper and deeper, till at last it arrives at the cavity of the tooth, and the mortification follows. Mortification is common to every part of the body; but in most other parts this tendency is owing in a great measure to the constitution, which being corrected, that disposition ceases; but here it is local, and as such it would appear that we have no power of resisting it. When gone thus far the decay makes a quicker progress, similar to those cases where the decay begins in the cavity; for then this disposition is given to the whole cavity of the tooth, which being a much larger surface than what the disease had before to act upon, the increase of the decay seems to be in the same proportion: at last it scoops out its inner substance, till almost nothing is left but a thin shell, which generally being broken by mastication, a smaller or larger open-ing is made, and the whole cavity becomes at length exposed.

The canal in the fang of the tooth is more slowly affected; the scooping process appears to stop there, for we seldom know a fang be-come very hollow to its point when in the form of a stump; and it sometimes appears sound, even when the body of the tooth is almost destroyed: hence I conclude that the fang of the tooth has greater living powers than the body, by which the process of the disease is re-tarded; and this part appears at last only to lose its living principle, and not to take on the mortifying process above described; for which reason it remains simply a dead fang: however, it does not remain per-fectly at rest[a].

This is the stage in which it is called a stump. It begins now to lose its sensibility, and is seldom afterwards the cause of pain.

Thus, in appearance, it will remain sometimes for many years, but there will be more or less of a change going on; Nature will be at-tempting to make up the deficiency by endeavouring to increase the stump; for in many cases we find the stumps thickened and lengthened at their terminations, or small ends; but it is a process she is not equal to, therefore no advantages accrue from it. When she either fails in this process, or is in such a state as not to attempt it, then by this condition of the tooth a stimulus is given to the alveolar processes which produces a filling up of the socket from the bottom, whereby the

---

[a] [The mortification and simple death of a part are exceedingly different things. On this subject the reader is referred to the Treatise on Inflammation: see Vol. III.]

stumps are gradually protruded. But although they are pushed out at the bottom, they seldom or never project further beyond the gum than at first; and that part of the tooth which projects seems to decay in proportion to its projection. Besides this decay at the external end of the stump, there is an absorption of the fang at the bottom, which is known by the following observation : the end of the stump, which was in the gum or jaw, becomes irregularly blunted, and often rough, and has not the appearance of the end of the fang of a sound tooth.

Such stumps are in general easily extracted, being attached often to little more than the gum, and that sometimes loosely.

Although the disease appears to be chiefly in the tooth itself, and but little to depend on external causes, yet in many cases the part which is already rotten seems to have some influence upon that which remains; for if the rotten part be perfectly removed before it has arrived at the canal of the tooth, a stop is sometimes put to the further progress of the decay, at least for a time.

However, this is not constantly so; it is oftener the contrary ; but it is expedient in most cases to make this trial, as it is always right to keep a tooth clean and free from specks.

This decay of the teeth does not seem to be so entirely the effect of accident as might be imagined; for it sometimes takes place in them by pairs, in which case we may suppose it owing to an original cause coming into action at its stated time; the corresponding teeth being in pairs with respect to the disease, as well as to situation, shape, &c.

This opinion is somewhat strengthened by the fore teeth in the lower jaw not being so subject to decay as those in the upper, although equally liable to all accidents arising from external influence which could produce the disease in general.

The fore teeth in the lower jaw appear to be less subject to this disease than any of the others ; the fore teeth in the upper jaw, and the grinders in both, are of course more frequently affected.

This disease and its consequences seem to be peculiar to youth and middle age; the shedding teeth are as subject to it, if not more so, than those intended to last through life; and we seldom or ever see any person whose teeth begin to rot after the age of fifty years.

This might be supposed to arise from the disproportion that the number of teeth after fifty bear to them before it; but the number of diseased teeth after fifty do not bear the same proportion.

This disease has not hitherto been accounted for : if it had been always on the inside of the cavity, it might have been supposed to be owing to a deficiency of nourishment from some fault in the vascular system; but as it begins most commonly externally, in a part where the teeth in their most sound state receive little or no nourishment, we cannot refer it to that cause.

It does not arise from any external injury, or from menstrua, which have a power of dissolving part of a tooth; for anything of that kind could not act so partially: and we can observe in those teeth where the disease has not gone deep, that from the black speck externally there is a gradual decay or alteration leading to the cavity, and becoming fainter and fainter. We may therefore reasonably suppose that it is a disease arising originally in the tooth itself; because when once the shell of the tooth has given way to the cavity, the cavity itself soon becomes diseased in the same way. That the disease spreads thus rapidly over the cavity as soon as the tooth has given way does not depend simply on the exposure; for if a sound tooth be broken by accident, so as to expose the cavity, no such quick decay ensues: however, sometimes we find in those cases that exposure of the cavity will produce a decay, and even pain, similar to an original disease; and in the diseased tooth we find that the exposure has a considerable effect in hastening the progress of the disease; for if the tooth be stopped so as to prevent its exposure to external injury, its cavity will not nearly so soon become diseased. Exposure, therefore, seems at least to assist the decay.

How far a rotten tooth has the power of contaminating those next to it, I believe, is not yet completely ascertained; some cases seem to favour this idea, and many to contradict it. We frequently see two teeth rotten in places exactly opposite to each other, and as one of them began first to decay, it gives a suspicion that the last diseased was infected by that which received the first morbid impression.

On the contrary, we often see one diseased, whilst another tooth, in contact with the decayed part, remains perfectly sound[a].

---

[a] [The reasoning which we find in the preceding section is not only inconclusive, but in many parts not wholly consistent with itself. Nor is it possible, with the vague notions entertained by Hunter, and even by some in the present day, who follow his words rather than his spirit respecting the peculiar character of the bony structure of these organs, to form a rational and consistent opinion on this difficult subject. Fox appears to have made an approach towards the truth; but by assuming the absolute identity of structure in the teeth and true bones, without taking into the account their remarkable and acknowledged discrepancies, he fell into the opposite error, of expecting to find in the morbid affections of the teeth the analogue of every disease to which the more highly organized bones are liable. The opinion that decay of the teeth is communicable by contact is now fast becoming obsolete. That we often see two teeth becoming decayed " at places exactly opposite to each other," as observed by Hunter, is a matter of almost proverbial notoriety; but it is not, I believe, difficult to account for this fact, without assuming a doctrine so inconsistent with all that is known of the

Symptoms of Inflammation.

Few or no symptoms are produced by this disease besides the above appearances till the cavity of the tooth is exposed : however, it often happens that a tenderness, or a soreness upon touch, or other external influences, takes place long before; but when the cavity is exposed, then pain and other symptoms often begin, which are generally very considerable : however, the exposure of the cavity of a tooth does not in all cases give pain. Some teeth shall moulder wholly away without ever having any sensation.

In many cases there will be very acute pain upon the cavity being exposed, which will subside and recur again without producing any other effect; but it more frequently happens that this pain is the first symptom of inflammation, and is in most cases very considerable, more so than that arising from such an inflammation in other places. The surrounding parts sympathize commonly to a considerable extent, viz. the gums, jaw-bones, and integuments covering them; they inflame and swell so much as to affect the whole of that side of the face where the affected tooth is situated. The mouth can hardly be opened; the glands of that side of the neck often swell; there is an increase of the saliva, and the eye is almost closed, the tooth not giving way to the swelling of the soft parts within it; and for this reason the local effects of the inflammation cannot be so visible as in the soft parts.

---

structure no less than of the chemical composition of these organs. As the enamel, when perfect, not only prevents the wearing away of the teeth by mastication, but also protects that part which is out of the gum from external causes of irritation and decay, whatever should tend to injure that substance and destroy the unity of its texture would be likely to occasion decay of the subjacent bony substance. When two teeth, therefore, are very strongly pressed together, either during their growth or afterwards, the crystallized structure of the enamel is frequently broken down, or at least the continuity of its texture injured, to such a degree as to admit of those external causes of inflammation and of subsequent loss of vitality which have just been alluded to. This would occur *at the point of contact*, and hence the frequency of the occurrence of this disease at that part. The prevalence of decay in contiguous teeth may also be accounted for by attributing it in both to the same general exciting cause, as cold, mechanical injury, &c. And, on the other hand, it appears impossible to imagine *infection* taking place through a substance so entirely inorganic, so dense, and so perfect and uniform in its structure, as this crystallized enamel. To which it may be added, that there is no chemical agent evolved during the decay of a tooth which can decompose this substance.

Notwithstanding the absurdity of the opinion, however, it is probable that at the time when Hunter wrote the doubt expressed in the text he was the only man in the profession who ventured to entertain such a doubt.]

This inflammation of the tooth often lasts a considerable time, and then gradually subsides. We may suppose, according to the general law of inflammation, that it is at first of the adhesive kind, and accordingly we sometimes find the teeth swelled at their ends, which is a character of the adhesive stage of inflammation; and sometimes two fangs are grown together. That we seldom find adhesions between the teeth and surrounding parts may be reasonably imputed to their less aptitude for such connexions. The suppurative inflammation succeeds; but as a tooth has not that power of suppuration which leads to granulations, so as to be buried, covered up, and made part of ourselves, as happens to other bones (which would destroy any use of a tooth), the inflammation wears out, or rather the parts not being susceptible of this irritation beyond a certain time, the inflammation gradually goes off, and leaves the tooth in its original diseased state. No permanent cure, therefore, can possibly be effected by such inflammations; but the parts being left in the same state as before, they are still subject to repetitions of inflammation till some change takes place, preventing future attacks, which I believe is generally, if not always, effected by the destruction of those parts which are the seat of it, viz. the soft parts within the tooth.

Nature seems in some measure to have considered the teeth as aliens, only giving them nourishment while sound and fit for service, but not allowing them when diseased the common benefits of that society in which they are placed. They cannot exfoliate, as no operations go on in them except growth; therefore, if any part is dead, the living has not the power of throwing it off, and forming an external surface capable of supporting itself, like the other parts of the body: indeed, if they had such a power no good purpose could be answered by it; for a piece of tooth simply dead is almost as useful as if the whole was living; which may be observed every day.

The pain, however, appears to take its rise from the tooth as a centre. That it should be more severe than what is generally produced by similar inflammations in other parts of the body, may, perhaps, be accounted for when we consider that these parts do not readily yield; as is likewise the case in whitloes.

It sometimes happens that the mind is not directed to the real seat of the disease, the sensation of pain not seeming to be in the diseased tooth, but in some neighbouring tooth which is perfectly sound. This has often misled operators, and the sympathizing tooth has fallen a sacrifice to their ignorance.

In all cases of diseased teeth the pain is brought on by circumstances unconnected with the disease; as, for instance, cold, wherefore they are more troublesome commonly in winter than in summer. Extraneous matter entering the cavity, and touching the nerve and vessels, will also bring on the pain.

This pain is frequently observed to be periodical; sometimes there being a perfect intermission, sometimes only an abatement of it. The paroxysm comes on once in twenty-four hours, and for the most part towards the evening. The bark has therefore been tried; but that failing, the disorder has been suspected to be of the rheumatic kind, and treated accordingly with no better success. At length, after a more particular examination of the teeth, one of them has been suspected to be unsound; and, being extracted, has put an end to the disorder. This shows how injudicious it is to give medicines in such cases, while the true state of the tooth is unknown.

This disease is often the cause of bad breath, more so than any other disease of those parts, especially when it has exposed the cavity of the tooth. This most probably arises from the rotten part of the tooth and the juices of the mouth and food all stagnating in this hollow part, which is warm, and hastens putrefaction in them.

I come now to the prevention and cure of this disease.

The first thing to be considered is the cure of the decaying state of the tooth, or rather the means of preventing the further progress of the decay; and more especially before it has reached the cavity, whereby the tooth may be in some degree preserved, the consequent pain and inflammations, commonly called tooth-ache, avoided, and often the consequent abscesses called gum-boils. I believe, however, that no such means of absolute prevention are as yet known. The progress of the disease, in some cases, appears to have been retarded by removing that part which is already decayed; but experience shows that there is but little dependence upon this practice. I have known cases where the black spot having been filed off and scooped entirely out, the decay has stopped for many years. This practice is supposed to prevent at least any effect that the part already rotten may have upon the sounder parts; however, if this is all the good that arises from this practice, I believe in most cases it might be as well omitted. Even if it were an effectual practice, it could not be an universal one; for it is not always in the power of the operator to remove this decayed part, either on account of its situation, or on account of its having made too great a progress before it is discovered. When it is on the basis of a grinder, or on the posterior side of its neck, it can scarcely be reached. It becomes also impracticable when the disease is still allowed to go on, and the cavity becomes exposed, so that the patient is now liable to all the consequences already described, and the tooth is making haste towards a total decay; in such a case, if the decay be not too far advanced, that is, if it be not rendered useless simply as a tooth, I would advise that it be extracted, then immediately boiled, with a view to make it perfectly clean, and also destroy any life there may be in the tooth; and then that it be restored to the socket: this will prevent any further decay of the tooth, as it is now dead, and not to be acted upon by any disease, but can only suffer chemically or mechanically.

This practice, however, I would only recommend in grinders, where we have no other resource on account of the number of fangs, as will be more fully explained hereafter. This practice has sometimes been followed with success; and when it does succeed, it answers the same end as the burning the nerve, but with much greater certainty.

If the patient will not submit to have the tooth drawn, the nerve may be burned: that this may have the desired effect, it must be done to the very point of the fang, which is not always possible. Either of the concentrated acids, such as the sulphuric, the nitric, or the muriatic, introduced as far into the fang of the tooth as possible, is capable of destroying its soft parts, which most probably are the seat of pain: a little caustic alkali will produce the same effect. But it is a difficult operation to introduce any of these substances into the root of the fang, till the decay has gone a considerable length, especially if it be a tooth of the upper jaw; for it is hardly possible to make fluids pass against their own gravity; in these cases, the common caustic is the best application, as it is a solid. The caustic should be introduced with a small dossil of lint, but even this will scarcely convey it far enough. If it be the lower jaw, the caustic need only be introduced into the hollow of the tooth, for by its becoming fluid, by the moisture of the part, it will then descend down the cavity of the fang, as will also any of the acids; but patients will often not suffer this to be done till they have endured much pain and several inflammations.

When there is no other symptom except pain in the tooth, we have many modes of treatment recommended, which can only be temporary in their effects. These act by derivation, or stimulus applied to some other part of the body. Thus, to burn the ear by hot irons has sometimes been a successful practice, and has relieved the tooth-ache.

Some stimulating medicine, as spirit of lavender, snuffed up into the nose, will often carry off the pain.

When an inflammation takes place in the surrounding parts, it often is assisted by an additional cause, as cold or fever: when the inflammation has taken place in a great degree, then it becomes more the object of another consideration; for it may be lessened like any other inflammation arising from similar causes, the pressure of an extraneous body, or exposure of an internal cavity.

If the inflammation be very great, it will be proper to take away some blood. The patient may likewise properly be advised to hold some strong vinous spirit for a considerable time in his mouth. Diluted acids, as vinegar, &c., may likewise be of use, applied in the same manner. Likewise preparations of lead would be advisable; but these might prove dangerous if they should be accidentally swallowed.

If the skin is affected, poultices, containing some of the above-mentioned substances, produce relief. The pain in many cases being often more than the patient can well bear, warm applications to the part have been recommended, such as hot brandy, to divert the mind; also spices, essential oils, &c., which last are, perhaps, the best. A little lint or cotton soaked in laudanum is often applied with success; and laudanum ought likewise to be taken internally to procure an interval of some ease. Blisters are of service in most inflammations of these parts, whether they arise from a diseased tooth or not. They cannot be applied to the part, but they divert the pain and draw this stimulus to another part; they may be conveniently placed either behind the ear or in the nape of the neck. These last-mentioned methods can only be considered as temporary means of relief, and such as only affect the inflammation. Therefore the tooth is still exposed to future attacks of the same disease[a].

---

[a] [In the foregoing passages there is much important and accurate observation evinced in the description of the symptoms either attending or succeeding inflammation in the teeth. There are, however, apparently no less than three distinct diseases confounded in this description. The first is the inflammation produced by the exposed pulp from decay of the tooth; the second, suppuration of the pulp, which often takes place independently of exposure; and the third, the inflammation and suppuration of the surrounding parts, which as frequently occur from the irritation produced by the existence of dead teeth or roots in the socket (as extraneous bodies) as from any other cause.

Many of the remarks on the treatment of these affections are replete with sound sense, and have undoubtedly laid the foundation for the best modes of practice in use since that day. A few observations of a more detailed nature may not, however, be wholly useless. When the disease termed caries, or more properly gangrene, has only just commenced under the enamel, so as only to exhibit the appearance of a brown opake mark, there can be no doubt that the entire excision of the spot will much retard the progress of decay by removing one cause of irritation to the surrounding healthy bone; but if the decay has extended to any distance from the surface, the file must be used to such an extent, in order to remove the whole of the diseased portion, as to expose a considerable part of the bone to external irritants, and consequently will hasten rather than retard the mischief.

The replacement of a decayed tooth after extraction, being first of all boiled to destroy its vitality, is recommended by Hunter only theoretically. An obvious and in-

The Stopping of the Teeth.

If the destruction of the life of the tooth, either by drawing and restoring it again, or by the actual or potential cauteries, has not been
effected, and only the core of the inflammation has been attempted,
another method of preventing inflammation is to be followed, which is
to allow as little stimulus to take place as possible. The cavity of the
tooth not being capable of taking the alarm like most other cavities in
the body, and of course not suppurating, as has been already observed,
often no more is necessary, either to prevent the inflammation from
taking place altogether, or extending further, than to exclude all extraneous irritating matter; therefore the stopping up the cavity becomes, in many cases, the means of preventing future attacks of the
inflammation, and often retards even the progress of the disease, that
is, the further decay of the tooth, so that many people go on for years
thus assisted : but it is a method which must be put in practice early,
otherwise it cannot be continued long; for if the disease has done considerable damage to the inside of the tooth, so as to have weakened it
much, the whole body of the tooth most probably will soon give way in
mastication : therefore, under such circumstances, the patient must be
cautioned not to make too free with the tooth in eating.

Gold and lead are the metals generally made use of for stopping teeth.
Gold being less pliable must be used in the leaf; lead is so soft in any
form as to take on any shape by a very small force.

---

surmountable objection exists to this operation, which is, that a dead extraneous body
is thus forced into the alveolus, still sore from the operation, which must necessarily
produce much irritation, and often suppuration, with all those severe symptoms which
so often arise from dead roots, or from teeth whose connexion with the socket has been
destroyed by a blow.

The burning of the nerve is deserving of no better eulogy than the operation just
mentioned. Hunter himself observes, with much *naïveté*, that " it must be done to the
very point of the fang, *which is not always possible.*" The truth is, that burning the
pulp of a tooth even superficially, to be of service at all, must be done when the cauter-
izing wire is at a white heat, or it otherwise only produces inflammation, and not the
instantaneous destruction of the surface; but when the small size of the instrument,
the distance which it must necessarily pass before it is brought into contact with the
pulp, and the time which must elapse before it is applied, are considered, the impossibility of effectually employing this remedy is obvious. The other remedies here alluded
to, and indeed all other caustic applications, are generally productive of more injury
than benefit, and exacerbate rather than diminish the inflammation and pain. Leeches,
purgative medicines, and the local application of narcotics, or camphor, &c., will often
be beneficial; but, the pulp being once exposed, the relief which these afford can be but
temporary, and the only remedy to be relied upon is the extraction of the tooth.]

Stuffing the hollow tooth with wax, galbanum, &c. can be but of very little service, as it is in most cases impossible to confine these substances, or preserve them from being soon worn away; however, they have their uses, as it is a practice which the patients themselves can easily put in execution.

It often happens from neglect, and much oftener in spite of all the means that can be used, that the tooth becomes so hollow as to give way, whereby the passage becomes too large to keep in any of the above-mentioned substances; however, in this case, it sometimes happens that a considerable part of the body of the tooth will still stand, and then a small hole may be drilled through this part, and after the cavity has been well stopped, a small peg may be put into the hole, so as to keep in the lead, gold, &c. But when this cannot be done, we may consider the broken tooth as entirely useless, or at least it will soon be so; and it is now open to attacks of inflammation, which the patient must either bear, or submit to have the tooth pulled out. If the first be chosen, and the repeated inflammations submitted to, a cure will be performed in time by the stump becoming totally dead; but it is better to have it pulled out, and suffer once for all.

Upon pulling out these teeth we may in general observe a pulpy substance at the root of the fang, so firmly adhering to the fang as to be pulled out with it. This is in some pretty large, so as to have made a considerable cavity at the bottom of the socket. This substance is the first beginning of the formation of a gum-boil, as it at times inflames and suppurates[a].

---

[a] [The operation of filling the teeth is much better understood in the present day than it was at the time when the foregoing directions were written. Notwithstanding the numerous experiments which have been made, and the innumerable quack nostrums which have been introduced to the public with promises which from their universality ought at once to be disbelieved, there is still no method of filling teeth with success where the pulp is exposed, and no substance which for durability and comfort can be compared to pure gold. All the amalgams, pastes, cements, or fusible metallic compositions, some of them ingenious and plausible, have insuperable disadvantages. It is not meant that they may not in some few cases partially succeed where a tooth will not bear the pressure necessary to render the gold sufficiently firm and solid, but in almost all cases where these are available gold would be much more so.

In order to employ this mode of retarding or preventing the progress of decay with the greatest effect, the pulp must not have been exposed. In fact the operation should be had recourse to as soon as the enamel has given way, or even earlier, and the decayed part can be drilled out of the tooth. When it has gone still further, the decayed portion must be entirely removed by means of little instruments adapted to this purpose, and the cavity being made perfectly dry, the gold, beaten of a proper thickness, is to be carefully pressed into the cavity until it is completely and solidly filled.]

§. 2. *The Decay of the Teeth by Denudation.*

There is another decay of the teeth, much less common than that already described, which has a very singular appearance. It is a wasting of the substance of the tooth very different from the former. In all the instances I have seen, it has begun on the exterior surface of the tooth, pretty close to the arch of the gum. The first appearance is a want of enamel, whereby the bony part is left exposed, but neither the enamel nor the bony part alters in consistence as in the above-described decay. As this decay spreads, more and more of the bone becomes exposed, in which respect also it differs from the former decay; and hence it may be called a denuding process. The bony substance of the teeth also gives way, and the whole wasted surface has exactly the appearance as if the tooth had been filed with a rounded file, and afterwards had been finely polished. At these places the bony parts, being exposed, become brown.

I have seen instances where it appeared as if the outer surface of the bony part, which is in contact with the inner surface of the enamel, had first been lost, so that the attraction of cohesion between the two had been destroyed, and as if the enamel had been separated for want of support, for it terminated all at once.

In one case, the two first incisors had lost the whole of the enamel; on their anterior surfaces they were hollowed from side to side, as if a round file had been applied to them longitudinally, and had the finest polish imaginable. The three grinders on each side appeared as if a round file had been used on them in a contrary direction to that on the incisors, viz. across their bodies close to the gum, so that there was a groove running across their bodies, which was smooth in the highest degree. Some of the other teeth in the same jaw had begun to decay in a similar manner; also the teeth in the lower jaw were become diseased.

I saw a case very lately where the four incisors of the upper jaw had lost their enamel entirely on their anterior surfaces, and there was scarcely a tooth in the mouth which had not the appearance of having had a file applied across it close to the gum.

Those whom I have known have not been able to attribute this disease to any cause; none of them had ever done anything particular to the teeth, nor was there in appearance anything particular in the constitution which could give rise to such a disease. In the first of these cases the person was about forty; in the last about twenty years of age.

From its attacking certain teeth rather than others in the same head, and a particular part of the tooth, I suspect it to be an original disease of the tooth itself, and not to depend on accident, way of life, constitution, or any particular management of the teeth[a].

§. 3. The Swelling of the Fang.

Another disease of the teeth is a swelling of the fang, which most probably arises from inflammation, while the body continues sound, and is of that kind which in any other bone would be called a spina ventosa[*]. It gives considerable pain, and nothing can be seen externally.

The pain may either be in the tooth itself or the alveolar process, as it is obliged to give way to the increase of the fang.

As a swelling of this kind does not tend to the suppurative inflammation, and as I have not been able to distinguish its symptoms from those of the nervous tooth-ache, it becomes a matter of some difficulty to the operator; for the only cure yet known is the extraction of the tooth, which has been often neglected on a supposition that the pain has been nervous.

These diseases of the teeth, arising from inflammation, become often the cause of diseases in the alveolar processes and gums, which I shall proceed to describe[b].

[*] Natural History of the Teeth, p. 17.

---

[a] [I have elsewhere mentioned a very curious case of an affection somewhat analogous to that here described. It consisted of the gradual truncation of the edges of the front teeth, both of the upper and lower jaw, extending back to the bicuspides. The exposed surface was perfectly smooth and polished, and the loss of substance extended so far that the cavities of the teeth must have been opened, but that they had become filled with a new solid bony substance, so transparent that it was only by touching it that its presence was ascertained. As the teeth never could have come in contact at the truncated part, and as no mechanical means had ever been used by which it could have been occasioned, the cause of this singular affection remains wholly unknown.]

[b] [The affection here described is nothing more than a deposit of bony matter around the fang, produced, doubtless, by inflammation of the periosteum. The new bone is rather yellower and less opake than the original structure. Hunter has alluded here to the occurrence of nervous pains, produced by these cases. It appears probable that the pressure of the new bone upon the nerves of the periosteum of the alveolus, or of the alveolar process itself, is the cause of this pain, for it cannot be distinguished from local neuralgia produced by any other similar cause. Cases of this description are detailed by Fox and by myself, in which the only means by which the true seat of pain could be ascertained was by striking the affected tooth, by which pain was produced; and the extraction of the tooth at once exhibited the cause of the pain and effected its cure.]

§. 4. *Gum-Boils*.

Although suppuration cannot easily take place within the cavity of a tooth, yet it often happens that the inflammation which is extended beyond it is so great as to produce suppuration in the jaw at the bottom of the socket where the diseased tooth is, forming there a small abscess, commonly called a gum-boil.

This inflammation is often very considerable, especially when the first suppuration takes place. It is often more diffused than inflammations in other parts, and affects the whole face, &c.

The matter, as in all other abscesses, makes its own way outwards, and as it cannot be evacuated through the tooth, it destroys the alveolar processes, and tumifies the gum, generally on the fore part, either pointing directly at the root of the tooth, or separating the gum from it, and is evacuated in one or other of these two ways, seldom on the inside of the gum; however, this sometimes happens.

Gum-boils seldom arise from other causes; however, it sometimes happens that they originate from a disease in the socket or jaw, having no connexion with the tooth, and only affecting it secondarily. Upon drawing such teeth, they are generally found diseased at or near the point, being there very rough and irregular, similar to ulcerating bones. There is no disease to appearance in the body of the tooth. These last-described gum-boils may arise wholly from such a cause, the appearance on the fang of the tooth being only an effect.

These abscesses, whether arising from the teeth or the sockets, always destroy the alveolar processes on that side where they open, as is very evident in the jaw-bones of many sculls; on which account the tooth becomes more or less loose. It may be perceived in the living body; for when the alveolar process is entirely destroyed on the outside of the tooth, if that tooth be moved, the motion will be observed under the gum along the whole length of the fang.

So far the teeth, alveolar processes, and gums become diseased by consent.

It is common for these abscesses to skin over, and in all appearance heal. This is peculiar to those which open through the gums; but those which discharge themselves between the gums and teeth can never heal up, because the gum cannot unite with the tooth; however, the discharge in them becomes less at times from a subsiding of the suppuration, which indeed is what allows the other to skin over. But either exposure to cold, or some other accidental cause, occasioning a fresh inflammation, produces an increased suppuration, which either opens the old orifice in the gum, or augments the discharge by the side of the tooth; however, I believe, the inflammation in this last case is not so violent as in the other, where a fresh ulceration is necessary for the passage of the matter.

Thus a gum-boil goes on for years, healing and opening alternately; the effect of which is that the alveolar processes are at length absorbed, and the tooth gets looser and looser, till it either drops out or is extracted.

Most probably in all such cases the communication between the cavity of the tooth and the jaw is cut off; yet it keeps in part its lateral attachments, especially when the gum grasps the tooth: but in those cases, where the matter passes between the gum and the tooth, these attachments are less; but some of them are still retained, particularly on the side opposite to the passage for the matter.

Gum-boils are easily known. Those which open through the gum may be distinguished by a small rising between the arch of the gum and the attachment of the lip: upon pressing the gum at the side of this point, some matter will commonly be observed oozing out at the eminence. This eminence seldom subsides entirely; for even when there is no discharge, and the opening is healed over, a small rising may still be perceived, which shows that the gum-boil has been there.

Those gum-boils which discharge themselves between the gum and the tooth are always discovered by pressing the gum, whereby the matter is pressed out, and is seen lying in the angle between the gum and tooth.

These abscesses happen much more frequently in the upper jaw than in the lower, and also more frequently to the cuspidati, incisores, and bicuspides in that jaw than to the molares; seldom to the fore teeth in the lower jaw.

As gum-boils are in general the consequence of rotten teeth, we find them in young and middle-aged people more frequently than in old; but they appear to be most common to the shedding teeth. This will arise from those teeth being more liable to become rotten; and perhaps there may be another reason, viz. the process of ulceration which goes on in these teeth*, in some cases falling into suppuration.

It sometimes happens in these gum-boils that a fungus will push out at the orifice, from a luxuriant disposition to form granulations in the inside of the abscess, and the want of power to heal or skin; the same thing frequently happens in issues, where the parts have a disposition

---

* Vide Natural History of the Teeth, for an explanation of this process in those teeth, pp. 43, 44.

to granulate, but have not the power of healing, on account of an extraneous body being kept there. The tooth in the present case acts as an extraneous body, and by the secretion of matter the abscess is prevented from healing.

In the treatment of gum-boils, the practice will be the same, whether the abscess has arisen from a diseased tooth, or a disease in the socket.

The teeth being under such circumstances in the animal machine that they cannot partake of all the benefits of a cure in the same manner as other parts do, on that account, when an abscess forms itself about the root of a tooth, the tooth, by losing its connexion with the other parts, loses every power of union, as it is not endowed with the power of granulating, and thereby it becomes an extraneous body, or at least acts here as an extraneous body, and one of the worst kind, such as it is not in the power of any operation of the machine to get rid of. This is not the case with any other part of the body, for when any other part becomes dead, the machine has the power of separating it from the living, called sloughing or exfoliation, and expelling it, whence a cure is effected; but in the case of gum-boils the only cure of them is the extraction of the tooth. As this is the last resource, everything is to be done to make the parts as easy under the disease as possible, so that this operation may be postponed.

When the abscess has opened through the gum, I believe the best method that can be tried with a view to prevent future gatherings is to prevent the closing up of the abscess; and this may be done by enlarging the opening, and keeping it enlarged till the whole internal surface of the cavity of the abscess is skinned over, or till the opening in the gum loses the disposition to close up, which will in a great measure prevent any future formation of matter, or at least whatever is formed will find an easy outlet, which will prevent these accumulations from taking place ever after. The end of the fang will indeed be hereby exposed, but under such circumstances it will not be in a worse situation than when soaked in matter.

One method of doing this is to open the gum-boils by a crucial incision, the full width of the abscess, and fill it well with lint, which should be dipped in lime-water, or a diluted solution of lunar caustic, made by dissolving one drachm of the caustic in two ounces of distilled water; and the wound should be dressed very frequently, as it is with difficulty that the dressing can be kept in. If this is not sufficient to keep the wound open, it may be touched with the lunar caustic, so as to produce a slough; and this may be repeated if it should be found necessary.

One considerable disadvantage occurs in this practice, which is the difficulty of keeping on the dressings; but constant attention will make up for the inconvenience of situation.

If the surface of the abscess be touched with the potassa fusa, and the lip kept from coming in contact with the part for one minute, it answers better than any other method; for this, within that space of time, will penetrate to the bottom.

The surface of the boil should be first wiped dry, as much as the nature of the part will allow, to prevent as much as possible the spreading of the caustic, which by care can be prevented, as the operator will watch it the whole time.

To extract the tooth, then to file off any diseased part of it, and immediately to replace it, has been practised, but often without the desired success; for it has often happened that a tooth has been introduced into a diseased jaw. This practice, however, now and then has succeeded.

When a gum-boil is formed on a back or molar tooth, such very nice treatment is not necessary as when it happens to the fore teeth, because appearances are there of less consequence; therefore the gum may be slit down upon the fang through its whole length, from the opening of the gum-boil to its edge, which will prevent any future union; and the whole cavity of the abscess skinning over will prevent any future collection of matter. The wound appears afterwards like the hare lip, and therefore this practice is not advisable where it would be much in view, as when the disease is in the fore teeth. In these cases, where the granulations push out through the small opening, they may be cured by the method above mentioned; but if it is not complied with, they may be very safely cut off with a knife or lancet. However, this does not effect a cure, for they commonly rise again. To slit the gum in this case has been common, but it is a bad method whenever the defect is in sight[a].

§. 5. *Excrescences from the Gum.*

From bad teeth there are also sometimes excrescences arising at once out of the gum, near, or in contact with, the diseased tooth.

In general they are easily extracted with a knife or whatever cutting instrument can be best applied; but this will vary, according to their situations and the extent of their base.

---

[a] [The practical surgeon who has seen much of the diseases of the teeth will see that the long detail of the treatment of gum-boil, or, as it may with more propriety be termed, alveolar abscess, is altogether supererogatory. The roots occasioning these gum-boils *must* be removed, or every other means will fail.]

They will often rise in a day or two after the operation as high as ever; but this newly generated matter generally dies soon, and the disease terminates well. They have often so much of a cancerous appearance as to deter surgeons from meddling with them; but where they arise at once from the gum, and appear to be the only diseased part, I believe they have no malignant disposition.

However, I have seen them with very broad bases, and where the whole could not be removed, and yet no bad consequences have attended their removal. These often rise again in a few years, by which means they become very troublesome.

After the extirpation of them, it is often necessary to apply the actual cautery to stop the bleeding; for arteries going to increased parts are themselves increased, and also become diseased, and have not the contractile power of a sound artery[a].

§. 6. *Deeply seated Abscesses in the Jaws.*

Sometimes deeper abscesses occur than those commonly called gumboils. They are often of very serious consequence, producing carious bones, &c. These commonly arise from a disease in the tooth, and more especially in the cuspidati, those teeth passing further into the jaw than the others. Their depth in the jaw being beyond the attachment of the lip to the gum, if an abscess forms at their points, it more readily makes its way through the common integuments of the face, than between the gum and lip, which disfigures the face; and when in the lower jaw looks like the evil.

In the upper jaw it makes a disagreeable scar on the face, about half an inch from the nose.

These, although they may sometimes arise from diseases of the teeth and gums, yet are properly the object of common surgery; and the surgeon must apply to the dentist, if his assistance is necessary, to pull out the tooth, or to perform any other operation which comes under his province.

---

a [Whenever the tumours here described are produced by the irritation arising from diseased or dead teeth, they will constantly recur after removal, until the cause is removed by the extraction of the teeth; and it often happens that after this operation they disappear spontaneously. It is not uncommon for a tumour of this description so completely to conceal the stump that has occasioned its growth, that it is only by the excision of the tumour that the cause can be ascertained. It is therefore necessary in all cases of this description that a root should be carefully searched for after the removal of such a tumour.]

It sometimes happens that the abscess is situated some way from the root of the diseased tooth both in the upper jaw and the lower; but, I think, more frequently in the lower. When it threatens to open externally on the skin of the face, great care should be taken to prevent it, and an opening very early made into the swelling on the inside of the lip; for it is generally very readily felt there. This practice of early opening these abscesses upon the inside of the mouth is more necessary when the abscess is in the lower jaw than when in the upper, because matter by its weight always produces ulceration more readily at the lower part. I have seen this practice answer, even when the matter had come so near the skin as to have inflamed it. If it is in the upper, the opening need not be so very large, as the matter will have a depending outlet.

To prevent a relapse of the disease, it will in most cases be necessary to pull out the tooth; which has either been the first cause, or has become diseased, in consequence of the formation of the abscess; and in either case is capable of reproducing the disease.

The mouth should be often washed; and while the water is within the mouth, the skin should be pressed opposite to the abscess.

If the life of the bone be destroyed, it will exfoliate; and very probably two or three of the teeth may come away with the exfoliation. Little should be done in such cases, except that the patient should keep the mouth as clean as possible by frequently washing it, and when the bones exfoliate, they should be removed as soon as possible. In these cases it is but too common for the dentist to be very busy, and perhaps do mischief through ignorance.

§. 7. *Abscess of the Antrum Maxillare.*

The antrum maxillare is very subject to inflammation and suppuration, in consequence of diseases of the neighbouring parts, and particularly of the duct leading to the nose being obliterated. Whether this is the cause, or only an effect, is not easily determined, but there is great reason to suppose it an attendant, from some of the symptoms. If it be a cause, we may suppose that the natural mucus of these cavities accumulating irritates and produces inflammation for its own exit, in the same manner as an obstruction to the passage of the tears through the lachrymal duct produces an abscess of the lachrymal sac.

This inflammation of the antrum gives a pain which will be at first taken for the tooth-ache, especially if there be a bad tooth in that side; however, in these cases, the nose is more affected than commonly in a tooth-ache.

The eye is also affected; and it is very common for people with such a disease to have a severe pain in the forehead, where the frontal sinuses are placed; but still the symptoms are not sufficient to distinguish the disease. Time must disclose the true cause of the pain; for it will commonly continue longer than that which arises from a diseased tooth, and will become more and more severe; after which a redness will be observed on the fore part of the cheek, somewhat higher than the roots of the teeth, and a hardness in the same place, which will be considerably circumscribed. This hardness may be felt rather highly situated on the inside of the lip.

As this disease has been often treated of by surgeons, I shall only make the following remarks concerning it.

The first part of the cure, as well as of that of all other abscesses, is to make an opening, but not in the part where it threatens to point: for that would generally be through the skin of the cheek.

If the disease is known early, before it has caused the destruction of the fore part of the bone, there are two ways of opening the abscess: one by perforating the partition between the antrum and the nose, which may be done; and the other by drawing the first or second grinder of that side, and perforating the partition between the root of the alveolar process and the antrum, so that the matter may be discharged for the future that way.

But if the fore part of the bone has been destroyed, an opening may be made on the inside of the lip, where the abscess most probably will be felt; but this will be more apt than the other perforation to heal, and thereby may occasion a new accumulation; which is to be avoided, if possible, by putting in practice all the common methods of preventing openings from healing or closing up: but this practice will rather prove troublesome; therefore the drawing the tooth is to be preferred, because it is not so liable to this objection[a].

---

a [The true nature of this affection is generally mistaken, and the error is perpetuated by the misapplication of the term *abscess*. It consists of nothing more than an altered secretion of the mucous lining of the antrum, produced by a condition of the part perfectly analogous to that of the lining of the urethra in gonorrhœa. It does not always happen that the opening into the nose becomes impervious in this disease. Yet even where this communication remains free, and allows of a ready exit for the muco-purulent secretion, no remedies can be applied to the diseased membrane without removing a tooth for the purpose of perforating the floor of the antrum. The usual mode of effecting this is by means of a small trocar; and the treatment is similar to that of gonorrhœa, as far as relates to the injection of stimulant or astringent applications, which are not of course liable to the same objections in the present instance as in the disease just mentioned.]

CHAPTER II.

OF THE DISEASES OF THE ALVEOLAR PROCESSES, AND THE CONSEQUENCES OF THEM.

HAVING thus far treated of the diseases of the teeth themselves, and those of the sockets and gums, which either arise from them or are similar to such as arise from them, I come now to consider the diseases which take place primarily in the sockets, when the teeth are perfectly sound. These appear to be two; and yet I am not sure but that they are both fundamentally the same, proceeding together from the same cause, or one depending on the other.

The first effect which takes place is a wasting of the alveolar processes, which are in many people gradually absorbed and taken into the system. This wasting begins first at the edge of the socket, and gradually goes on to the root or bottom.

The gum, which is supported by the alveolar process, loses its connexion, and recedes from the body of the tooth, in proportion as the socket is lost; in consequence of which, first the neck, and then more or less of the fang itself, becomes exposed. The tooth of course becomes extremely loose, and at last drops out.

The other effect is a filling up of the socket at the bottom, whereby the tooth is gradually pushed out. As this disease seldom happens without being attended by the other, it is most probable that they generally both arise from the same cause. The second in these cases may be an effect of the first. Both combine to hasten the loss of the tooth; but it sometimes happens that they act separately; for I have seen cases where the gum was leaving the teeth, and yet the tooth was not in the least protruded: on the other hand, I have seen cases where the tooth was protruding, and yet the gum kept its breadth; but where this is not the case, and the gums give way, the gums generally become extremely diseased; and as they are separated from both the teeth and the alveolar process, there is a very considerable discharge of matter from those detached surfaces.

Though the wasting of the alveoli at their mouths, and the filling up at their bottoms, are to be considered as diseases, when they happen early in life, yet it would appear to be only on account of a natural effect taking place too soon; for the same thing is very common in old age* : and also, as this process of filling up the bottom, and wasting of

---

* Natural History of the Teeth, p. 4.

the mouths of the alveolar processes, takes place in all ages, where a tooth has been drawn, and the connexion between the two parts is destroyed, this might lead us to suspect that the original cause of these diseases may be a want of that perfect harmony which is required between the tooth and socket, whereby a stimulus may be given in some degree similar to the loss of a tooth; and by destroying that stimulus upon which the absorption of the process and the filling up of the socket depend, the natural disposition may be restored. This last opinion is strengthened by the following case.

One of the first incisores of the upper jaw of a young lady was gradually falling lower and lower. She was desirous of having a tooth transplanted, which might better fit the shallow socket, as it was now become. She consulted me: I objected to this, fearing that the same disposition might still continue; in which case the new tooth would be probably pushed out in about half a year; that the time since the old one began to sink, and a relief of so short a continuance, would be all the advantage gained by the operation; but I observed, at the same time, that the operation might have the effect of destroying the disposition to filling up, so that the new tooth might keep its ground. This idea turned the balance in favour of the operation; and it was performed. Time showed that the reasoning was just: the tooth fastened, and has kept in its situation for some years.

These diseases arise often from visible causes. Anything that occasions a considerable and long-continued inflammation in those parts, such particularly as a salivation, will produce the same effect. The scurvy also, when carried to a great height, attacks the gums and the alveolar processes, which becomes a cause of the dissolution of those parts. This is most remarkable in the scurvy at sea.

When the disease arises from these two last causes, the gums are either affected with the same disease, together with the alveolar processes, or they sympathize with them. They swell, become soft and tender, and upon the least pressure or friction bleed very freely.

How far these diseases can be prevented and cured is, I believe, not known.

The practice has principally been to scarify the gums freely; and this with a view to fasten the teeth made loose by the disease, which has therefore generally made a considerable progress before even an attempt towards a cure has been made. This scarification has certainly a good effect in some cases, the teeth thereby becoming much faster; but how far the alveolar processes have been destroyed in such instances cannot be determined. Perhaps only a general fullness of the attaching membrane between the tooth and the process had taken place, as in a slight salivation, so as to push the tooth a little way out of the bony socket; which having subsided by the plentiful bleeding, the tooth of course becomes fast. Or perhaps, by producing an inflammation of another kind, the first inflammation, or disposition to inflame, is destroyed; which evidently appeared in the case of the young lady above mentioned.

If the above practice is unsuccessful, and the tooth continues to protrude, it will either become very troublesome or a great deformity. A front tooth may not, indeed, be at first so troublesome as a grinder, because these teeth frequently overhang, but it will be extremely disagreeable to the eye.

If the cause cannot be removed, the effect must be the object of our attention. To file down the projecting part is the only thing that can be done; but care must be taken not to file into the cavity, otherwise pain, inflammation, and other bad consequences may probably ensue. This practice, however, will be very troublesome, because it will be difficult to file a loose tooth. At last the tooth will drop out, which will put an end to all further trouble.

If the alveoli have really been destroyed in those cases of loose teeth which have become firm again, it would be difficult to ascertain whether they have a power of renewing themselves analogous to that power by which they first grow, or whether the fastening be effected by a closing of the gum and process to the teeth. When the disease arises from the scurvy, the first attempt must be to cure that disease, and afterwards the above local treatment may be of service.

Together with drawing blood from the gums, astringents have always been used to harden them. But when the disease does not arise from a constitutional cause, which may be removed, (such as the sea-scurvy or salivation,) but from a disposition in the parts themselves, I have seen little relief given by them.

The tincture of myrrh, tincture of Peruvian bark, and sea-water are some of the applications which have been recommended.

In such cases I have seen considerable benefit from the use of the tincture of bark and laudanum, in the proportion of two parts of the tincture of bark to one of the laudanum : and this to be used frequently, and at each time to be kept in the mouth during ten, fifteen, or twenty minutes.[a]

---

[a] [The practice here recommended of filing a tooth which is descending in the alveolus, is, on more than one account, exceedingly injurious. The immediate cause of such a descent of the tooth is, as Hunter observes, a deposit of bone in the alveolus; and, as this deposit takes place in consequence of some irritation in the periosteum, everything should be avoided that could increase this irritation. Filing, however, would certainly

CHAPTER III.

OF THE DISEASES OF THE GUMS, AND THE CONSE-QUENCES OF THEM.

§. 1. *The Scurvy in the Gums (vulgarly so called).*

THE gums are extremely subject to diseases, the symptoms of which, in an advanced state of them, are in general such as were described in the preceding chapter.

They swell, become extremely tender, and bleed upon every occasion; which circumstances being somewhat similar to those observable in the true scurvy, the disease has generally been called a scurvy in the gums.

But as this seems to be the principal way in which the gums are affected, I suspect that the same symptoms may arise from various causes, as I have often seen the same appearances in children evidently of a scrofulous habit, and have also suspected the same cause in grown people : they likewise frequently appear in persons who are in all other respects perfectly healthy.

When the gums first begin to have a tenderness, we may observe it first on their edges : the common smooth skin of the gum is not continued to its very edge, but becomes at the edge a little rough like a border, and somewhat thickened. The part of the gum between two teeth swells, and often pushes out like luxuriant flesh, which is frequently very tender.

The inflammation is often carried so far as to make the gums ulcerate, so that the gums in many cases have a common ulcer upon them, by which process a part of the teeth is denuded. This is often on one part only, often only on one jaw, while in some cases it is on the whole gums on both jaws.

In this case it often happens that the alveolar process disappears,

---

increase it to a great degree. It would also tend greatly to lessen the attachment of the tooth to the socket, and the support which the latter affords to it. The best mode of treatment appears to be, to apply leeches occasionally, particularly when there is any unusual sensation produced by touching the tooth, indicating a degree of inflammation in the periosteum of the socket. This plan may be followed up by the use of astringent lotions. It is unnecessary to add, that any force applied to the tooth, and even frequently touching it, should be avoided. Ligatures are especially improper.]

after the manner above described (see page 80), by taking part in the inflammation, either from the same cause, or from sympathy. In such cases there is always a very considerable discharge of matter from the inside of the gum and alveolar process, which always takes the course of the tooth for its exit.

In many of these cases we find that while the gums are ulcerating in one part, they are swelling and becoming spongy in another, and hanging loose upon the teeth; and this often takes place where there is no ulceration in any part.

The treatment proper in this disease, where the gums become luxuriant from a kind of tumefaction, is generally to cut away all the redundant swellings of the gum. I have seen several instances where this has succeeded; but still I am inclined to think that this is not the best practice; for it is not that an adventitious substance is thus removed, as in the case of luxuriant granulations from a sore, but a part of the gum itself is destroyed, in like manner as a part enlarged by inflammation may be reduced by the knife to its natural size; which would certainly be bad practice. I should suspect that the good arising from such practice is owing to the bleeding which takes place, especially as I have found from experience that simply scarifying the gums has answered the same purpose. Where there are reasons for supposing it to arise from a peculiarity in the constitution, the treatment should be such as will remove this peculiarity.

If the constitution is scorbutic, it must be treated with a view to the original disease. If scrofulous, local treatment, by wounding the parts, may do harm; but sea-bathing, and washing the mouth frequently with sea-water, are the most powerful means of cure that I know.[a]

§. 2. *Callous Thickenings of the Gums.*

The gums are also subject to other diseases, abstracted from their connexion with the alveoli and teeth, which do not wholly belong to our present subject.

---

[a] [In the most severe cases of this disease which have ever come under the notice of the editor, after every other means had failed to produce any permanent benefit, the two remedies mentioned in the text, sea-bathing and washing the mouth with sea-water, have proved, as Hunter observes, the most powerful means of cure. It is very probable that the general tonic effect of change of air and of scene, and the absence of all the debilitating tendencies of close application to business and of a town residence and town habits, may have greatly assisted the means alluded to; but there appears also to have been much direct benefit derived from the local application of sea-water.]

A very common one is the thickening of the gum in some particular place, of a hard callous nature, similar to an excrescence. Many of these have a cancerous appearance, which deters the surgeon from meddling with them; but in general without reason.

They may be often removed by the knife, but not always. The bleeding which follows is generally so considerable that it is frequently necessary to apply the actual cautery.

They sometimes grow again, which subjects the patient to the same operation. I have known them extracted six times; but in such cases I suspect that they really have a cancerous disposition; at least, it has been so in two cases which have fallen under my observation.

But here the skill of the surgeon rather than that of the dentist is required.

CHAPTER IV.

OF NERVOUS PAINS IN THE JAWS.

THERE is one disease of the jaws which seems in reality to have no connexion with the teeth, but of which the teeth are generally suspected to be the cause. This deserves to be taken notice of in this place because operators have frequently been deceived by it, and even sound teeth have sometimes been extracted through an unfortunate mistake.

This pain is seated in some one part of the jaws. As simple pain demonstrates nothing, a tooth is often suspected, and is perhaps drawn out; but still the pain continues, with this difference, however, that it now seems to be in the root of the next tooth: it is then supposed either by the patient or the operator that the wrong tooth was extracted, whereupon that in which the pain now seems to be is drawn, but with as little benefit. I have known cases of this kind where all the teeth of the affected side of the jaw have been drawn out, and the pain has continued in the jaw; in others it has had a different effect, the sensation of pain has become more diffused, and has at last attacked the corresponding side of the tongue. In the first case I have known it recommended to cut down upon the jaw, and even to perforate and cauterize it, but all without effect.

Hence it should appear that the pain in question does not arise from any disease in the part, but is entirely a nervous affection.

It is sometimes brought on, or increased, by affections of the mind, of which I once saw a remarkable instance in a young lady.

It often has its periods, and these are frequently very regular.

The regularity of its periods gives an idea of its being a proper case for the bark, which however frequently fails.

I have seen cases of some years' standing, where the hemlock has succeeded when the bark has had no effect; but sometimes all attempts prove unsuccessful. Sea-bathing has been in some cases of singular service.[a]

CHAPTER V.

OF THE EXTRANEOUS MATTER UPON THE TEETH.

There are parts of the tooth which lie out of the way of friction, viz. the angles made by two teeth, and the small indentation between the tooth and gum.

Into these places the juices are pressed, and there stagnate, giving them at first the appearance of being stained or dirty. A tooth in this stage is generally clean for some way from its cutting edge towards

---

[a] [The disease here treated of is evidently that which has since the time of Hunter been so often treated of under the terms Neuralgia and Tic douloureux. It is unnecessary here to say much on the subject of this disease when arising from constitutional causes, in which case, I believe, the periodical character will almost always distinguish it; but it may not be useless to offer a few observations on those cases of local neuralgia which are more or less connected with the teeth, and which more or less nearly simulate tic douloureux, especially when occurring in a constitution predisposed to that affection. It appears that the pressure of any extraneous body on the fibre of a nerve will produce the peculiar pain in question. Hence it not unfrequently happens that the deposit of bony matter on the extremity of the root of a tooth, the existence of a dead tooth, and any other similar cause will produce it. I have seen a case in which every constitutional remedy, usually employed in tic douloureux, had been employed without effect for an affection of this kind, which had become excessively violent in its attacks; and on learning that it had existed ever since the extraction of a tooth, the part was carefully examined, and a small spicula of the alveolar process was discovered under the edge of the gum, on touching which the paroxysm of pain was instantly excited. The removal of this spicula was at once successful. This case is here mentioned to show how trifling a cause may produce the most severe pains of this description, and to point out the necessity for a careful and even minute examination of the part in which the pain appears to commence.]

the gum, on account of the motion of the lips upon it, and the pressure of the food, &c. It is also pretty clean close to the gum from the motion of the loose edge of the gum upon that part; but this circumstance is only observable in those who have their gums perfectly sound, for in others this loose edge of the gum is either lost, or no longer retains its free motion.

If art be not now used, as the natural motion of the parts is not sufficient, the incrustation increasing covers more and more of the teeth. As mastication generally keeps that part clear which is near to the edges and grinding surfaces, and as the motion of the lips in some measure retards its growth outwards, it accumulates on the parts above mentioned till it rises almost as high as the gum; its growth being now retarded in that direction, it accumulates on the edge next to the gum, so that in time it passes over the gum, of which it covers a greater or less portion. When it has increased so much as to touch the gum, (which very soon happens, especially in the angle between the teeth,) it produces ulceration of that part, and a train of bad consequences. Often the gums, receding from this matter, become very tender, and subject to hæmorrhage.

The alveolar processes frequently take part with the gums, and ulcerate, so that the teeth are left without their support, and at last drop out, similarly to the diseases of these parts already described.

All our juices contain a considerable quantity of calcareous earth, which is dissolved in them, and which is separated from them upon exposure, which continues mixed with the mucus; so that the extraneous matter consists of earth and the common secreted mucus*.

This disposition of the juices of the mouth to abound so much with earth, seems to be peculiar to some people, perhaps to some constitutions; but I have not been able to ascertain what these are. We find persons who seem to have nothing particular either in constitution or way of life so subject to this accumulation that the common methods of prevention, such as washing and brushing the teeth, have not the desired effect.

The disposition is so strong in some people that the concretion forms on the whole body of the tooth; I have seen it even on the grinding surface of the molares, and often two or three teeth are cemented together with it. This I think could only happen to those who seldom or never use these teeth. It is very apt to accumulate on a tooth the opposite of which is lost.

I once saw a case of this kind where the accumulation, which was on a grinder, appeared like a tumour on the inside of the mouth, and

* Vide Natural History, page 55, in the note, for a further description of this.

made a rising in the cheek, which was supposed by every one that felt it to be a scirrhous tumour forming on the cheek; but it broke off and discovered what it was.

This accumulation is very apt to begin during a fit of sickness, when the extraneous juices are allowed to rest; and perhaps the juices themselves may have at this time a greater tendency to produce the incrusting matter.

It may also arise from any circumstance which prevents a person from eating solids, whereby the different parts of the mouth have less motion on each other. Lying-in women are instances of this; not to mention that the assistance of art in keeping the teeth clean is commonly wanting under such circumstances.

The adventitious substance, as was said before, is composed of mucus, or animal juices, and calcareous earth; the earth is attached to and crystallized upon the tooth, and the mucus is entangled in these crystals.

The removal of this adventitious matter is a part in which the dentist ought to be very cautious; he should be perfectly master of the difference between the natural, or original, tooth and the adventitious matter; and he should be sensible of the propriety of saving as much as possible of the tooth, and at the same time take pains to remove all that which is not natural. Many persons have had their teeth wholly spoiled by an injudicious treatment of them in this respect.

As the cause of this incrustation is not either a known disease of the constitution or of the parts, but depends on a property of the matter secreted, simply as inanimate matter, the remedy of course becomes either mechanical or chemical.

The mechanical remedies are friction, filing, and picking. The first is sufficient when the teeth are only beginning to be discoloured; or, when already clean, they may be thus kept clean. Various are the methods proposed: to wash them with cold water, and at the same time to rub them with a piece of cloth on the fore finger, has been thought sufficient by some; others have recommended the dust of a burnt cork, burnt bread, &c., with a view to act with more power on the adventitious matter than what can be applied by the means of a soft brush or cloth.

In cases where this incrustation has been more considerable, powders of various kinds have been employed, such as tartar, bole, and many others.

Cream of tartar is often used, which at the same time that it acts mechanically, has likewise a chemical power, and dissolves this matter.

Other mechanical means are instruments to pick, scrape, and file off the calcareous earth; these should only be made use of when it is in large quantities, and with great caution, as the teeth may be somewhat loose; or a part of the tooth may be broken off with the incrustation.

The chemical means are solvents: these are either alkalies or acids; the alkaline salt will answer very well early in the disease, for the crust in the first stage consists chiefly of mucus, which the alkali will remove very readily; but it should not be used too freely, as it rather softens the gums, and makes them extremely tender.

Acids are also employed with success, as they dissolve the earth, but are attended with this disadvantage, that they act with more force upon the tooth itself, dissolving part of it; which is to be avoided, if possible, for no part of a sound tooth can be spared.

We may observe that people who eat a good deal of salad or fruit have their teeth much cleaner than common, which is owing to the acids in those fruits; and for the same reason people's teeth are commonly cleaner in summer than winter in those countries where there is a great plenty of fruit. When the accumulation has been considerable, the teeth and gums will feel tender on the removal of this matter, and even be affected by cold air; but this will not be of long continuance.

CHAPTER VI.

OF THE IRREGULARITY OF THE TEETH.

As that part of each jaw which holds the ten fore teeth is exactly of the same size when it contains those of the first set as when it contains those of the second, and as these last often occupy a much larger space than the first*, in such cases the second set are obliged to stand very irregularly.

This happens much oftener in the upper jaw than in the lower, because the difference of the size of the two sets is much greater in that jaw.

This irregularity is observed almost solely in the incisores and cuspidati; for they are the only teeth which are larger than their predecessors.

It most frequently happens to the cuspidati, because they are often

* Natural History, p. 45.

formed later than the bicuspides; in consequence of which the whole space is taken up before they make their appearance: in such cases they are obliged to shoot forwards or outwards over the second incisor. However, it frequently happens to the incisores, but seldom to such a degree. This arises often from the temporary cuspidatus of one or both sides standing firm. I have seen the irregularities so much as to appear like a double row.

The bicuspides generally have sufficient room to grow, because even more space than what they can occupy is kept for them by the temporary grinders*. This, however, is not universally the case; for I have seen where the bicuspides were obliged to grow out of the circle, very probably from their being later in growing than common.

That it is from want of room in the jaw, and not from any effect that the first set produces upon them, is evident; first, because in all cases of irregularity we find that there is really not room in the jaw to allow of placing all the teeth properly in the circle; so that some are necessarily on the outside of the circle, others within it, while others are turned with their edges obliquely, as it were, warped; and secondly, because the bicuspides are not out of the circle, although they are as much influenced by the first set as any of the others.

As they are not influenced by the first set, it cannot be of any service to draw the first possessor, for that gives way in the same proportion as the other advances. As the succeeding tooth, however, is broader, it often interferes with a shedding tooth next to it, the fang of which not being influenced by the growth of its own succeeding tooth, it does not decay in proportion as the other advances, and therefore the drawing of the adjoining shedding tooth is often of service†.

In cases of considerable irregularity for want of room, a principal object is to remove those which are most out of their place, and thereby procure room for the others which are to be brought into the circle.

To extract an irregular tooth would answer but little purpose if no alteration could be made in the situation of the rest; but we find that the very principle upon which teeth are made to grow irregularly is capable, if properly directed, of bringing them even again. This principle is the power which many parts (especially bones) have of moving out of the way of mechanical pressure.

The irregularity of the teeth is at first owing to mechanical pressure; for one tooth getting the start of another, and fixing firmly in its place, becomes a resistance to the young, loose, forming tooth, and gives it an oblique direction. The same principle takes place in a completely formed tooth whenever a pressure is made upon it. Probably a tooth

* Natural History, p. 36. † Ibid., p. 47.

might by slow degrees be moved to any part of the mouth, for I have seen the cuspidati pressed into the place of the incisores. However, it is observed that the teeth are easier moved backwards than forwards, and when moved back that they are permanent, but often when moved forwards that they are very apt to recede.

The best time for moving the teeth is in youth, while the jaws have an adapting disposition; for after a certain time they do not so readily suit themselves to the irregularity of the teeth. This we see plainly to be the case when we compare the loss of a tooth at the age of fifteen years and at that of thirty or forty. In the first case we find that the two neighbouring teeth approach one another, in every part alike, till they are close; but in the second the distance in the jaw between the two neighbouring teeth remains the same, while the bodies will in a small degree incline to one another from want of lateral support.

And this circumstance of the bodies of the teeth yielding to pressure upon their base, shows that even in the adult they might be brought nearer to one another by art properly applied.

As the operation of moving the teeth is by lateral pressure upon their bodies, these bodies must first have passed through the gum sufficiently for a hold to be taken.

The best time seems to be, when the two grinders of the child have been shed; for at this time a natural alteration is taking place in that part of the jaw.

The means of making this pressure I shall only slightly describe, as they will greatly vary according to circumstances, so considerably, indeed, that scarcely two cases are to be treated alike, and in general the dentists are tolerably well acquainted with the methods.

In general, it is done with ligatures or plates of silver. The ligatures answer best when it is only required to bring two teeth closer together, which are pretty much in the circle. The trouble attending this is but trifling, as it is only that of having them tied once a week or fortnight.

Where teeth growing out of the circle are to be brought into it, curved silver plates, of a proper construction, must be used. These are generally made to act on three points, two fixed points on the standing teeth, and the third on the tooth which is to be moved. That part of the plate which rests on the two standing teeth must be of a sufficient length for that purpose, while the curved part is short, and goes on the opposite side of the tooth to be moved. Its effect depends very much on the attention of the patient, who must frequently press hard upon it with the teeth of the opposite jaw; so that this method is much more troublesome to the patient than the ligature.

It is impossible to give absolute directions what tooth or teeth ought to be pulled out. That must be left to the judgment of the operator; but the following general hints may be of service.

1. If there is any one tooth very much out of the row, and all the others regular, that tooth may be removed, and the two neighbouring ones brought closer together.

2. If there are two or more teeth of the same side very irregular (as, for instance, the second incisor and cuspidatus), and it appears to be of no consequence, with respect to regularity, which of them is removed, I should recommend the extraction of the furthest back of the two, viz. the cuspidatus; because, if there should be any space not filled up when the other is brought into the row, it will not be so readily seen.

3. If the above-mentioned two teeth are not in the circle, but still not far out of it, and yet there is not room for both, in such a case I would recommend the extraction of the first bicuspis, although it should be perfectly in the row, because the two others will then be easily brought into the circle, and if there is any space left, it will be so far back as not to be at all observable.

The upper jaw is often rather too narrow from side to side, near the anterior part which supports the fore teeth, and projects forwards considerably over the lower, giving the appearance of the rabbit-mouth, although the teeth be quite regular in the circle of the jaw.

In such a case it is necessary to draw a bicuspis of each side, by which means the fore part of the circle will fall back; and if a cross-bar was to be stretched from side to side across the roof of the mouth, between cuspis and cuspis, it would widen the circle. The fore teeth might also be tied to this bar, which would be a means of assisting nature in bringing them back. This has been practised, but it is troublesome.

As neither the bodies nor the fangs of the teeth are perfectly round; we find that this circumstance often becomes a cause of their taking a twist; for, while growing, they may press with one edge only on the completely formed tooth, by which means they will be turned a little upon their centre.

The alteration of these is more difficult than of the former, for it is, in general, impossible to apply, so long and constantly as is necessary for such an operation, any pressure that has the power of turning the tooth upon its centre. However, in the incisores, it may be done by the same powers which produce the lateral motion; but where these cannot be applied, as is frequently the case, the tooth may be either pulled out entirely, and put in again even, or it may be twisted round sufficiently to bring it into a proper position, as has been often practised.

It may not be improper, in this place, to take notice of a case which frequently occurs. It is a decay of the first adult grinder at an early age, viz. before the temporary grinders are shed, and before the second grinder of the adult has made its appearance through the gum. In this case, I would recommend removing the diseased tooth immediately, although it may occasion no kind of trouble; for, if it be drawn before the temporary grinders are shed, and before the second adult grinder has cut the gum, it will in a short time not be missed; because the bicuspis of that side will fall a little back, and the second and third grinders will come a little forward, by which means the space will be filled up, and these teeth will be well supported. Besides, the removal of this tooth will make room for the fore teeth, which are often very much wanted, especially in the upper jaw.[a]

CHAPTER VII.

OF IRREGULARITIES BETWEEN THE TEETH AND JAW.

CERTAIN disproportions between the teeth and jaw sometimes occur, one of which is, when the body of the lower jaw is not of sufficient length for all the teeth. In such cases, the last grinder never gets perfectly from under the coronoid process, its anterior edge only being uncovered; and the gum, which still in part lies upon the tooth, is

---

[a] [The foregoing observations on irregularity are generally very judicious; and it would have been well if many writers on this subject had imitated the moderation which characterizes the mode of treatment here recommended. It is in the treatment of the teeth of children during the second dentition that we have in the present day chiefly to deplore the continual interference of interested ignorance, in the early removal of the temporary teeth, under the pretence of *making room* for the permanent ones. It is impossible too often or too forcibly to deprecate this practice. Cruel as it is, this is perhaps its least evil, for the pain and apprehension which are occasioned by it are but temporary; but a great permanent disadvantage follows this practice, which is, that if the temporary teeth be removed before the permanent ones are ready to fall into their place, the jaw will considerably contract during the growth of the child, and thus create a discrepancy between the size of the new teeth and the extent of the arch which they are to occupy. I feel assured that, upon the whole, more injury is at present done, with regard to irregularity, by the interference of dentists, than would accrue were the teeth of children at this period never examined or meddled with at all.

rubbed against the sharp points of the tooth, and is often squeezed between the tooth upon which it lies and the corresponding one of the upper jaw. This occasions so much uneasiness to the patient, that it becomes necessary to relieve the gum, if possible, by dividing it freely in several places, that it may shrink and leave this surface of the tooth wholly uncovered. If this does not answer, which is sometimes the case, it is advisable to draw the tooth.

Sometimes, although but seldom, an inconvenience arises from the dentes sapientiæ being in the upper jaw and not in the lower; these teeth pressing upon the anterior part of the root of the coronoid process when the mouth is shut; for the coronoid processes are further forwards in such cases than when the lower jaw also has its dentes sapientiæ; in short, the exact correspondence between the two jaws is not kept up.

In such cases, I know of no other remedy but the extraction of the tooth.

Of Supernumerary Teeth.

When there are supernumerary teeth*, it will in general be proper to have them drawn, for they are commonly either troublesome, or disfigure the mouth.

CHAPTER VIII.

OF THE UNDER JAW.

IT is not uncommon to find the lower jaw projecting too far forwards, so that its fore teeth pass before those of the upper jaw when the mouth is shut†; which is attended with inconvenience, and disfigures the face.

This deformity can be greatly mended in young people. The teeth in the lower jaw can be gradually pushed back, in those whose teeth are not close, while those in the upper can be gently brought forward; which is by much the easiest operation.

These two effects are produced by the same mechanical powers.

* Natural History, p. 46.   † Ibid. p. 30.

While this position of the jaw is only in a small degree, so that the edges of the under teeth can be by the patient brought behind those of the upper, it is in his own power to increase this till the whole be completed, that is, till the grinders meet; and it is not necessary to go further. This is done by frequently bringing the lower jaw as far back as he can, and then squeezing the teeth as close together as possible.

But when it is not in the person's power to bring the lower jaw so far back as to allow the edges of its fore teeth to come behind those of the upper, artificial means are necessary.

The best of these means is an instrument of silver, with a socket or groove shaped to the fore teeth of the lower jaw to receive them, so as to become fast to them, and sloped off as it rises to its upper edge, so as to rise behind the fore teeth in the upper jaw in such a manner that, upon shutting the mouth, the teeth of the upper jaw may catch the anterior part of the slanting surface, and be pushed forward with the power of the inclined plane. The patient who wears such an instrument must frequently shut his mouth with this view.

These need not be continued longer than till the edges of the lower teeth can be got behind those of the upper, for it is then within the power of the patient, as in the first-stated case.

CHAPTER IX.

OF DRAWING THE TEETH.

The extraction of teeth is in some cases an operation of considerable delicacy, and in others no operation is less difficult.

As this is often not thought of till an inflammation has come on, it becomes an object of consideration whether it be proper to remove the tooth while that inflammation continues, or to wait till it has subsided. I am apt to believe it is better to wait even till the parts have perfectly recovered themselves, because the state of irritation renders them more susceptible of pain. The contrary practice might also appear reasonable, for by removing the tooth it might be imagined that we should remove the cause; but when the inflammation has once begun, the effect will go on independently of the cause; and to draw the tooth, in such a situation, is rather to produce a fresh cause, than to remove the present. Of this I think an instance has occurred to me. However, most teeth are drawn in the height of inflammation; and, as we do not find any mischief from the operation, it is perhaps better to do it when the resolution of the patient is the greatest. The sensibility of the mind may even be less at this time.

Teeth are easy or difficult of extraction, according as they are fast or loose in their sockets; in some degree according to the kind of tooth, and also in some degree with reference to their situation*.

They are naturally so fast as to require instruments, and the most cautious and dextrous hand; and yet are sometimes loose enough to be pulled out by the fingers.

When the sockets and gums are considerably decayed, and the tooth or teeth very loose, it would in most cases be right to perform extraction; for when they are allowed to stay, and perhaps are kept in their proper place by being tied to the neighbouring teeth, they then act upon the remaining gum and socket as extraneous bodies, producing ulceration there, and making those parts recede much further than they naturally would have done if the tooth had been drawn earlier; which produces two bad effects—it weakens the lateral support of the two neighbouring teeth, and it renders it more difficult to fix an artificial tooth. But unless these two last circumstances are forcibly impressed upon the patient, it is hardly possible to persuade him to consent to the loss of a tooth while it has any hold, especially a tooth which appears sound.

The extraction should never be done quickly; for this often occasions great mischief, breaking the tooth or jaw; on the same principle as a bullet going against an open door with great velocity will pass through it, but with little velocity will shut it.

This caution is most necessary in adults, or in the permanent teeth†; for in young subjects, where there are only the temporary teeth‡, the jaw not being so firm, the tooth is not in much danger of being broken§.

It is a common practice to divide the gum from the tooth before it is drawn, which is attended with very little advantage, because at best it can only be imperfectly done, and that part of the gum which adheres to the tooth decays when it is lost. But if such a separation as

---

* For further directions, see Natural History, p. 54.
† Natural History, p. 36.   ‡ Ibid., Pl. VIII. f. 16, 17, 18.
§ I must do Mr. Spence the justice to say, that this method appears to be peculiar to him, and that he is the only operator I ever knew who would submit to be instructed, or even allow an equal in knowledge; and I must do the same justice to both his sons.

can be made saves any pain in the whole of the operation, I should certainly recommend it; and at least, in some cases, it might prevent the gum from being torn. It is also a common practice to close the gum, as it is termed: this is more for show than use; for the gum cannot be made so close as to unite by the first intention, and therefore the cavity from which the tooth came must suppurate like every other wound. But, as the sensations of these parts are adapted to such a loss, and as a process very different from that which follows the loss of so much substance in any other part of the body is to take place, the consequent inflammations and suppurations are not so violent*. We may be allowed to call this a natural operation which goes on in the gum and alveoli, and not a violence; as we see that the delivery of a young animal before its time, which is similar to the drawing of a fixed tooth, in happening before all the containing parts are prepared for the loss, produces considerable local violence, without doing proportionable mischief. Therefore in general it is very unnecessary to do anything at all to the gum.

There are some particular circumstances which naturally, and others which accidentally, attend and follow the drawing of teeth; but they are in general of no great consequence.

There follows a bleeding from the vessels of the socket and those passing between it and the teeth†. This commonly is but trifling; however, instances have occurred where it has been very considerable, and the awkwardness of the situation makes it very difficult to stop it. In general it will be sufficient to stuff the socket with lint, or lint dipped in the oil of turpentine, and to apply a compress of lint, or a piece of cork thicker than the bodies of the adjacent teeth, so that the teeth in the opposite jaw may keep up a pressure.

It has been advised to stuff into the socket some soft wax, on a supposition that it would mould itself to the cavity, and so stop the bleeding; this perhaps may sometimes answer better than the other method, and therefore should be tried when that fails.

It is scarcely possible to draw some teeth without breaking the alveolar processes. This in general is but of little consequence, because, from the nature of the union between the teeth and sockets, these last can scarcely be broken further than the points of the fang, and in very few cases so far; therefore little mischief can ensue, as the fracture extends no further than the part of the socket which will naturally decay after the loss of the tooth; and that part which does not decay will be filled up as a basis for the gum to rest upon. It has been supposed that

---

* Vide Natural History, on decay of the Alveoli, p. 4.
† Natural History, pp. 19, 20, Pl. VIII. f. 1—8.

the splinters do mischief: I very much doubt this; for if they are not so much detached as to lose the living principle, they still continue part of our body, and are rounded off at their points, as all splinters are in other fractures, and particularly here, for the reasons already assigned, viz. because this part has a greater disposition for wasting. And if they are wholly detached they will either come away before the gum contracts entirely, or after it is closed will act as an extraneous body, form a small abscess in the gum, and come out.

It sometimes happens that the tooth is broken, and its point or more of the fang is left behind, which is very often sufficient to continue the former complaints; and therefore it should be extracted, if it can be done, with care. If it cannot be extracted the gum will in part grow over it, and the alveoli will decay as far as where it is. The decaying principle of the socket will produce the disposition to fill up at the bottom, whereby the stump will be pushed out; but, perhaps, not till it has given some fits of the tooth-ache. However, this circumstance does not always become a cause of the tooth-ache.

Transplanting Teeth.

Although this operation is in itself a matter of no difficulty, yet upon the whole it is one of the nicest of all operations, and requires more chirurgical and physiological knowledge than any that comes under the care of the dentist. There are certain cautions necessary to be observed, especially if it be a living tooth which is to be transplanted, because in that case it is meant to retain its life, and we have no great variety of choice. Much, likewise, depends upon the patient; he should apply early, and give the dentist all the time he thinks necessary to get a sufficient number of teeth that appear to be of a proper size, &c. Likewise he must not be impatient to get out of his hands before it is advisable.

The incisores, cuspidati, and bicuspides can alone be changed, because they have single fangs. The success is greater in the incisores and cuspidati than the bicuspides, these last having frequently the ends of their fangs forked, from which circumstance the operation will become less perfect.

It is hardly possible to transplant the grinders, as the chance of fitting the sockets of them is very small. When indeed a grinder is extracted, and the socket sound and perfect, the dentist may, perhaps, be able to fit it by a dead tooth.

Of the State of the Gums and Sockets.

The first object of attention is the sockets and gums of the person who is to have the fresh tooth. If the tooth which is to be removed be not wholly diseased, there is great probability that the socket will be as sound and complete as ever; but if the body of the tooth has been destroyed some time, and the fang has been in the state of what is commonly called a stump, it has most probably begun to decay on its outer surface and point, in which case the socket will be filled up in the same proportion; if so, there is no possibility of success. But as, in the operation of transplanting, the diseased tooth is to be first drawn, it will show the state of the socket; and the scion* tooth is to be left or drawn, according to the appearance on the diseased one.

If the appearance be not favourable, and it therefore be not probable that the scion tooth can be introduced, so as to unite in the place of the stump, I would recommend to every dentist to have some dead teeth at hand, that he may have a chance to fit the socket. I have known these sometimes last for years, especially when well supported by the neighbouring teeth. Indeed this very practice is recommended by some dentists in preference to the other. But even this should not be attempted unless the socket is sound and pretty large, as the tooth can otherwise have but very little hold.

Whenever there are gum-boils I would not recommend transplanting, as there is always in such cases a diseased socket, although the disease has originated in the tooth. In one or two instances, indeed, which I have seen, the boil has been cured by such an operation.

If the gums are diseased, and become spongy, as has been described, it will be very improper to transplant, as there will be but little chance of success; also, if the sockets have a disposition to waste, and the tooth becomes in some degree loose; in short, the sockets and gums should be perfectly sound. No person should have a tooth transplanted while taking mercury, even although the gums are not affected by it at the time, for they may become affected by that medicine before the tooth is fixed. I would carry this still further: no one should have a tooth transplanted who has any complaint that may subject him to the taking of mercury before the tooth is well fixed. For this reason, those who have teeth transplanted ought particularly to avoid for some time the chance of contracting any complaint for the cure of which mercury may be necessary.

I would not recommend transplanting, even where mercury has been taken lately. How soon mercury may be taken after a tooth has been transplanted is not easily ascertained. I have known it fail from this

* As the transplanting of teeth is very similar to the ingrafting of trees, I thought that term might be transferred from gardening to surgery, finding no other word so expressive of the thing.

cause (as-it seemed) after six weeks, where there was every reason to suppose that it might have been attended with success.

Of the Age of the Person who is to have the Scion Tooth.

The socket should be of its full size, and one or two grinders on each side of each jaw should be full grown, to keep the two jaws at a proper distance, which will allow the transplanted tooth to be undisturbed by the motion of the jaw while fastening. This will be at the age of eighteen or twenty years.

It sometimes, however, happens that a fore tooth decays before this age, and even before it is completely formed; and therefore all the above-mentioned advantages cannot be had. In such cases it is not very material whether transplanting is practised or not, as simply to draw the diseased tooth will in most cases be sufficient, for the two neighbouring teeth may be brought together, so as to fill up the space, the others following in a less degree, as has been already observed upon irregularities of the teeth.

Of the Scion Tooth.

The scion tooth, or that which is to be transplanted, should be a full-grown young tooth; young, because the principle of life and union is much stronger in such than in old ones.

It will be scarcely necessary to observe, that the new teeth should always be perfectly sound, and taken from a mouth which has the appearance of that of a person sound and healthy; not that I believe it possible to transplant an infection of any kind from the circulating juices, although we know from experience that it may be done by a matter secreted from them. The scion tooth should be less than what the tooth was, the place of which it is to supply. This cannot at first be known with certainty, but it may in most cases be nearly ascertained, and that is by judging from the size of the bodies of the two teeth; but as the fangs do not always bear an exact proportion to the body, it sometimes happens that this method fails. Also it is not always in our power to judge after this manner, for in some cases the body of the tooth of the person who is to have one transplanted shall be quite destroyed, the fang only remaining : in these cases we must judge from its correspondent on the opposite side; but even that tooth is sometimes destroyed.

It has been supposed that we run no risk by taking the scion tooth from a young subject; but this is no security, for a complete tooth is of the same size in the young as the old*. To remedy this inconvenience as much as possible, the scion tooth should be that of a female, for female teeth are in general smaller than those of men; but the inconvenience still remains whenever a female is the subject of this operation. Some women have such small teeth that it is almost impossible to fit them. When the fang of the scion tooth is larger than that which it is intended to supply, it must be made smaller, and only in that part where it exceeds. But the necessity of this should be avoided if possible, for a tooth that is filed has lost all those inequalities which allow it to be held much faster. If, however, some part must be removed, it should be done so as to imitate the old tooth as much as possible. The best remedy is to have several people ready whose teeth in appearance are fit, for if the first will not answer, the second may. I am persuaded this operation has failed, from a tooth being forced in too tight, for let us reflect what must be the consequence of such practice. A part of the soft covering of the tooth, or lining of the socket, is squeezed between two hard bones, so that all circulation of juices is prevented; a mortification in that part takes place; and in consequence of that a gum-boil, and the loss of all union between tooth and socket, so that the tooth drops out.

It will be hardly necessary to mention that the sooner the scion tooth is put into its place the better, as delay will perpetually lessen the power upon which the union of the two parts depends†.

Of replacing a sound Tooth when drawn by mistake.

It sometimes happens that a tooth is drawn on an idea that it is diseased, because it gives pain, but appears after the extraction to be perfectly sound. In such a case I would recommend the replacing it, that there may be no loss by the operation; and the seat of the pain will probably be removed to the next tooth. A tooth beat out by violence should be replaced in the same manner. This ought to be done as soon as possible; however, I would even recommend the experiment twenty-four hours after the accident, or as long as the socket will receive the tooth, which may be for some days.

If the tooth be replaced at any time before its life is destroyed, it will reunite with the cavity of the socket, and be as fast as ever.

No tooth is excepted from this practice, for although in the grinders

* Natural History, p. 49, on the Growth of Teeth.

† See Natural History of Teeth, pp. 55, 56, for an explanation of the principle upon which the success of this operation depends.

there are more fangs than one, yet these fangs will as readily go into their respective sockets as one fang would ; and most probably when the tooth has been beat out, the sockets are enlarged by their giving way.

However, the grinders are not so subject to such accidents as the fore teeth, both from their situation and from their firmness in the sockets.

Where a tooth has been only loosened, or shoved out in part, the patient must not hesitate, but must replace it immediately. As a proof of the success to be expected from replacing teeth, I will relate the following case.

A gentleman had his first bicuspis knocked out, and the second loosened. The first was driven quite into his mouth, and he spit it out upon the ground, but immediately picked it up and put it into his pocket. Some hours afterwards he called upon me, mentioned the accident, and showed me the tooth. Upon examining his mouth, I found the second bicuspis very loose, but pretty much in its place. The tooth which had been knocked out was not quite dry, but very dirty, having dropped on the ground, and having been some time in his pocket. I immediately put it into warm water, let it stay there to soften, washed it as clean as possible, and then replaced it, first having introduced a probe into the socket to break down the coagulated blood which filled it. I then tied these two teeth to the first grinder, and the cuspidatus with silk, which was kept on some days, and then removed. After a month they were as fast as any teeth in the head, and if it were not for the remembrance of the circumstances above related, the gentleman would not be sensible that his teeth had met with any accident. Four years have now passed since it happened.

Of transplanting a dead Tooth.

The insertion of a dead tooth has been recommended, and I have known them continue for many years. If this always succeeded as well as the living I would give it the preference, because we are much more certain of matching them, as a much greater variety of dead teeth can be procured than of living ones. But they do not always retain their colour, but are susceptible of stain. However, I have known them last for years without any alteration ; and some have appeared rather to acquire a transparency, which dead teeth in general have not.

Of the immediate Fastening of a transplanted Tooth.

When a tooth has been transplanted, the next thing to be done is to fix it in that position in which it is intended to remain, that is, in general, to the two neighbouring teeth, by means of silk or sea-weed. If it is an incisor or cuspidatus, the silk should first be tied to the neck of one of the neighbouring teeth, as near the gum as possible; then the two ends of the silk should be brought round upon the body of the scion tooth, but not so near the gum as in the former, and tied there; then it should be brought round the neck of the other neighbouring tooth, as near the gum as possible, as in the first, and tied there. The reason of the difference of the heights of the silk recommended must appear evident, it being our intention to keep the tooth close to the bottom of the socket.

If the transplanted tooth be a bicuspis, the same mode of tying may be followed; but the silk may be brought over its grinding surface between the two points, by which it will be better confined than in any other way. It sometimes happens that the body of the scion tooth is either too long, too thick, or in such a position as to be pressed upon by the teeth of the opposite jaw. Great care should be taken to prevent this, as the opposite teeth constantly oppose the fastening of those which are transplanted, in every motion of the jaw. To remedy this inconvenience, we have recommended smaller teeth than those lost; but even when they are of a proper size in other respects they will in some cases still touch the opposite teeth. When this arises from length of the tooth, a small portion may be filed off from the cutting edge with great safety. If it is owing to the thickness of the scion tooth, and in the upper jaw, some part may be filed off the hollow or concave surface of the tooth directly opposed to it. When it is owing to the position of the teeth, the same thing may be done with propriety. By attending to this circumstance in the tying, this inconvenience may in many cases be prevented: however, if it should not be in the power of the dentist to prevent it by the above-mentioned method, then he should bring them forwards by tying them to a silver plate, a little more bent than the circle of the teeth, and resting at each end upon the neighbouring teeth.

Where a tooth does not exactly fit, but is too short, then there arises a difficulty with the patient whether he ought to consult propriety or beauty. The tooth should be as much in the socket as it can be with ease, for although in that case it is too short, appearances must give way.

The patient must now finish the rest. He must be particularly attentive at first, and give it as little motion as possible. In many cases a soreness will continue some days, and the gums will swell; in others there will neither be soreness nor swelling.

The patient must take great care not to catch cold, or expose himself to any of the other common causes of fever, for such accidents are very likely to prevent the success of this operation. This caution is more necessary in the winter than the summer.

The tooth in some will begin to be fast in a few days, and the gum will cling close to it; while in others many weeks will pass before this happens, though the tooth may become fixed at last.

I have seen the transplanted tooth come a little way out of the socket, and, without any art being used, retire into it as far as at first. The silk is to be removed sooner or later, according as the tooth is more or less fast; in some people after a fortnight, in others not till some months after the operation.

This operation, like all others, is not attended with certain success. It sometimes happens that the two parts do not unite, and in such cases the tooth often acts as an extraneous body*, and instead of fastening, the tooth becomes looser and looser, the gum swells, and a considerable inflammation is kept up, often terminating in a gum-boil. In some cases, where it is also not attended with success, there are not these symptoms: the parts appear pretty sound, only the teeth do not fasten, and sometimes drop out.

It also happens that transplanted teeth have a very singular operation performed on them while in the socket; the living socket and gum finding this body kept in by force, so that they cannot push it out, set about another mode of getting rid of it, by eating away the fang till the whole is destroyed, exactly similar to the wasting of the fangs of the temporary teeth in the young subject†.

I have all along supposed, that where this practice is attended with success there is a living union between the tooth and socket, and that they receive their future nourishment from this new master. My reasons for supposing it were founded on experiments on other parts‡, in animals, and also observations made on the practice itself; for first I observed that they kept their colour, which is very different from that of a dead tooth; for a living tooth has a degree of transparency, while a dead one is of an opake chalky white.

* I say often, because I do not suppose that it always acts as an extraneous body; because we know that dead teeth have stood for years without affecting the sockets or gums in the least. We may therefore suppose that it is sometimes the case with transplanted living teeth.

† Natural History, p. 43, Pl. VIII. f. 16, 17.   ‡ Natural History, p. 55.

Secondly, there are instances of their becoming diseased, in the same manner as an original living tooth; at least the following case favours strongly this opinion.

In October 1772, a gentleman of the city of London had a tooth transplanted, which was perfectly sound, and fixed in its new socket extremely well; about a year and a half after two spots were observed on the fore part of the body of the tooth, which threatened a decay; they were exactly similar to specks, or the first appearance of decay, which come upon natural living teeth. Pain is also sometimes felt in the transplanted tooth.

But what puts it beyond a doubt is, that a living tooth, when transplanted into some living part of an animal, will retain its life; and the vessels of the animal shall communicate with the tooth, as is shown by the following experiments.

I took a sound tooth from a person's head; then made a pretty deep wound with a lancet into the thick part of a cock's comb, and pressed the fang of the tooth into this wound, and fastened it with threads passed through other parts of the comb. The cock was killed some months after, and I injected the head with a very minute injection; the comb was then taken off and put into a weak acid, and the tooth being softened by this means, I slit the comb and tooth into two halves, in the long direction of the tooth. I found the vessels of the tooth well injected, and also observed that the external surface of the tooth adhered everywhere to the comb by vessels, similar to the union of a tooth with the gum and sockets*.[a]

* I may here just remark, that this experiment is not generally attended with success. I succeeded but once out of a great number of trials.

---

[a] [It is unnecessary in the present day to enter into any discussion on the merits of on operation now, I believe, wholly discontinued. From the experiments which Hunter made on the transplanting of teeth from the jaw to other situations, and the successful result of several of them, the operation in question became a favourite one with him; and it appears to have been very frequently performed either by himself or under his directions. The frequent failures which occurred, even in the operation itself, and still more the severe results which very often succeeded its performance at different periods, have very properly induced almost all subsequent practitioners to abandon its employment. Nothing but the sanguine expectations created in an ardent mind, by the interesting results which followed his first experiments, could account for a man of so sound a judgment having followed up a practice so obviously objectionable.

The experiment with which this section is closed has, however, an interest attached to it far more important than its having given rise to the temporary adoption of an objectionable operation. In the result of this experiment may be found an interesting collateral argument in favour of the organized structure of the teeth, and their actual living connexion with the body. The vessels of the tooth, we are told, were well injected, and the external surface adhered everywhere to the comb by vessels. To what

Of Dentition.

Teeth, at their first formation, and for some time while growing, are completely inclosed within the sockets and gums*, and in their growth they act upon the inclosing parts in some degree as extraneous bodies; for while the operation of growth is going on in them, another operation is produced, which is a decay of that part of the gum and socket that covers the tooth, and which becomes the cause of the very disagreeable and even dangerous symptoms which attend this process. As the teeth advance in size, they are in the same proportion pressing against these sockets or gums, from whence inflammation and ulceration are produced.

That ulceration which takes place in dentition is one of the species which seldom or never produces suppuration : however, in some few cases I have found the gums ulcerated, and the body of the tooth surrounded with matter; but I believe this seldom happens till the tooth is near cutting the skin of the gums.

As this is a disease of an early age, and indeed almost begins with life, its symptoms are more diffused, more general, and more uncertain at such an early period than those of any disorder of full-grown people, putting on the appearance of a great variety of maladies; but these symptoms become less various and less hazardous as the child advances in years, so that the double teeth of the child, and still more so the second set of teeth, or those of the adult, are usually cut without producing much disturbance.

These symptoms are so various in different children, and often in the same child, that it is difficult to conceive them to be from the same origin, and the varieties are such as seem to be beyond our knowledge.

They produce both local and constitutional complaints, with local sympathy.

The local symptoms we may suppose to be attended with pain, which appears to be expressed by the child when he is restless, uneasy, rubs his gums, and puts everything into his mouth. There is gene-

---

* Natural History, pp. 33 and 34, Pl. VIII. f. 15.

---

purpose are these vessels formed, what object can possibly be fulfilled by the existence of a vascular pulp in the internal cavity, and a vascular periosteum covering the external surface,—so obviously vascular that it was *well* injected from the vessels of a cock's comb, into which it had been transplanted,—unless they are intended to *nourish* the bony substance of which the tooth consists, and to form the medium of its connexion with the general system?]

rally inflammation, heat, and swelling of the gums, and an increased flow of saliva.

The constitutional or general consequential symptoms are fever and universal convulsion. The fever is sometimes slight and sometimes violent. It is very remarkable both for its sudden rise and declension; so that in the first hour of this illness the child shall be perfectly cool, and in the second flushed and burning hot, and in the third temperate again.

The partial or local consequential symptoms are the most various and complicated; for the appearance they put on is in some degree determined by the nature of the parts they affect: wherefore they imitate various diseases of the human body. These symptoms we shall describe in the order of their most frequent occurrence.

Diarrhœa, costiveness, loss of appetite, eruptions on the skin, especially on the face and scalp, cough, shortness of breath, with a kind of convulsed respiration, similar to that observable in the hooping cough, spasms of particular parts, either by intervals or continued, an increased secretion of urine, and sometimes a diminution of that secretion, a discharge of matter from the penis, with difficulty and pain in making water, imitating exactly a violent gonorrhœa.

The lymphatic glands of the neck are at this time apt to swell; and if the child has a strong tendency to the scrofula, this irritation will promote that disease.

There may be many other symptoms with which we are not at all acquainted, the patients in general not being able to express their feelings. Many of the symptoms of this disease are dangerous, namely, the constitutional ones, and also those local symptoms which attack a vital part. The fever, indeed, seldom lasts so long as to be fatal; but the convulsions, especially when universal, frequently are so. Local convulsions, if not in a vital part, although often very violent, do not kill; and when any part not vital sympathizes, the patient is generally free from danger; a security to the whole being obtained by the sufferings of a part which is of little consequence to life.

Universal sympathy seems to be the first effect of irritation, and in general appears as such in those whose local and partial sensation, and irritability, are not yet formed; for in such subjects, when one part is irritated, the whole sympathizes, and general convulsions ensue. But as the sensations and partial irritability begin to be formed, each part, in some degree acting for itself, acquires its own peculiarities; so that when a local disease takes place in a patient that is very young, it is capable of giving a general disposition to sympathize; but as the child advances, the power of sympathy becomes partial, there not being now in the constitution that universal consent of parts; but some one part is found which has a greater aptitude than the rest to fall in with the local irritation ; therefore the whole disposition for sympathy is directed to some particular part, and it sympathizes according to its own peculiar action. This arises from the different organs acquiring more and more their own independent sensations as the child grows older, and gradually losing the power of sympathizing with one another, so that by the age of six years few parts suffer but those immediately affected; and in adults, who cut their teeth, we almost always find the pain and other symptoms confined to the part, or only local sympathy taking place, such as a swelling of the side of the face.

But as the symptoms become more confined, the suffering part is often much more violently affected than where it has a power of taking in the other parts. Therefore we find that in adults the pain of cutting a grinder is frequently excessive, and that the local inflammation is very considerable, and often of long continuance*. This is not the case with children; their pain does not appear to be so very considerable, and we are certain that the local inflammation is not great; that it is confined to the very parts which suffer, and is not diffused over the face ; so that in children the symptoms of sympathy are often more violent than those of the parts themselves. Though it is generally a fact that the symptoms of dentition in adults are confined to the parts immediately injured, it is not always or certainly so; for sometimes, as will appear from Case the fourth, there will be the strongest symptoms imaginable from sympathy, which seems to be owing to a peculiar aptitude in the constitution to universal sympathy. These pains in the adult are often periodical, having their regular and fixed periods, from which circumstance they are often supposed to be aguish, and the bark is administered, but without effect. Medicines for the rheumatism are likewise given, with as little success, when a tooth will appear, and disclose the cause of the complaint; and by lancing the gums the cure often is performed, but the disease will recur if the gum happens to heal over the tooth, which it will very readily do if the tooth is pretty deep. As these teeth are generally slower in their growth than the others, and more especially those which come very late, they become the cause of many returns of the symptoms. How far children under this circumstance are subject to paroxysms of the disease is not an easy thing to determine; but from many of their sympathetic symptoms going off and returning, it would appear that they have also their exacerbation.

* Vide Case the third.

Of the Cure.

The cure of diseases arising from dentition, from their nature, can only be temporary and local, even when it is directed to the real seat of the disease; and certainly every method of cure which is not so directed must prove ineffectual, as it can only operate by destroying the effect. Opiates, indeed, will in some degree take off the irritation, by destroying the sensibility of the part; but surely it would be better at once to remove the cause than to be attempting from time to time to remove or palliate the effect. When the sympathy is partial, and not in a vital part, it would be better to allow it to continue than cure it, because it may by such means become universal; for instance, if it is a diarrhœa, the best way is to allow it to go on, or at least only correct it if too violent, which is often the case. I have seen cases where the stomach and intestines have sympathized so much as almost to threaten death. The small quantity of nourishment that the stomach could admit of was hurried off by the intestines.

Of cutting the Gums.

As far as my experience has taught me, to cut the gum down to the teeth appears to be the only method of cure. It acts either by taking off the tension upon the gum, arising from the growth of the tooth, or by preventing the ulceration which must otherwise take place.

It often happens, particularly when the operation is performed early in the disease, that the gum will reunite over the teeth; in which case the same symptoms will be produced, and they must be removed by the same method.

I have performed the operation above ten times upon the same teeth, where the disease had recurred so often, and every time with the absolute removal of the symptoms.

It has been asserted that to cut the gum once will be sufficient, not only to remove the present but to prevent any future bad symptoms from the same cause. This is contrary to experience and the known laws of the animal œconomy; for frequently the gum, from its thickness over the tooth, or other causes, must necessarily heal up again; and the relapse is as unavoidable as the original disease.

A vulgar prejudice prevails against this practice, from an objection that if the gum is lanced so early as to admit of a reunion, the cicatrized part will be harder than the original gum, and therefore the teeth will find more difficulty in passing, and give more pain. But this is also contrary to facts; for we find that all parts which have been the seat either of wounds or sores are always more ready to give way to pressure or any other disease which attacks either the part itself or the constitution. Therefore each operation tends to make the passing of the teeth easier.

When the teeth begin to give pain, we find them generally so far formed as to be easily discerned through the gum.

The fore teeth are to be observed at first, not on the edge of the gum, but on the fore part, making risings there, which appear whiter than the other parts; and it may be observed that the gums are broader than usual. At this period the incisions must be made pretty deep, till the tooth be felt with the instrument, otherwise little effect will be produced by the operation; and this is the general rule with respect to the depth of the incision in all cases.

When the grinders shoot into the gum, they flatten the edge of the gum, and make it broad. These teeth are more easily hit by the instrument than the fore teeth.

The operation should not be done with a fine-pointed instrument, such as a common lancet, because most probably the point will be broken off against the tooth, which will make the instrument unfit for going on further, if more incisions are required.

A common lancet with its point rounded is a very good instrument, but an instrument something like a fleam, would be of the most convenient shape.

There is no need of any great delicacy in the operation, the gums being very insensible parts; and to cut through the whole gum down to the teeth with certainty, when they are pretty deep, requires some force.

The gums will bleed a little, which may be of service in taking off the inflammation. I never saw a case where the bleeding either proved inconvenient or dangerous. If it ever should be troublesome, I think there could be no great difficulty in stopping it. In general, no application is necessary: the gums soon unite at the most distant part from the tooth, if it lies deep; and if it be more superficial, the thin gum soon shrinks back over the tooth, leaving it bare, and decays.

The cutting of the dentes sapientiæ is often attended with an inconvenience which does not attend the others; and this happens, I believe, only when they come very late, viz. when the jaws have left off growing. This arises from the want of room in the jaws for these late teeth; a circumstance which produces an addition to the other inconveniences arising from dentition. When it takes place in the upper jaw, the tooth is often obliged to grow backwards; and in such a position it sometimes presses on the interior edge of the coronoid process, in shutting the mouth, and gives great pain. When it takes place in the lower jaw, some part of the tooth continues to lie hid under that process, and covered by the soft parts, which are always liable to be squeezed between that tooth and the corresponding tooth in the upper jaw. To open very freely, is absolutely necessary in these cases; but even that is often not sufficient. Nothing but drawing the tooth, or teeth, will remove the evil in many cases.

CASES.

It would be endless to give histories of cases exemplifying each symptom of dentition: I shall only relate a few which are singular, and which, being extraordinary, will the better enforce the propriety, in all cases, of the cure I have recommended.

Case I.—A young child was attacked with contractions of the flexor muscles of the fingers, and also of the toes. These contractions were so considerable as to keep her fingers and thumb constantly clenched, and so irregularly that they appeared distorted. All the common antispasmodic medicines were given, and continued for several months, but without success.

I scarified the gums down to the teeth, and in less than half an hour all the contractions had ceased. This, however, only gave relief for a time. The gums healed; the teeth continued to grow, and filled up the new space acquired by the scarifications; and the same symptoms appeared a second time.

The former operation was immediately performed, and with the same success.

Case II.—A boy, about two years of age, was taken with a pain and difficulty in making water, and voided matter from the urethra. I suspected that, by some means or other, this child might possibly be affected by the venereal poison; and the suspicion naturally fell on the nurse.

These complaints sometimes abated, and would go off altogether, and then return again. It was observed at last that they returned only upon his cutting a new tooth. This happened so often, regularly and constantly, that there was no reason to doubt that it was owing to that cause.

Case III.—A lady, about the age of five or six and twenty years, was attacked with a violent pain in the upper jaw, which at last extended through the whole side of the face, similar to a violent toothache from a cold, and was attended with consequent fever.

It was treated at first as a cold; but, from its continuance, was afterwards supposed to be nervous.

The case was represented to me from the country, and I gave the best directions that I could, on a representation of the symptoms.

She came to London some months after, still labouring under the same complaint. Upon examining the mouth, I observed one of the points of the dens sapientiæ ready to come through. I lanced the gums, and the disorder gave way immediately.

A lady, about the same age, was attacked with a violent pain in the left side of her face. It was regularly periodical, coming on at six o'clock in the evening. She took the Peruvian bark, which had no effect. She took antimonials, and Dover's powder, which also were equally ineffectual. But one of the points of the dens sapientiæ of the upper jaw of the same side appearing, showed the cause, and indicated the remedy. The gums were lanced, and the pain ceased.

A

TREATISE

ON THE

VENEREAL DISEASE.

BY

JOHN HUNTER, F.R.S.

WITH NOTES

BY

GEORGE G. BABINGTON,

SURGEON OF ST. GEORGE'S HOSPITAL; FORMERLY SURGEON OF
THE LOCK HOSPITAL, &c.

CONTENTS.

PART VI.

CHAP. I.

OF THE LUES VENEREA.

1. Of the Nature of the Sores or Ulcers proceeding from the Lues Venerea.—2. Of the Matter from Sores in the Lues Venerea compared with that from Chancres and Buboes.—3. Of the Local Effects arising from the Constitution considered as critical—Symptomatic Fever.—4. Of the Local and Constitutional Forms of the Disease never interfering with one another.—5. Of the supposed Termination of the Lues Venerea in other Diseases.—6. Of the Specific Distance of the Venereal Inflammation.—7. Of the Parts most susceptible of the Lues Venerea.—Of the Time and Manner in which they are affected—what is meant by Contamination, Disposition, and Action—Summary of the Doctrine.

CHAP. II.

OF THE SYMPTOMS OF THE LUES VENEREA.

1. Of the Symptoms of the first Stage of the Lues Venerea.—2. Experiments made to ascertain the Progress and Effects of the Venereal Poison.—3. Of the Symptoms of the Second Stage of the Lues Venerea.—4. Of the Effects of the Poison on the Constitution.

CHAP. III.

GENERAL OBSERVATIONS ON THE CURE OF THE LUES VENEREA.

1. Of the Use of Mercury in the Cure of the Lues Venerea.—2. Of the Quantity of Mercury necessary to be given.—3. Of the sensible Effects of Mercury upon Parts.—4. Of the Action of Mercury.—5. Of the different Methods of giving Mercury—Externally—Internally.—6. Of the Cure of the Disease in the Second or Third Stage.—7. Of Local Treatment.—8. Of Abscesses—Exfoliation.—9. Of Nodes on Tendons, Ligaments, and Fasciæ.—10. Of Correcting some of the Effects of Mercury.—11. Of the form of the different Preparations of Mercury when in the Circulation.—12. Of the Operation of Mercury on the Poison.—13. Of Gum Guaiacum, and Radix Sarsaparillæ, in the Venereal Disease.

PREFACE.

OF all the works of John Hunter, there is none on which he bestowed more labour, or which he was more solicitous to perfect, than his treatise on the Venereal Disease. "I am resolved," said he to a friend, "that it shall not be a mere bookseller's job, every subsequent edition rendering the former useless. The truth of the doctrines I have proved so long as to reduce them to conviction; and, in order to render the language intelligible, I meet a committee of three gentlemen*, to whose correction every page is submitted." It would seem that this correction of style was adopted in the second edition. On comparing it with the first we find numberless verbal alterations, which were evidently intended to render the expressions more lucid and more elegant. It is doubtful whether much has been gained by the change. The language is certainly less rugged, but it is also less forcible, and occasionally less distinct and decided. However, as the corrections have extended in some instances to points of more consequence than style, the second edition must undoubtedly be

---

* The three gentlemen were, Dr. (afterwards Sir Gilbert) Blane, Dr. George Fordyce, and Dr. David Pitcairn, and with these Mr. Marshall appears to have been associated.

considered as containing the latest experience and ultimate conclusions of the author. The third edition
was published after his death by Sir Everard Home,
who has in general followed the text of the first edition,
and has introduced some passages which were certainly
never written by John Hunter. For these reasons the
text of the second edition has been followed as the most
genuine : but as the alterations by Sir E. Home profess
to be derived from materials left by the author, it has
been thought best not to omit them entirely, and consequently such of them as are more than verbal have
been added in notes at the bottom of the page.

It cannot be disputed that the work thus produced
bears marks of the mind that gave it birth. To form
a just estimate of its merits, it is necessary to compare
it with the books on the same subject which had previously appeared in this country. These seem, for the
most part, to have been written less with the design of
increasing the knowledge of the disease, than with a
view to temporary notoriety, and to the emoluments
which such notoriety might bring. John Hunter always had higher objects. He has laboured to apply to
this disease the general principles of pathology, and to
subject it to the same scrutinizing analysis which generally guided his philosophical researches. The facts
he has selected from his daily experience are valuable,
not for their singularity, but for the inferences to which
they lead. Where the practice was previously uncertain
and contradictory, he has often established systematic
principles of treatment ; and where the practice was

right, he has placed it on a sure foundation, by substituting the deductions of reason for the habits of empiricism. With respect especially to diseases of the bladder and urethra, the observations contained in this work first threw light on those affections, and formed the basis on which our present accurate knowledge of them has been founded.

Yet at the same time it must be admitted that this treatise is not without defects, and that the reputation of John Hunter rests more on his other works than on this. Many of the remarks are rather theoretical than practical, and some of the doctrines have not obtained that general assent which has crowned most of his other labours. The causes of these imperfections are to be found in the nature of the subject and the character of the author.

A little reflection will show that the Venereal Disease was less adapted than many other subjects to the peculiar genius of John Hunter. The faculties which chiefly distinguished him from other men of science, and which generally insured his success, were an ardour and an energy which nothing could damp, and an industry which nothing could tire. Under the influence of these qualities he pushed his investigations with unexampled activity, and brought to light a multitude of facts, which the less energetic inquiries of other philosophers had failed to discover. Wherever our previous knowledge was partial and indistinct, the new facts which he collected by observation, or discovered by dissection, or established by experiment, illuminated the whole subject, and substituted the clear distinctness of the day for the obscurity and uncertainty of twilight. His view was always large and comprehensive; and by combining these new discoveries with what was known before, he deduced without difficulty laws which had eluded previous research, and then verified his deductions by a further observation and a more extended experiment. It is more to the activity of his inquiries than to the strength of his reasoning powers that we owe his discoveries. Indeed, his powers of reasoning were scarcely on a level with his other faculties; but the errors of his logic were perpetually corrected by the variety and accuracy of his experiments.

Now it so happens that in the Venereal Disease he had little opportunity for the exercise of his usual means of investigation. Experiments on animals are impossible in this case, as the disease seems to be confined to the human species. Dissections give little information, for the virus itself altogether eludes our sight; and such of its effects as are not obvious, are for the most part too minute to be distinguished by the eye. As most syphilitic symptoms occur in parts which are superficial and exposed to view, their general form and character have long been familiar to surgeons: the minuter changes are not discoverable by simple inspection, nor easily demonstrable to the senses. The casual observations of every day were open to John Hunter as to others, but he was exposed to the same difficulties which had checked the progress of his predecessors, and was liable to be misled by the same causes of error. In the Venereal Disease we have abundance of facts, of a certain kind, on record. It is not additional experience that we want, but a more correct discrimination, which would enable us better to understand our experience, to disentangle its perplexities, and reconcile its apparent contradictions. The facts noticed by John Hunter are not sufficiently novel or important to throw of themselves much additional light on the pathology of the malady. He was therefore reduced to the necessity of reasoning from the old experience, and of endeavouring, by subjecting it to a more correct process of induction, to correct the errors and improve on the knowledge of those who had preceded him. Consequently it is not surprising that his labours should have been less successful here than in some other branches of pathology, and that he should often have failed in removing the obscurity which envelops this malady. It may even be doubted whether his natural appetite for generalization has not sometimes misled him, and whether, in his desire to ascertain a general law, he has not sometimes abandoned his hold of the acknowledged facts of the disease, and left it even more obscure than before.

There was one way in which the investigation might have been conducted, which would have promised higher results. The symptoms of the Venereal Disease, though very obvious, are at the same time infinitely various, and even to this day they have never been accurately discriminated. If the Author had bent the full powers of his keen and penetrating mind to tracing out in the first instance a correct description of each sepa-

rate symptom ; if he had then pursued the research so
as to have ascertained in each case the particular structure affected, and the particular nature of the morbid
alteration, he would have laid a firm basis for his reasoning, and could not have failed to elucidate both this
malady and many which resemble it. It is probable
that he would have so ascertained the laws which regulate the peculiar action of the venereal virus, as to
have left no room for confounding its effects with diseases from other causes. It is probable that he would
have explained the apparent contradictions in the effect
of remedies, and, by appropriating each to its peculiar
class of affections, have rendered the system of treatment no longer dubious and empirical, but clear and
intelligible. It is certain that he would have opened
the way for subsequent discoveries to an extent which
cannot be calculated, and that, not only in the disease
under consideration, but also in other maladies which
have hitherto been little studied by pathologists, especially in eruptions and other diseases of the skin.

That such a task as this was well adapted to the
powers of John Hunter cannot be questioned. The
descriptions he has given in the work before us are sufficient of themselves to establish his reputation. In
accuracy and distinctness they have never been surpassed, and they remain at the end of half a century
the standard definitions to which all subsequent writers
have referred. But the plan here sketched out would
have been toilsome and long. It would have required
the labour of a life. The fruit which it promised was

remote and uncertain. It might never have been gathered by the author, but might have remained to be
the spoil of a future generation. He followed his natural inclination. He preferred the more delusive,
apparently the more direct road which has seduced so
many philosophers. He sought to arrive at the general laws of nature at once by conjecture ; rather than,
by a close and detailed study of her inferior operations,
to ascend, step by step, through a slow and gradual induction to those laws which govern her general proce-
dure. " Altera (via) a sensu et particularibus advolat
" ad axiomata maximè generalia, atque ex iis principiis
" eorumque immotâ veritate judicat et invenit axio-
" mata media ; altera a sensu et particularibus excitat
" axiomata, ascendendo continenter et gradatim, ut ul-
" timo loco perveniatur ad maximè generalia*."

But though this treatise is tainted more than any
other of the works of John Hunter with the vice of a
too hasty generalization, yet it is full of practical observations of the highest value, and must always form
an essential part of the study of every surgeon who
wishes to make himself acquainted with the disease of
which it treats. In the present Edition it has been
attempted to render it more generally useful by en-
grafting on it the labours of other surgeons. The
opinions of the author have been treated with the respect which is due to his high reputation ; but where
important facts have been brought to light by others,
either in confirmation or in correction of his principles,

* Bacon, Aphorism xix.

they have been presented to the reader, in order that he may have before him in one view the present state of the science, and that by comparing the reasoning of others with that of the author, he may be enabled to form a just opinion of the truth or the error of his conclusions.

G. G. BABINGTON.

Golden Square, June 13, 1835.

N.B. The Editor's Notes are distinguished from the Author's by being placed below the line, within brackets. They are also further distinguished by initial letters instead of the usual marks of reference.

The various readings of the text, according to the third edition, by Sir Everard Home, are placed above the line, with that gentleman's name affixed.

A TREATISE

ON THE

VENEREAL DISEASE.

INTRODUCTION.

TWO motives have induced me to publish the following treatise. In the first place, I am not without hope that several new observations contained in it will be deemed worthy of the public attention; in the next place, I am desirous to have an opportunity of showing, from whom some opinions that have made their way into the medical world originated.

But as much of the theory which will often be referred to in the course of this work is peculiar to myself, it seems necessary to give an introductory explanation of some parts of it, in order that the terms used may be the more intelligible to the reader.

§. 1. *Of Sympathy.*

I divide sympathy into two parts, *universal* and *partial*.

Universal sympathy is an affection wherein the whole constitution sympathizes with some sensation or action. Partial sympathy is an affection wherein one or more distinct parts sympathise with some local sensation or action.

The universal sympathies are different in different diseases; but those that occur in the venereal disease are principally two, the symptomatic fever and the hectic fever. The symptomatic fever is an immediate effect of some local injury, and seldom takes place in the venereal disease in any great degree under any of its forms, except in the case of a swelled testicle, which is itself an instance of a partial sympathy; the

symptomatic fever here, therefore, is an universal sympathy arising from
a partial one.   The hectic fever is an universal sympathy with a local
disease, which the constitution is not able to overcome.   This takes
place oftener and in a greater degree in the lues venerea than in any
other form of the disease.

I divide partial sympathy into three kinds; the *remote*, the *contiguous*,
and the *continuous*.   The remote is where there appears to be no visible
connexion of parts from whence we can account for such effects, as in
the case of pain of the shoulder in an inflammation of the liver.   The
contiguous is that which appears to have no other connexion than what
arises from vicinity or contact of separate parts, an instance of which
we have in the stomach and intestines sympathising with the integuments of the abdomen.   The continuous is where there is no interruption of parts, and the sympathy runs along from the irritating point, as
from a centre, which is the most common of all sympathies.   We have
an example of this in the spreading of inflammation.

§. 2. *Of Morbid Actions being incompatible with each other.*

The venereal disease is not only suspected to be present in many
cases where the nature of the disorder is not well marked, but it is supposed that it can be combined with other diseases, such as the itch and
the scurvy.   Thus, we hear of pocky itch and of scurvy and the venereal disease combined; but this supposition appears to me to be founded
in error.   I have never seen any such cases, nor do they seem to be consistent with the principles of morbid action in the animal œconomy.   It
appears to me, beyond a doubt, that no two actions can take place in
the same constitution, or in the same part, at one and the same time.
No two different fevers can exist in the same constitution, nor two local
diseases in the same part, at the same time; yet as the venereal disease,
when it attacks the skin, bears a resemblance to those symptoms which
are vulgarly called scorbutic, they are often supposed to be mixed, and
to exist in the same part.

What has been called a scorbutic constitution is no more than a constitution very susceptible of an action producing eruptions on the skin
whenever an immediate cause takes place; and there are some parts of
the body more susceptible of this than others, in which, therefore, a
slighter immediate cause is sufficient to excite the action; but the easy
susceptibility with respect to one disease is not a reason why a constitution should not likewise be susceptible of other diseases. A man may
have the pox and the smallpox at the same time; that is, parts of his

body may have been contaminated by the venereal poison, and the smallpox may take place, and both diseases may appear together, but not in the same parts. If both were consequences of fever, and each followed the fever nearly about the same time, it would be impossible for each to have its respective eruption, even in different parts, at the same time; two fevers, antecedent to these different diseases, cannot be co-existent.

From this principle I think I may fairly put the following queries. Does not the failure of inoculation, and the power of resisting many infections, sometimes arise from the person's having at the same time some other disease, and therefore being incapable of a new action? Does not the great difference in the time, from the application of the cause to the appearance of the effect, in many cases, depend upon·the same principle? It has been sometimes observed that the puncture in the arm has shown no sign of inflammation in fourteen days after the application of the variolous poison. Has there not been another disease in the constitution at the time of inoculation? Does not the cure of some diseases depend upon the same principle? The suspension or cure of a gonorrhœa by a fever may be an instance of this.

Let me illustrate this principle still further, by one of many cases which have come under my own observation. On Thursday, March 16, 1775, I inoculated a gentleman's child, in whose arms it was observed I made large punctures. On the Sunday following he appeared to have received the infection, a small inflammation or redness appearing round each puncture, and a small tumour above the surface of the skin having been observed. On the 20th and the 21st the child was feverish, but I declared that the fever was not variolous, as the inflammation had not at all advanced since the 19th. On the 22nd a considerable eruption appeared, which was evidently the measles: upon this the sores on the arms appeared to go back, becoming less inflamed. On the 23rd he was very full of the measles, the punctures on the arms being in the same state as on the preceding day. On the 25th the measles began to disappear. On the 26th and 27th the punctures began again to look a little red. On the 29th the inflammation increased, and there was a little matter formed. On the 30th he was seized with fever. The smallpox appeared at the regular time, went through its usual course, and terminated favourably. In like manner, it may be observed that the venereal disease makes its appearance at different periods after infection. Is not this explicable on the same principle?

§. 3. *Of the comparative Powers of different Parts of the Body—from Situation—from Structure.*

We shall have occasion to observe, that the parts affected assume the morbid action more readily and continue it more rapidly when near to the source of the circulation than when far from it; for the heart exerts its influence upon the different parts of the body in proportion to their vicinity to it; and the more distant that the parts are, the weaker are their powers.

This is perhaps better illustrated by disease than by any actions in health, for in health we have no comparative trials, as no two parts of the machine, at unequal distances from the heart, can be thrown into equal action, and therefore no conclusions can be drawn. It may be observed that all the vital parts are near the heart.

In diseases we see mortification arising from debility, in the extremities oftener than in other parts, more especially if the person is tall; the heart not propelling the blood to these distant parts with equal force. In such a state of constitution, those who labour under a hemiplegia are often found to die at last from a mortification in the extremities of the paralytic side. In some of these cases the arteries give way, and allow of an extravasation of the blood, and therefore we may reasonably suppose that they are proportionally weak in health. We also find that such extravasation commonly begins in the extremities. This principle is not only evident in these two diseases, but also in every disease that can affect an animal body. It appears in the readiness with which diseases come on and proceed in parts distant from the source of the circulation, and also in the steps towards a cure.

Parts differ not only in their powers, in proportion as they are nearer or further from the heart, but likewise according to their peculiar structure, whereby they vary as much in the progress of morbid actions as in the operations of health.

An animal body is composed of a variety of substances, as muscle, tendon, cellular membrane, ligament, bone, nerve, &c. We have therefore an opportunity of observing the comparative progress of diseases in them, and their comparative powers of performing a cure; and we find that they differ very much from one another in those respects. How far these differences take place in all diseases, I have not been able to determine; but should suppose, that in specific diseases, as scrofula and cancer, there is in general no difference in the mode of action in any of the structures*, these diseases producing the same specific effects in all the parts that are capable of being affected by them; but in diseases arising from accident a great difference in the degrees of action takes place, the parts from such a cause being allowed to act according to their natures; which observation holds good also in the venereal disease. This difference appears to be chiefly in the degrees of strength and weakness in resisting morbid action. The less the natural powers of action are in any particular structure of parts, the less they are able to resist disease; therefore bone, tendon, ligament, and cellular membrane go through their morbid actions more slowly than muscle or skin; and this principle is applicable to the venereal disease.

§. 4. *Of Parts susceptible of particular Diseases.*

There are some parts much more susceptible of specific diseases than others. Poisons take their different seats in the body as if allotted for them. Thus we have the skin attacked with what are vulgarly called scorbutic eruptions, and many other diseases; it is also the seat of the smallpox and the measles; the throat is the seat of the hydrophobia and the hooping-cough. The scrofula attacks the absorbent system, especially the glands. The breasts, testicles, and the conglomerate glands are the seat of cancer. The skin, throat, and nose are more readily affected by the lues venerea than the bones and periosteum; which, on the other hand, suffer sooner than many other parts, particularly the vital parts, which perhaps are not at all susceptible of the disease.

§. 5. *Of Inflammation.*

I consider common inflammation to be an increased action of the smaller vessels of a part, joined with a peculiar mode of action, by which they are enabled to produce the following effects: to unite parts of the body to each other, to form pus, and to remove parts of the solids. These effects are not produced by a simple increase of action or enlargement of the vessels, but by a peculiar action, which is at present perhaps not understood.

These three effects of inflammation I have called distinct species of inflammation. That which unites parts I have called the adhesive in-

---

* Here it is to be understood, that we do not include those parts which have a greater tendency to specific diseases than what many others have; as the lymphatics to the scrofula, the breast to the cancer.

flammation; that which forms pus, the suppurative inflammation; and that which removes parts, the ulcerative inflammation.

In the adhesive inflammation the arteries throw out coagulable lymph, which becomes the bond of union. This, however, is not simply extravasated, but has undergone some change before it leaves the arteries, since in inflamed veins it is found lying coagulated upon the internal surface of the vessel, which could not have happened if simply extravasated. In the suppurative inflammation a still greater change is produced upon the blood before it is thrown out by the arteries, whereby it is formed into pus; which change is probably similar to secretion. In the ulcerative inflammation, the action of the arteries does not remove the parts: that office is performed by the absorbent vessels which are brought into action.

In the two first species of inflammation there must be a change in the disposition and mode of action of the arteries; for the suppurative species cannot be considered as simply an increase of the action of the adhesive, as its effects are totally different; but in the third species there is probably no change of action in the arteries from that of the second: the action only of the absorbents being superadded, by which solid parts, and of course the arteries themselves, are removed.

§. 6. *Of Mortification*.

Mortifications are of two kinds, one preceded by inflammation, the other not. But as the cases of mortifications which will be mentioned in this work are all of the first kind, I shall confine my observations to that species.

I consider inflammation as an increased action of that power which a part is naturally in possession of. This increased action, in healthy inflammations at least, is probably attended with an increase of power; but in inflammations which terminate in mortification there is no increase of power. On the contrary, there is a diminution of power, which, joined to an increased action, becomes the cause of mortification, by destroying the balance which ought to subsist between the power and action of every part.

If this account of mortifications be just, we shall find it no difficult matter to establish a rational practice. But, before we attempt this, let us just take a view of the treatment hitherto recommended, and see how far it agrees with our theory.

It is plain, from the common practice, that the weakness has been attended to, but it is as plain that the increased action has been over looked; and therefore the whole aim has been to increase the action, with a view to remove the weakness. The Peruvian bark, confectio cardiaca, serpentaria, &c., have been given in as large quantities as the case appeared to require, or the constitution could bear : by which means an artificial or temporary appearance of strength has been produced, while it was only an increased action. The cordials and wine, upon the principle on which they have been given, are rationally administered; but there are strong reasons for not recommending them, arising from the general effect which all cordials have of increasing the action without giving real strength; and the powers of the body are afterwards sunk proportionally as they have been raised : by which nothing can be gained, but a great deal may be lost; for, in all cases, if the powers are allowed to sink below a certain point, they are irrecoverable.

The local treatment has been as absurd as the constitutional. Scarifications have been made quite to the living parts, that stimulating and antiseptic medicines might be applied to them, such as turpentines, the warmer balsams, and sometimes the essential oils. Warm fomentations have been also applied as congenial to life · but warmth always increases action, and stimulants are improper where the actions are already too violent.

Upon the principles here laid down, the bark is the only medicine that can be depended upon, as it increases the powers and lessens the action. Upon many occasions opium will be of singular service by lessening the action, although it does not give real strength. I have seen good effects from it, both when given internally in large doses, and when applied to the part. To keep the parts cool is proper; and all the applications should be cold. The above-mentioned practice is to be kept in view in mortifications that happen in the venereal disease.

PART I.

CHAPTER I.

OF THE VENEREAL POISON.

THE Venereal Disease arises from a poison, which, as it is produced by disease, and is capable of again producing a similar disease, I call a morbid poison, to distinguish it from the other poisons, animal, vegetable, and mineral.

The morbid poisons are many, and they have different powers of contamination. Those which infect the body either locally or constitutionally, but not in both ways, I call *simple*. Those which are capable of affecting the body both locally and constitutionally, I call *compound*. The venereal poison, when applied to the human body, possesses a power of propagating or multiplying itself; and as it is also capable of acting both locally and constitutionally, it is a compound morbid poison. Like all such poisons, it may be communicated to others in all the various ways in which it can be received, producing the same disease in some one of its forms.

§. 1. *Of the first Origin of the Poison.*

Though the first appearance of this poison is certainly within the period of modern history, yet the precise time and manner of its origin has hitherto escaped our investigation, and we are still in doubt whether it arose in Europe or was imported from America. I shall not attempt to discuss this question; and those who wish to examine at length the facts, authorities, and arguments brought in favour of the latter opinion, may consult Astruc; and for the former, a short treatise* published in 1751, without a name. The author of this treatise appears to have

---

* Intitled "A Dissertation on the Origin of the Venereal Disease; proving that it was not brought from America, but began in Europe from an epidemical Distemper. Translated from the original Manuscript of an eminent Physician. London, printed for Robert Griffiths, 1751."

considered the subject very fully, and, as far as reasoning goes on a subject of this kind, proves that the disease was not brought from the West Indies. Not contented with this, he goes on to account for its first rise in Europe; but in this he is not equally successful. The subject is a difficult one, and the want of a sufficient number of facts leaves too much room for conjecture.

We shall not, therefore, enter further into this question; nor is it material to know at what period, and in what country, this disease arose; but we may in general affirm, that as animals are not naturally formed with disease, or so as to run spontaneously into morbid actions, but with a susceptibility of such impressions as produce such actions, diseases must always arise from impressions made upon the body; and as man is probably susceptible of more impressions that become the immediate cause of disease than any other animal, and is besides the only animal which can be said to form artificial impressions upon himself, he is subject to the greatest variety of diseases. In one of those self-formed situations, therefore, the impression most probably was given which produced the venereal disease.

§. 2. *It began in the Human Race, and in the Parts of Generation.*

In whatever manner it arose, it certainly began in the human race, as we know no other animal that is capable of being infected with this poison. It is probable, too, that the parts of generation were the first affected; for if it had taken place in any other part of the body, it might probably never have gone further than the person in whom it first arose, and therefore never have been known; but being seated in the parts of generation, where the only natural connexion takes place between one human being and another, except that between the mother and child, it was in the most favourable situation for being propagated; and as we shall find hereafter, in the history of the disease itself, that no constitutional effect of this poison can be communicated to others, we are led of necessity to conclude that its first effects were local.

§. 3. *Of the Nature of the Poison.*

We know nothing of the poison itself, but only its effects on the human body. It is commonly in the form of pus, or united with pus, or some such secretion, and produces a similar matter in others, which shows that it is most generally, although not necessarily, a consequence of inflammation. It produces or excites, therefore, in most cases, an inflammation in the parts contaminated; besides which inflammation, the parts so contaminated have a peculiar mode of action superadded, different from all other actions attending inflammation; and it is this specific mode of action which produces the specific quality in the matter. It is not necessary that inflammation should be present to keep up this peculiar mode of action, because the poison continues to be formed long after all signs of inflammation have ceased. This appears from the following facts : men having only what is called a gleet, or healing chancre, give the disease to sound women; and many venereal gonorrhœas happen without any visible signs of inflammation.

In women the inflammation is frequently very slight, and often there is not the least sign of it, for they have been known to infect men though they themselves have had no symptoms of inflammation, or of the disease in any form. Therefore the inflammation and suppuration, when present, are only attendants on the peculiar mode of action, the degree in which they take place depending more on the nature of the constitution than on that of the poison.

The formation of matter also, though a very general, is not a constant attendant on this disease, for we sometimes find inflammation produced by the venereal poison which does not terminate in suppuration; such inflammation I suspect to be of the erysipelatous kind. It is the matter produced, with or without inflammation, which alone contains the poison, for without the formation of matter no venereal poison can exist. Therefore a person having the venereal irritation in any form, not attended with a discharge, cannot communicate the disease to another. To communicate the disease, therefore, it is necessary that the venereal action should first take place, that matter should be formed in consequence of that action, and that the matter should be applied to a sound person or part.

That the venereal disease is to be propagated only by matter is proved every day by a thousand instances. Married men contract the disease, and not suspecting that they have caught it, cohabit with their wives, even for weeks. Upon discovering symptoms of the disease they of course desist; yet in all my practice I never once found that the complaint was communicated under such circumstances, except where they had not been very attentive to the symptoms, and therefore continued the connexion after the discharge had appeared. I have gone so far as to allow husbands while infected, but before the appearance of discharge, to cohabit with their wives in order to save appearances, and always with safety. I could carry this still further, and even allow a man who has a gonorrhœa to have connexion with a sound woman, provided that great care be taken to clear all the parts of any matter, by first syringing the urethra, making water, and washing the glans* [a].

* The last sentence omitted.—*Home.*

---

[a] [The omission of the last sentence in Sir Everard Home's edition is not without reason, since the truth of the doctrine is, to say the least, very questionable, and the practice which is deduced from it is undoubtedly most mischievous and reprehensible.

The author's doctrine is, that the virus resides in pus, or some such secretion, and hence he draws two practical conclusions:

1. That when there is no pus, or puriform secretion, the disease cannot be communicated. So that before the appearance of a gonorrhœa, or after the healing of a chancre, there is no possibility of infection.

2. That even when pus actually exists, yet if particular care be taken to remove it in the first instance, by very careful ablution, the individual may have connexion with a sound woman without danger of infecting her.

The second conclusion cannot be too strongly reprobated. It is opposed to every day's experience; and from the omission of the passage in Sir E. Home's edition, it may be supposed that further observation had led the author himself to change his opinion before the termination of his life.

The former position also is by no means free from danger, as will be seen by the following instances, which are far from singular:

A married woman was seized with the usual symptoms of gonorrhœa, which greatly surprised her, as her husband was free from complaint. On questioning, however, the husband, he confessed that he had had connexion with a common girl about a week before his wife complained; but he positively asserted that he had had no discharge or uneasiness whatever, and certainly then showed no signs of disease. In about four days afterwards, that is to say, nearly a fortnight after the impure connexion, and a week after he must have communicated the disease to his wife, a gonorrhœal discharge appeared on him.

A gentleman, when absent from home, exposed himself to the hazard of infection. At the end of three days he returned home, and in about four days afterwards his wife had a gonorrhœa. On the tenth day after the connexion the gentleman first perceived a discharge, and the other symptoms of gonorrhœa.

But it may be said, that though such cases show that the conclusion at which the author has arrived is practically unsafe, they by no means disprove the truth of the general principle on which it was founded. It may be said, that in these cases it is an error to suppose that there is no purulent secretion; that in the very early stage of a gonorrhœa it is probable thàt the pus is too small in quantity to flow from the urethra; that it lodges in the lacunæ, and is washed out by the urine, and is thus concealed from observation, but that it not less really exists; and that the position therefore remains untouched,—that where there is no matter there can be no infection.

However, there is another class of cases which go still further to throw doubts on the truth of this doctrine.

A gentleman was exposed to infection when in London. A day or two afterwards he set off for Ireland, where his family resided. He made some stay at Cheltenham, and while there, there appeared on the inner prepuce two or three small indurations or tubercles. He showed them to a surgeon, who convinced himself that there was no ulceration, and did not believe the affection to be venereal. After a short interval he returned to Ireland, these indurations still existing, and infected his wife, who suffered from primary sores.

A gentleman had an induration on the penis, which remained after the healing of a

The matter which is impregnated with this poison, when it comes in contact with a living part, irritates that part, and inflammation is the common consequence. It must be applied either in a fluid state, or rendered fluid by the juices of the part to which it is applied. There is no instance where it has given the infection in the form of vapour, as is the case in many other poisons.

§. 4. *Of the greater or less Acrimony of the Poison.*

Venereal matter must in all cases be the same : one quantity of matter cannot have a greater degree of poisonous quality than another ; and if there is any difference it is only in its being more or less diluted, which produces no difference in its effects. One can conceive, however, that it may be so far diluted as not to have the power of irritation. Thus any fluid taken into the mouth, capable of stimulating the nerves to taste, may be so diluted as not to be tasted. But if the poison can irritate the part to which it is applied to action, it is all that is required ; the action will be the same, whether from a large or small quantity, from a strong or a weak solution*.

We find from experience that there is no difference in the kind of matter ; and no variation can arise in the disease from the matter's being of different degrees of strength, for it appears that the same matter affects very differently different people. Two men having been connected with one woman, and both catching the disease, one of them shall have a violent gonorrhœa, or chancre, while the other shall have merely a slight gonorrhœa. I have known one man give the disease to different women, and some of the women have had it very severely, while in others it has been very slight. The same reasoning holds good with regard to chancres. The variations of the symptoms in different persons depend upon the constitution and habit of the patient at the time.

* These words added, " Since those men who have taken great pains in washing the parts immediately after connexion have caught the disease, and the symptoms have been equally severe as in others who used no such precaution."—*Home.*

___

chancre. He suffered repeatedly from secondary symptoms, which were as often removed by appropriate treatment, but the induration always remained. At length, when a considerable interval had passed without a relapse, and he believed himself to be finally cured, he married, though the induration was not removed. His wife was infected.

Cases of this kind might be multiplied without difficulty, and almost necessarily lead to the inference that infection may take place from the contact of a simple chancrous thickening, although no ulceration whatever is present. A misconception of this truth has often led to consequences which are most lamentable. In a considerable proportion of those cases in which a wife has been infected in consequence of marriage with a man labouring under syphilis, the communication seems to have taken place from the cicatrix of a sore which has been healed.]

What happens in the inoculation of the smallpox strengthens this opinion. Let the symptoms of the patient from whom the matter is taken be good or bad; let it be from one who has had a great many pustules, or from one who has had but few; let it be from the confluent or distinct kind, applied in a large quantity or a small one, it produces always the same effect. This could only be known by the great numbers that have been inoculated under all these different circumstances[a].

§.5. *Of the Poison being the same in Gonorrhœa and in Chancre.*

It has been supposed by many that the gonorrhœa and the chancre arise from two distinct poisons; and their opinion seems to have some foundation, when we consider only the different appearances of the two symptoms, and the different methods of cure; which, with respect to the nature of many diseases, is too often all we have to lead our judgement. Yet, if we take up this question upon other grounds, and also have recourse to experiments, the result of which we can absolutely depend upon, we shall find this notion to be èrroneous.

If we attend to the manner in which the venereal poison was communicated to the inhabitants of the islands of the South Seas, there are many circumstances which tend to throw light upon the present question. It has been supposed, as no mention is made of a gonorrhœa at Otaheite, that it must have been the chancre that was first introduced into that island, and that of course nothing but a chancre could be propagated there; for as no gonorrhœa had been communicated, no such disease could take place. But if we were to reason upon all the probable circumstances attending the voyages to that part of the world, we should conclude the contrary: for it was almost impossible to carry a chancre so long a voyage without its destroying the penis; while we know from experience that a gonorrhœa may continue for a great length of time. It is mentioned in Cook's voyage, that the people of Otaheite who had this disease went into the country and were cured; but when it became a pox it was then incurable. This shows that the disease which they had must have been a gonorrhœa, for we know that it is only a gonor-

---

[a] [Sir E. Home has here added a note, in which he calls in question the truth of this doctrine, as far as regards smallpox. He says that he has in many instances diluted variolous matter, and always found that the disease produced from such matter was milder than when employed for inoculation in an undiluted state. However, in the venereal disease it must be acknowledged that there are no facts which prove the existence of a similar difference in the virulence of the contagion, or would justify the conclusion that the variations in the symptoms depend on any other cause than the constitution and habit of the recipient.]

rhœa that can be cured by simple means; and further, if it had been a chancre, and they had been acquainted with the means of curing it, they could also have cured the lues venerea.

Wallis left Plymouth in August 1766, and arrived at Otaheite in July 1767, eleven months after his embarkation; and, if none of his men had the disease when he sailed, there was hardly a possibility of their contracting it anywhere afterwards in the voyage. This appears to be too long for a gonorrhœa to last. But let us suppose even that Wallis carried it thither in his ship, one or two of his crew having the disease: as he stayed there five weeks, it was very possible, even very probable, that such person or persons might have communicated it so quickly as to have become the cause of contamination of the whole crew of his ship. But as this did not happen, it is a presumptive proof that Wallis did not carry it thither.

Bougainville left France in December 1766; but he touched at several places where some of his people might have got the disease, the last of which places was Rio de la Plata, which he left in November 1767, and arrived at Otaheite in April 1768, five months after. This interval of time agrees better with the usual continuance of the disease than the length of Wallis's voyage; and, therefore, from this circumstance it becomes more probable that Bougainville carried it thither. Besides, it is likely that he could guard his people less against the disease than Wallis; for Wallis could have his choice of men at his first setting out, which was all that was necessary to prevent his carrying the disease with him, for he ran no risk of contracting it afterwards; but although Bougainville had the same advantage at first, yet he had it not afterwards, for his men were in the way of infection in several places, and he had no opportunity of changing them, and probably no great chance of having them cured. The circumstance of the disease being found by Bougainville at Otaheite soon after his arrival is a kind of proof that he carried it thither himself: for I observed before, that if Wallis had carried it by one man only, this man could in a very few days have so far propagated it as to have spread it through the whole ship's crew; and as Bougainville arrived at the island ten months after Wallis, there was a sufficient time for the inhabitants of the whole island to have been infected, and the ravages of the disease must have been evident to them immediately upon their arrival. Bougainville remained only nine days at the island of Otaheite, and observed nothing of the disease till some weeks after his departure, when it was found that several of the crew were infected, which most probably must have happened in consequence of the poison being carried there by some of his own people. It is also mentioned by Cook that the Otaheiteans ascribed the introduction of the disease to Bougainville; and we can hardly suppose that they would be so complaisant to our countrymen as to accuse Bougainville, when they must have known whether the disease was imported by Wallis or not, especially as they had no reason to be partial in favour of the people who accompanied the latter. But as we find in Cook's last voyage that the disease in every form is now there, and as we have no new intelligence of a gonorrhœa being since introduced, we must suppose that every form of the disease has been propagated from one root, which most probably was a gonorrhœa.

If any doubt still remain with respect to the two diseases being of the same nature, it will be removed by considering that the matter produced in both is of the same kind, and has the same properties: the proofs of which are, that the matter of a gonorrhœa will produce either a gonorrhœa, a chancre, or the lues venerea; and the matter of a chancre will also produce either a gonorrhœa, a chancre, or the lues venerea*.

The following case is an instance of a gonorrhœa producing a lues venerea. A gentleman twice contracted a gonorrhœa, of which he was cured both times without mercury. About two months after each, he had symptoms of the lues venerea. Those in consequence of the first infection were ulcers in the throat, which were removed by the external application of mercury; the symptoms in consequence of the second were blotches on the skin, for which also he used the mercurial ointment, and was cured. With regard to the lues venerea proceeding from chancres, instances occur so frequently to every one's observation as to require no further proof here.

Since, then, it appears that the gonorrhœa and chancre are the effects of the same poison, it may be worthy of inquiry to what circumstances two such different forms of the disease are owing.

To account for these two very different effects of the same poison, it is only necessary to observe the difference in the mode of action of the parts affected when irritated, let the irritation be what it may. The gonorrhœa always proceeds from a secreting surface†, and the chancre

---

* The following paragraph is here inserted:

" That chancre is sometimes the consequence of gonorrhœa is rendered probable by the following case: A. B. had a gonorrhœa about the beginning of January 1788; the inflammation went off, the discharge continued: about a month after, a chancre appeared on the glans penis, for which he took mercury, and it got well in about a month."— Home.

† By secreting surfaces I mean all the passages for extraneous matter, including also the ducts of glands, such as the mouth, nose, eyes, anus, and urethra; and by nonsecreting surfaces, the external skin in general. To which I may add a third kind of surface, leading from the one to the other, as the glans penis, prolabium of the mouth, the inside of the lips, the pudendum; which surfaces, partaking of the properties of each,

is formed on a non-secreting surface; and in this last the part to which the poison is applied must become a secreting surface before matter can be produced. All secreting surfaces in the body being probably similar, one mode of application only is necessary to produce this disease in them all, which is by the poisonous matter simply coming in contact with them. But to produce the chancre, the venereal matter may be applied in three different ways: the first and most certain is by a wound, into which it may be introduced; the second is by applying the matter to a surface with a cuticle, and the thinner that is, it allows the matter to come more readily to the cutis; and the third is by applying the matter to a common sore already formed.

The poison, then, being the same in both cases, why do they not always happen together in the same person? For one would naturally suppose that the gonorrhœa, when it has appeared, cannot fail to become the cause of a chancre; and that this, when it happens first, must produce a gonorrhœa. Although it does not often happen so, yet it sometimes does; at least there is great reason to believe so. I have seen cases where a gonorrhœa came on; and in a few days after in some, in others in as many weeks, a chancre has appeared: and I have also seen cases where a chancre has come first; and in the course of its cure, a running and pain in making water have succeeded. It may be supposed that the two diseases arose from the original infection, and only appeared at different times; and their not occurring oftener together would almost induce us to believe it was so, since the matter is the same in both, and therefore capable of producing either the one or the other.

I suspect that the presence of one irritation in these parts becomes in general a preventive of the other. I have already observed, that the two parts sympathise in their diseases; and it is possible that that very sympathy may prevent the appearance of the real disease; for if an action has already taken place which is not venereal, it is impossible that another should take place till that ceases; and it is probable that this sympathy will not cease while the cause exciting it exists; and therefore when both happen in the same person at the same time, I suspect that either the urethra never had sympathised with the chancre, or if it did at first, that the sympathy had ceased, and then the venereal matter might stimulate the parts to action[a].

but in a less degree, are capable of being affected in both ways, sometimes by being excited to secretion, and at other times to ulceration.

---

[a] [There is yet a stronger argument than any which is here given. The author inoculated himself with the matter of gonorrhœa, and the consequence was the produc-

§. 6. *Of the Cause of the poisonous Quality—Fermentation—Action.*

As the consideration and explanation of this point will throw some light upon the disease and cure, I may be allowed to dwell a little upon

---

tion of chancres, followed by bubo, and by secondary symptoms. The experiment is related, at length, in Part VI., Chap. ii., Sect. 2, of the present work.

But, nevertheless, the identity of the poison of gonorrhœa with that of chancre has been disputed, and that on no slight grounds.

In reply to the argument drawn from the transfer of the venereal disease to the islands in the South Seas, it has been denied that the disease exists there at all. Mr. Wilson, surgeon to His Majesty's ship Porpoise, visited Otaheite in 1801, and, after a careful investigation, came to the conclusion that the venereal disease was then unknown in that island.

It may also be alleged, that even if the disease actually prevails there, as has been reported by others, it by no means follows that it must have been originally carried thither in the form of gonorrhœa. The facts stated by John Hunter do not bear out his conclusion. Bougainville left the Rio de la Plata in November 1767, and arrived at Otaheite in April 1768. It is very possible that a chancre might have existed during the five months which intervened. Cases frequently occur in which primary sores continue for a much longer period, without occasioning any remarkable destruction, and certainly without at all rendering the subject incapable of sexual intercourse.

The author affirms that cases occur in which true chancres are produced in those parts which are steeped in the discharge of a gonorrhœa. At the same time he acknowledges that such a circumstance is extremely rare. Yet nothing is more common than that excoriations should arise on the surface of the glans, or on the inside of the prepuce, from the contact of gonorrhœal matter. These excoriations, if neglected, will last for an indefinite period; but if the irritating matter is carefully removed by very frequent ablution, they will heal in two or three days, without the least necessity for the exhibition of mercury. Why do they not assume the characters of chancres, or infect the system? Surely their innocence affords a negative proof of the diversity of the virus, more strong than the very rare occurrence of true chancres can be supposed to give of its identity. For it must not be forgotten, that in these cases the chancre may be attributed to another cause. It may be that the patient has again exposed himself to infection, and that the chancre has arisen from this second exposure. The patient under such circumstances is naturally disposed to conceal his misconduct. Still he may often be induced to confess it on a strict examination; and in those cases where no such avowal can be elicited, it is perhaps most reasonable to suspect that it is only prevented by shame.

It cannot be denied that there are cases in which secondary symptoms appear to be the consequence of gonorrhœa; but these are so rare, that they must rather be considered as anomalies which we cannot as yet account for, than be admitted in contradiction to the general current of experience. The secondary symptoms in such instances are rarely of an indubitable character. It may be doubted whether distinct copper tubercles ever followed simple gonorrhœa. We have generally a mottled state of the skin, or the lighter and more fugitive forms of lichen, or slight excoriation of the surface of the tonsil.

It has been asserted that women who are affected with gonorrhœa alone, will fre-

it. It has been supposed by some that the poisonous quality of the matter arises from a fermentation taking place in it as soon as it is formed.

---

quently produce chancres in those men that are connected with them.   Without ven-
turing to give a positive denial to this statement, it may be suggested that its truth has
seldom, if ever, been satisfactorily ascertained.   The investigation of the surgeon has
evidently been confined to the external parts.   The interior of the vagina has not been
examined : yet it is certain that chancres do occur here, though more rarely, so as to
be discovered only by the use of a speculum.   When to this consideration is added all
the deception which is constantly practised in regard to sexual intercourse, it must be
allowed that these statements are deserving of very little confidence.

There still remains the experiment of John Hunter; and if such experiments were
multiplied, it cannot be denied that they would be decisive.   That in his case the system was infected with the venereal virus can scarcely be questioned; but it may be
doubted whether the virus might not have been derived from some other source than
inoculation with the matter of gonorrhœa.   The chances of falling into error are so
numerous, that such experiments should be frequently repeated.   As it is, the case
stands alone; opposed to the general course of experience, and opposed to a series of
other experiments which rest on the authority of Mr. Benjamin Bell.   The subjects
were medical students, who instituted the experiments with the view of de-
ciding this question.   They are thus related by Mr. Bell (Bell on Venereal Disease,
vol. i. p. 439.) :

" ' Matter,' says one of these individuals, ' was taken upon the point of a probe, from
a chancre on the glans penis before any application was made to it, and completely introduced into the urethra, expecting thereby to produce gonorrhœa.   For the first eight
days I felt no kind of uneasiness, but about this period I was attacked with pain in passing water.   On dilating the urethra as much as possible, nearly the whole of a large chancre was discovered, and in a few days thereafter, a bubo formed in each groin.   No
discharge took place from the urethra during the whole course of the disease ; but another chancre was soon perceived in the opposite side of the urethra, and red precipitate
was applied to it as well as to the other, by means of a probe previously moistened for
the purpose.   Mercurial ointment was at the same time rubbed on the outside of each
thigh, by which a profuse salivation was excited.   The buboes, which, till then, had continued to increase, became stationary, and at last disappeared entirely ; the chancres became clean, and by a due continuance of mercury a complete cure at last was obtained.'

" The next experiment was made with the matter of gonorrhœa, a portion of which
was introduced between the prepuce and glans, and allowed to remain there without
being disturbed.   In the course of the second day, a slight degree of inflammation was
produced, succeeded by a discharge of matter, which in the course of two or three days
disappeared.

" The same experiment was, by the same gentleman, repeated once and again, after
rendering the parts tender to which the matter of gonorrhœa was applied; but no chancre
ever ensued from it.

" Two young gentlemen, while prosecuting the study of medicine, became anxious to
ascertain the point in question ; with which view they resolved on making the following
experiments, at a time when neither of them had ever laboured under either gonorrhœa
or syphilis; and both in these and in the preceding experiments, the matter of infection
was taken from patients who had never made use of mercury.

" A small dossil of lint soaked in the matter of gonorrhœa was by each of them inserted between the prepuce and glans, and allowed to remain on the same spot for the
space of twenty-four hours.   From this they expected that chancres would be produced ;

But whether this poisonous quality arises from that cause, or whether the animal body has a power of producing matter according to the irritation given, whereby the living powers, whenever irritated in a particular manner, produce such an action in the parts as to generate a matter similar in quality to that which excited the action, is what I am now to consider.

In the examination of this subject I shall confine myself to the gonorrhœa. In support of either of the two opinions it must be supposed that the venereal matter has, by its specific properties, a power of irritation beyond common matter. I have already observed that it has the power of exciting inflammation even on the common skin, and of forming a chancre, which power is not possessed by common matter. In the first opinion it must be supposed that there is no specific inflammation or suppuration produced by the application of the venereal mat-

---

but in the one a very severe degree of inflammation ensued over the whole glans and preputium, giving all the appearances of what is usually termed gonorrhœa spuria ; a considerable quantity of fœtid matter was discharged from the surface of the inflamed parts; and for several days he had reason to fear that an operation would be necessary for the removal of a paraphimosis. By the use of saturnine poultices, however, laxatives, and low diet, the inflammation abated, the discharge ceased, no chancres took place, and he soon got entirely well.

" The other gentleman was not so fortunate. The external inflammation, indeed, was slight, but by the matter finding access to the urethra, he, on the second day, was attacked with a severe degree of gonorrhœa, which continued for a considerable time to give him a great deal of distress ; nor did he for upwards of a year get entirely free from it.

" By this he was convinced of the imprudence and hazard of all such experiments; nor could he be prevailed on to carry them further, although they were keenly prosecuted by his friend, who, soon after the inflammation arising from his first experiment was removed, inserted the matter of gonorrhœa on the point of a lancet beneath the skin of the preputium, and likewise into the substance of the glans ; but although this was repeated three different times, no chancres ensued. A slight degree of inflammation was excited, but it soon disappeared, without anything being done for it. His last experiment was attended with more serious consequences. The matter of a chancre was inserted on the point of a probe to the depth of a quarter of an inch, or more, in the urethra. No symptoms of gonorrhœa ensued; but in the course of five or six days a painful inflammatory chancre was perceived on the spot to which the matter was applied. To this succeeded a bubo, which ended in suppuration, notwithstanding the immediate application of mercury ; and the sore arising from this proved both painful and tedious. Ulcers were at last perceived in the throat; nor was a cure obtained till a very large quantity of mercury was given, under a state of close confinement, for a period of thirteen weeks."

These experiments, which strictly accord with the general results of experience, must be admitted to disprove altogether the argument derived from the difference between a secreting and a non-secreting surface, and to afford a very strong presumption that, at least in the great majority of cases, the poison of gonorrhœa is not identical with that of chancre.]

ter, but only a common inflammation and suppuration; and that the matter capable of producing these effects acts as a ferment upon the new-formed matter, rendering it venereal as soon, or nearly as soon, as it is formed; and as there is a succession of secretions, there immediately follows a succession of fermentations. Now let us see how far this idea agrees with all the variety of phænomena attending the disease. First, it may be asked, what becomes of this ferment in many cases where the suppuration does not come on for some weeks after the irritation and inflammation have taken place? In such cases we can hardly suppose the original venereal matter to remain, and to act as a ferment. Secondly, when there is a cessation of the discharge, and no matter formed, which sometimes happens for a considerable time, and yet all the symptoms recur, what is it that produces this fermentation a second time? Nothing can, but a new application of fresh venereal matter. When, for example, the irritation is translated to the testicle, and the discharge is totally stopped, as often happens, what becomes of the virus; and how is a new virus formed when the irritation falls back upon the urethra? Thirdly, if the poisonous quality were produced by fermentation taking place in the matter already formed, it would not be an easy matter to account for the symptoms ever ceasing, for, according to my idea of a ferment, it would never cease to act if new matter were continually added; nor could anything possibly check it but a substance immediately applied to the part, which could stop or prevent the fermentation in the new matter. But as the venereal inflammation in this species of the disease is not kept up beyond a certain time, the production of the poison cannot depend on fermentation. Fourthly, if it depended on a fermentation in the secreted matter, all venereal cases would be alike, nor would one be worse than another, except from a greater or smaller number of fermenting places. Upon this supposition also all cases would be equally easy of cure, for the fermentation would be equally strong in a slight case as in a bad one. It can only be fermentation in the matter after it has left the vessels.

When the venereal matter has been applied to a sore, so as to irritate, it produces a venereal irritation and inflammation. But even this does not always take place, for the common matter from the sore may remove the venereal matter applied, before it can affect the sore so as to produce the venereal inflammation and suppuration there. This experiment I have made several times, and have only once produced the venereal inflammation. But if the venereal matter were capable of acting as a ferment, then it would in all cases produce venereal matter without altering the nature of the sore.

The effects produced by venereal poison appear to me to arise from its peculiar or specific irritation, joined with the aptness of the living principle to be irritated by such a cause, and the parts so irritated acting accordingly. I shall therefore consider it as a poison, which by irritating the living parts in a manner peculiar to itself, produces an inflammation peculiar to that irritation, from which a matter is produced peculiar to the inflammation. Let us consider how far this opinion agrees with the various phænomena attending the disease.

First, the venereal matter having a greater power of irritating than common matter, conveys more the idea of irritation than of fermentation. Secondly, its producing a specific disease with specific symptoms and appearances, shows that it has a specific power of irritation, the living powers necessarily acting according to that irritation. Thirdly, the circumstance of the inflammation having its stated time of appearance and termination, is agreeable to the laws of the animal œconomy in most cases, as it is a circumstance that takes place in other diseases that have a crisis; and when the disease is longer of duration in some than in others, it is because they are much more susceptible of this kind of irritation; and there may be perhaps other concurrent circumstances. Fourthly, the venereal inflammation being confined to a specific distance, is more agreeable to the idea of a specific irritation than that of a fermentation. Fifthly, we have a further proof of this opinion, from the appearance of the disease being translated from one part of the body to another, as in the case of the swelled testicle, in which the discharge is often stopped or otherwise affected. Sixthly, the discharge often stops from the constitution being attacked by a fever, and returns after some days or weeks, or not at all, according to the continuance of the fever. Now we can plainly see why the fever should put a stop to the discharge, as the disposition produced by it in a part, is very different from that disposition which formed the matter; and we can plainly see why the same disposition to form matter should often return; but how that return should be venereal, upon the principles of fermentation, we do not see. Seventhly, the production by art of an irritation of another kind, which is not specific, removes the specific irritation: now an irritation of another kind cannot prevent the fermentation from going on, but may destroy the venereal irritation. Eighthly, the circumstance of particular parts of our body being much more readily irritated than others by the venereal poison, when in the constitution, shows that it arises from an irritation, and that of a particular kind. Ninthly, we know of no other animal that is susceptible of the venereal irritation, for repeated trials have shown that it is impossible to give it to a dog, a bitch, or an ass*. It is much easier to suppose that a dog or an ass is not suscep-

* I have repeatedly soaked lint in matter from a gonorrhœa, chancre, and bubo, and introduced it into the vagina of bitches, without producing any effect. I have also in-

tible of many irritations of which the human body is susceptible, as we find to be the case in all other specific diseases, and most poisons, than that the matter of the human body is susceptible of a change, of which that of the dog or ass is not.

This argument is still further supported by comparing the venereal poison with other morbid poisons. The animal poison productive of the hydrophobia seems to be produced by a particular irritation affecting certain parts, which shows that if the body, or any part of the body, is irritated, it takes a disposition to act in a peculiar manner, and that this mode of action is capable of secreting such juices as will throw another animal into the same action. In the hydrophobia the throat and its glands are particularly affected; and how the saliva should become of such a nature from the same kind of matter being either carried into the constitution, or perhaps only by the general sympathy of the constitution with a local infection, and more particularly with the parts about the throat, is not easily to be accounted for, without a supposition either that the absorbed poison circulating can produce a specific constitutional action capable of affecting the throat and glands there, just as the poison of the smallpox affects the skin, or that the circulating poison has power to affect or irritate the glands of the mouth only, or that those parts only are capable of immediately sympathising with the part irritated, as the muscles of the lower jaw are when they produce the locked jaw.

If this theory be just, it explains why epidemical diseases, arising from particular seasons, particular constitutions of air, &c., irritate in such a manner as to produce a fever, the effluvia of which shall irritate in the same manner: for it is not in the least material how the original irritation arises; it is only necessary that there should exist in the animal a power of acting according to the stimulus given by that irritation.

CHAPTER II.

THE MODE OF VENEREAL INFECTION.

EVERY infectious disease has its peculiar manner of being caught; and among mankind there is generally something peculiar in the way of life,

troduced it into the vagina of asses without any effect. I have introduced it under the prepuce of dogs without any effect. I have also made incisions and introduced it under the skin, and it has only produced a common sore. I have made the same experiments upon asses, with the same result.

or some attending circumstance, which exposes them at one time or other to contract such diseases, and which, if avoided, would prevent their propagation. The itch, for instance, is generally caught by a species of civility, the shaking of hands; therefore the hand is most commonly the part first affected. And as the venereal infection is generally caught by the connexion between the sexes, the parts of generation commonly suffer first. From this circumstance people do not suspect this disease when the symptoms are anywhere else, while they always suspect it in every complaint of those parts.

In the lower class of people, one as naturally thinks of the itch when there is an eruption between the fingers, as in young men of the venereal disease whose genitals are affected; but as every secreting surface, whether cuticle or not cuticle, (as was explained before,) is liable to be infected by the venereal poison when it is applied to it, it is possible for many other parts besides the genitals to receive this disease. Therefore it appears in the anus, mouth, nose, eyes, ears, and, as has been said, in the nipples of women who suckle children affected by it in their mouths, which children have been infected in the birth from the diseased parts of the mother.

CHAPTER III.

OF THE DIFFERENT FORMS OF THE DISEASE.

THE venereal poison is capable of affecting the human body in two different ways; locally, that is, in those parts only to which it is first applied; and constitutionally, that is, in consequence of the absorption of the venereal pus which affects parts while diffused in the circulation.

Between the first and second kind, or the local and constitutional*, certain intermediate complaints take place in the progress of absorption; these are, inflammations and suppurations, forming what are called buboes, in which the matter is of the same nature as that of the original disease.

When the matter has got into the constitution, and is circulating

* I have called this form of the disease constitutional; yet it is not strictly so, for every complaint in consequence of it is truly local, and is produced by the simple application of the poison to the parts.

with the blood, it there irritates to action. There are produced from that irritation many local diseases, as blotches on the skin, ulcers in the tonsils, thickening of the periosteum and bones.

The local, or first kind, is what I have called *immediate*, arising immediately upon the application of venereal pus. Of this kind there are two sorts, seemingly very different from one another. In the first there is a formation of matter without a breach of the solids, called a gonorrhœa; in the second there is a breach in the solids, called a chancre. Neither of these two ways in which the disease shows itself is owing to anything peculiar in the kind of poison applied, but to the difference in the parts contaminated.

The readiness with which the parts run into violent action in this species of inflammation, is greater or less, according to the nature of the parts affected, which perhaps does not arise from any specific difference in the parts, but is according to the common principle of sensibility and irritability; for we find that the vagina is not so much disposed to inflammation in this disease as the urethra is in the same sex, because it is not so sensible. However, it is possible that there may be some specific disposition to irritation and inflammation in the urethra in man; and what would incline me to think so is, that this canal is subject to be more frequently out of order than any other, producing a great variety of symptoms.

§. 1. *Varieties in different Constitutions.*

This disease, when it appears in the form either of a gonorrhœa or a chancre, differs very much in the violence of its symptoms in different people. In some it is extremely mild, in others extremely violent. When mild, it is generally simple in its symptoms, having but few, and those of no great extent, being much confined to the specific distance; but when violent, it becomes more complicated in its symptoms, having a greater variety, and extending itself beyond the specific distance. This does not arise from any variety in the specific virtue of the poison, but from a difference in the disposition and mode of action of the body, or parts of the body, some being hardly susceptible of this or any irritation, others being very susceptible of it, and of every other irritation, so as readily to run into violent action.

The venereal irritation, however, does not always follow these rules; for I have known young men, in whom a sore from common accident has healed up readily, yet the irritation attending a gonorrhœa has been violent, and a chancre has inflamed and spread itself with great rapidity, and even has mortified. On the other hand, I have known young men, in whom a sore from common violence has been healed with great difficulty, yet when they had contracted a gonorrhœa or chancre, the disease has been mild and easily curable.

In particular people it is either mild or severe, for the most part, uniformly. In the first-stated dispositions it is not invariably so; but then I believe there is some indisposition at the time. I have known several gentlemen who had their gonorrhœas so slight in common that they frequently cured themselves. But it has so happened that a gonorrhœa has been remarkably severe, and has obliged them to apply for assistance: but then they were soon attacked with the symptoms of a fever; and when the fever has gone off, the symptoms of the gonorrhœa have immediately become mild. I may now also observe, that when the disease is in the form of a lues venerea, different constitutions are differently affected. In some its progress is very rapid, in others it is very slow.

CHAPTER IV.

OF THE LUES VENEREA BEING THE CAUSE OF OTHER DISEASES.

EVERY animal may be said to have natural tendencies to morbid actions, which may be considered as predisposing causes; and these may be called into action whenever the immediate cause takes place, which may be such as to have no connexion with these tendencies, and cannot therefore be considered as the cause of the disease. One disease excites another, and therefore is supposed to be the sole cause of it. Thus, slight fevers, or colds, smallpox, and measles, become frequently the immediate cause of scrofula; and certain derangements of the natural actions of the body often bring on the gout, agues, and other diseases: but these diseases will be always more or less, according to the constitution and parts; and the constitutions will differ according to circumstances, which may be numerous; two of these, however, will be, local situation and age.

In this country the tendency to scrofula arises from the climate, which is in many a predisposing cause, and only requires some derangement to become an immediate cause and produce the whole disease.

The venereal disease also becomes often the immediate cause of other disorders, by calling forth latent tendencies to action. This does not happen from its being venereal, but from its having destroyed the natural actions, so that the moment the venereal action and disposition have terminated, the other takes place; and I have seen in many cases the tendency so very strong that it has taken place before the venereal has been entirely subdued; for by pursuing the mercurial course the symptoms have grown worse; but by taking up the new disposition, and rendering it less active than the venereal, the venereal has come into action anew; and these effects have taken place alternately several times. In such cases it is a lucky circumstance when the two modes of treatment can be united; but where they act in opposition it is very unfortunate. If the venereal disease attacks the lungs, although that disposition may be corrected, consumption may ensue; and in like manner where the bones are affected, or the nose, scrofulous swellings or fistula lachrymalis may be the consequence, though the disease may have been cured.

Many of the diseases arising from this source appear to be peculiar to such causes, and seem to be formed out of the constitution, the disease, and method of cure. It is therefore difficult to say of what nature such a disease may be; but it will in general have a particular tendency from the constitution; and if we are acquainted with the general tendency of a constitution, we are to suspect that as the strongest cause, and that the disease will partake more of it than the other. In this country these complaints have most commonly a scrofulous tendency, and are often truly scrofulous, the disease partaking more of that disposition than any other.

Parts have also their peculiar tendency to diseases, which are stronger than those of the constitution at large, and when injured they will of course fall into the morbid action arising from such tendencies. Therefore, when parts have had their natural actions destroyed by a venereal irritation, those tendencies will be brought into action; and, therefore, the diseases arising from the tendencies of such parts are to be kept in view. They will be assisted likewise by local situation and age.

In particular countries, and in young people, the tendency to scrofula will be predominant; therefore buboes in them will more readily become scrofulous. In old people they may form cancers; and when in parts of the body which have a particular tendency to cancer, that disease will more readily take place.

The want of knowledge and of attention to this subject has been the cause of many mistakes, for whenever such effects have been produced in consequence of the venereal disease, it has immediately been blamed, and not only as a cause, but it has been supposed to be the disease itself. This is an inference natural enough to those who cannot see that a variety of causes are capable of producing one effect, or, in other words, that where the predisposing cause is the same, a variety of immediate causes may produce the same action. It shows great ignorance, however, to suppose the venereal disease can be both the predisposing and immediate cause.

When the venereal disease attacks the urethra, it often becomes itself the predisposing cause of abscesses and many other complaints; when it attacks the outside of the penis, forming chancres, they often ulcerate so deep as to communicate with the urethra, producing fistula in the urethra, and often a continued phimosis.

In describing diseases which, like the venereal disease, admit of a great variety of symptoms, we should keep a middle line, first giving the most common symptoms of the disease in each form, then the varieties which most commonly occur, and last of all the most uncommon; but it will not be easy to take notice of every possible variety. Therefore, when a variety occurs not mentioned, it is not to be supposed that the author is leading his readers astray, or is unacquainted with the disease at large. If his general principles are just, they will help to explain most of the singularities of the disease.

PART II.

CHAPTER I.

OF GONORRHŒA.

WHEN an irritating matter of any kind is applied to a secreting surface. it increases that secretion, and changes it from its natural state (whatever that be) to some other. This, in the present disease, is pus.

When this takes place in the urethra, it is called a gonorrhœa; and as it arises from the matter being applied to a non-cuticular surface, which naturally secretes some fluid, it is of no consequence in what part of the body this surface is; for if in the anus, it will produce a similar discharge there, and a similar effect on the inside of the mouth, nose, eyes, and ears. It is conceived by some that gonorrhœas may take place without the above-mentioned immediate cause, that is, that they may arise from the constitution; if so, they must be similar to what is supposed to be a venereal ophthalmia. But, from the analogy of other venereal affections proceeding from the constitution, I very much suspect the existence of either the one or the other; for when the poison is thrown upon the mouth, throat, or nose, it produces ulcers, and not an increased secretion like a gonorrhœa. But we never find an ulcer on the inside of the eyelids in those ophthalmiæ; and gonorrhœas in the urethra are too frequent to proceed from such a cause.

Till about the year 1753, it was generally supposed that the matter from the urethra in a gonorrhœa arose from an ulcer or ulcers in that passage; but from observation it was then proved that this was not the case.

It may not be improper to give here a short history of the discovery that matter may be formed by inflammation without ulceration. In the winter, 1749, a child was brought into the room used for dissection in Covent Garden; on opening of whose thorax a large quantity of pus was found loose in the cavity, with the surface of the lungs and the pleura furred over with a more solid substance, similar to coagulable lymph. On removing this from those surfaces, they were found entire.

This appearance being new to Dr. Hunter, he sent to Mr. Samuel Sharp, desiring his attendance; and to him it also appeared new. Mr. Sharp afterwards, in the year 1750, published his Critical Enquiry, in which he introduced this fact, " That matter may be formed without a breach of substance;" not mentioning whence he had derived this notion. It was ever after taught by Dr. Hunter in his lectures. We, however, find writers adopting it without quoting either Mr. Sharp or Dr. Hunter. So much being known, I was anxious to examine whether the matter in a gonorrhœa was formed in the same way. In the spring of 1753 there was an execution of eight men, two of whom I knew had at that time very severe gonorrhœas. Their bodies being procured for this particular purpose, we were very accurate in our examination, but found no ulceration. The two urethras appeared merely a little blood-shot, especially near the glans. This being another new fact ascertained, it could not escape Mr. Gataker, ever attentive to his emolument, who was then attending Dr. Hunter's lectures, and also practising dissection under me. He published soon after, in 1754, a treatise on this disease, and explained fully that the matter in a gonorrhœa did not arise from an ulcer, without mentioning how he acquired this knowledge; and from that time successive writers have repeated the same doctrine. Since the period mentioned above I have constantly paid particular attention to this circumstance, and have opened the urethra of many who at the time of their death had a gonorrhœa, yet have never found a sore in any; but always observed that the urethra, near the glans, was more bloodshot than usual, and that the lacunæ were often filled with matter. I have indeed seen an instance of a sore a little within the urethra; but this sore was not produced by any ulceration of the surface, but from an inflammation taking place, probably in one of the glands, which produced an abscess in the part, and that abscess opened its way into the urethra. The very same sore opened a way through externally at the frænum, so that there was a new passage for the urine. Indeed, the method of curing a gonorrhœa might have shown that it could not depend upon a venereal ulcer, for there is hardly an instance of a venereal ulcer being cured by anything but mercury, escharotics excepted. We know, however, that most gonorrhœas are curable without mercury, and, what is still more, without any medical assistance; which, I believe, is never the case with a chancre. This doctrine that a gonorrhœa does not depend on ulcers, was first taught publicly by Dr. Hunter, at his lectures, in the year 1750; but he did not attempt to account for it.

§. 1. *Of the Time between the Application of the Poison, and Effect.*

In most diseases there is a certain time between the application of the cause and the appearance of the effect. In the venereal disease this time is found to vary considerably, owing probably to the state of the constitution when the infection was received. Each form of the disease also varies in this respect; the gonorrhœa and chancre being earlier in their appearance after contamination than the lues venerea, and of the two former, the gonorrhœa appearing sooner than the chancre. In the gonorrhœa, the times of appearance are very different: I have had reason to believe that in some the poison has taken effect in a few hours, while in others it has been six weeks; and I have had examples of it in all the intermediate periods. So far, however, as we can rely upon the veracity of our patients, (and further evidence we cannot have,) six, eight, ten, or twelve days should appear to be the most common period, though it is capable of affecting some people much sooner, and others much later. I was informed by a married gentleman, who came from the country, and left his wife behind him, that in a frolic he went to a bagnio and had connexion with a woman of the town. The next morning he left her; and he had no sooner got to his lodging than he felt a moisture of the part, and upon inspection he found a beginning gonorrhœa, which proved a very troublesome one. I was told by another gentleman that he had been with a woman overnight, and in the morning the gonorrhœa appeared; and that the same happened to him twice. I was informed by a third gentleman that the discharge appeared in six-and-thirty hours after the application of the poison. In the above-mentioned patients the infection must have arisen from the poison applied at those stated times, as neither of these patients is supposed to have had an opportunity of receiving the infection for many weeks before*.

These assertions from men of veracity, and where there could be no temptation to deceive, not even an imaginary one, are sufficient evidences. On the other hand, upon equally good authority, I have been informed that six weeks after the application had passed before any symptom appeared. The patient had strange and uncommon complaints preceding the running, such as an unusual sensation in the parts, with

* The following case added:
"A gentleman had a chancre, which was cured by the internal use of mercury: when the chancre was nearly well, a gonorrhœa made its appearance; this was nearly five weeks after the chancre."—*Home.*

most of the other symptoms of gonorrhœa, except the discharge. He
had the same complaint about twelve months afterwards,. and then it
was four weeks from the application of the poison before it appeared,
giving for some part of that time the former disagreeable sensations;
but from his late experience he suspected what was coming. From this I
am inclined to believe that it seldom or never lies perfectly quiet so long,
and that the inflammatory state may take place for some considerable time
before the suppurative; and in these cases there is less disposition for
a cure, as the very disposition which forms a running is in general a
salutary one, and is an intermediate step between the disease, which is
the inflammation, and the cure; for in the time of suppuration a change
has taken place in the vessels, producing the formation of matter. If
this change should never take place, it is not certain what would be the
consequence. Whether the inflammation would go off without suppuration, as in many common inflammations, I have not been able to determine, but should suspect that it would continue much longer than
usual, because the parts have not completed their actions; and I also
suspect that such cases always arise from some peculiarity of constitution.

§. 2. *Of the Difficulty of distinguishing the virulent from the
simple Gonorrhœa.*

The surface of the urethra is subject to inflammation and suppuration from various other causes besides the venereal poison; and sometimes discharges happen spontaneously when no immediate cause can
be assigned. Such may be called simple gonorrhœas, having nothing
of the venereal infection in them; though those persons that have been
formerly subject to virulent gonorrhœas are most liable to them. It is
given as a distinguishing mark between the simple and the virulent gonorrhœa that the simple comes on immediately after copulation, and is
at once violent; whereas the virulent comes on some days after, and gradually. But the simple is not in all cases a consequence of a man's
having had connexion with women; it does not always come on at once,
nor is it always free from pain. On the other hand, we see many venereal gonorrhœas that begin without any appearance of inflammation,
and I have been very much at a loss to determine whether they were
venereal or not; for there is a certain class of symptoms common to
almost all diseases of the urethra, from which it is difficult to distinguish
the few that arise solely from the specific affection. I have known the
urethra sympathize with the cutting of a tooth* producing all the sym-

* Natural History of the Teeth, Part II. p. 110.

ptoms of a gonorrhœa. This happened several times to the same patient. The urethra is known to be sometimes the seat of the gout*; I
have known it the seat of the rheumatism. The urethra of those who
have had venereal complaints is more apt to exhibit symptoms similar
to gonorrhœa than the urethra of those who never had any such complaint; and it is generally in consequence of the parts having been hurt
by that disease that the simple gonorrhœa comes on, which, perhaps,
is also a reason why they are in some measure similar. A discharge,
and even pain, attacks the urethra: and strange sensations are every
now and then felt in these parts, which may be either a return of the
symptoms of the venereal disease without virus, may arise as it were
spontaneously, or may be a consequence of some other disease. When
it happens in consequence of some former venereal gonorrhœa, it is seldom constant, and may be called a temporary gleet, ceasing for a time
and then returning; but in such cases the parts seldom swell, the glans
does not change to the ripe cherry colour, nor does it sweat a kind of
matter. Such a complaint as a discharge without virus is known to
exist, by its coming on when there has been no late connexion with
women, and likewise by its coming on of its own accord where there
had never been any former venereal complaint, nor any chance of infection. From its commonly going off soon, both in those who have had
connexion with women and those who have not, it becomes very difficult in many cases to determine whether or not it is venereal: for it is
often thought venereal when it really is not so; and, on the other hand,
it may be supposed to be only a return of the gleet when it is truly venereal. But, perhaps, this is not so material a circumstance as might
at first be supposed. These diseases, when they are a consequence of
former venereal complaints, may be considered only as an inconvenience
entailed on those who have had the venereal gonorrhœa. No certain
cure for them is known: they are similar to the fluor albus in women.

§. 3. *Of the common final Intention of Suppuration not answering in the present Disease.*

When a secreting surface has once received the inflammatory
action, its secretions are increased and visibly altered. Also when
the irritation has produced inflammation and an ulcer in the solid
parts, a secretion of matter takes place, the intention of which in both
seems to be to wash away the irritating matter; so that it is the end of

* Essays and Observations, Physical and Literary, of Edinburgh, vol. iii. p. 425.

irritations to produce their own destruction, like a mote in the eye, which, by increasing the secretion of tears, is itself washed away. But in inflammations arising from specific or morbid poisons this effect cannot be produced : for although the first irritating matter be washed away, yet the new matter formed has the same quality with the original; and therefore, upon the same principle, it would produce a perpetual succession of irritations, and of course secretions, even if there were no other cause for the continuance than its own matter. But the venereal inflammation is not kept up by the pus which is formed ; but, like many other specific diseases, by the specific quality of the inflammation itself. This inflammation, however, it would appear, can only last a limited time, the symptoms peculiar to it vanishing of themselves by the parts becoming less and less susceptible of irritation. This circumstance is not peculiar to this particular form of the venereal disease; it is, perhaps, common to almost every disease that can affect the human body. From hence it will appear that the consequent venereal matter has no power of continuing the original irritation; and indeed if this were not the case there would be no end to the disease.

As the living principle in many diseases is not capable of continuing the same action, it also loses this power in the present, when the disease is in the form of a gonorrhœa; and the effect is at last stopped, the irritation ceasing gradually. This cessation will vary according to circumstances : for if the irritated parts are in a state very susceptible of such irritations, in all probability their actions will be more violent and continue longer; but in all cases the difference must arise from the difference in the constitution, and not from any difference in the poison itself.

The circumstance of the disease ceasing spontaneously only happens when it attacks a secreting surface, and when a secretion of pus is produced; for when it attacks a non-secreting surface, and produces its effects there, that is, an ulcer, the parts so affected are capable of continuing the disease, or this mode of action, for ever, as will be taken notice of when we shall hereafter consider chancre. But this difference between spontaneous and non-spontaneous cure seems to depend more on the difference in the two modes of action than on the difference in the two surfaces; for when the disease produces an ulcer on a secreting surface, which it often does from the constitution, as on the tonsils, it has no disposition to cure of itself; nor in the urethra, if ulcers are formed there, would they heal more readily than when formed in any other part.

The common practice proves these facts : we every day see gonorrhœas cured by the most ignorant ; but in chancre, or the lues venerea, more skill is necessary. The reason is obvious : gonorrhœa cures it-self, whilst the other forms of the disease require the assistance of art.

It sometimes happens that the parts which become irritated first get well, while another part of the same surface receives the irritation, which continues the disease, as happens when it shifts from the glans to the urethra.

From this circumstance of all gonorrhœas ceasing without medical help, I should doubt very much the possibility of a person getting a fresh gonorrhœa while he has that disease, or of his increasing the same by the application of fresh matter of its own kind. And this ob-servation holds in all the forms of the disease ; for it has been proved that the application of the matter from a gonorrhœa to a bubo does not in the least retard the cure of that bubo : nor does the matter of a chancre applied to a bubo, nor the matter of a bubo applied to a chancre, produce any bad effect ; though if venereal matter is applied to a com-mon sore it will often produce the venereal irritation. By all which I am led to believe that the venereal matter formed in a gonorrhœa does not assist in keeping up that gonorrhœa ; for it is only an application of matter, the poison and effects of which are exactly similar to the effects upon the solids already produced ; and that nothing could increase or continue the effect but something that is capable of increasing the disposition of the parts themselves to such inflammation, or of making them more susceptible of it. We find, besides, that a gonorrhœa may be cured while there is a chancre, and *vice versâ* : now if fresh venereal matter were capable of keeping up the disease, no gonorrhœa could ever get well while there is this supply of venereal matter*. From all this it is reasonable to suppose that such a surface of an animal body is not capable of being irritated by its own matter ; nor is it capable of being irritated beyond a certain time ; and therefore if fresh venereal matter were continued to be applied to the urethra of a man having a gonor-rhœa, that it would go off just as soon as if no such application had been made, and get as soon well as if great pains had been taken to

---

* When treating of pus, in my lectures, I observed that I was inclined to be-lieve that no matter, of whatever kind, can produce any effect upon the part that formed it: nor do I believe that the matter of any sore, let it be what it will, ever does or can do any hurt to that sore ; for the parts which formed the matter are of the same nature, and cannot be irritated by that which they produced, except extraneous matter is joined with it. The gland which forms the poison of the viper, and the duct which conveys it to the tooth, are not irritated by the poison ; and it would appear from Abbé Fontana's experiments that the viper cannot be affected by its own poison. Vide Traité sur le Venin de la Vipère, par M. F. Fontana, vol. i. p. 22. If what I have now ad-vanced is true, wiping or washing away matter, under the idea of keeping the parts clean, is in every case absurd.

wash its own matter away. The same reasoning holds good in chancres.

I carry this idea still further, and assert that the parts become less susceptible of the venereal irritation ; and that not only a gonorrhœa cannot be continued by the application of either its own or fresh matter, but that a man cannot get a fresh gonorrhœa, or a chancre, if he applies fresh venereal matter to the parts when the cure is nearly completed, and continues the application ever after, or at least at such intervals as are within the effect of habit. I can conceive that in time the parts may become so habituated to this application as to be insensible of it; for by a constant application the parts would never be allowed to forget this irritation, or rather never become unaccustomed to it ; and therefore this supply of fresh matter could not affect the parts so as to renew the disease till they first recovered their original and natural state, and then they would be capable of being affected again.

This opinion is not derived from theory only, but is founded on experience and observation. A man, immediately after having suffered a gonorrhœa, shall have frequent connexions with women of the town, and that for years successively, without being infected ; yet a fresh man shall contract it immediately from the very same woman : and if the first-mentioned man were to be out of the habit of this irritation for some time, he then would be as easily infected as the other. Where this habit is not so strong as to prevent altogether the parts from being affected, still it will do it in part ; and it is a strong proof of this that most people have their first gonorrhœa the most severe, and the succeeding ones generally become milder and milder, till the danger of infection almost vanishes.

This seems to be explained by the following facts. A married man, who had had a communication with his wife only for several years, slept with a woman with whom he had formerly cohabited. She gave him a severe gonorrhœa, and declared that she was not conscious of being diseased. He put himself and her under my care ; and while they were going on with their cures they still continued their intercourse, which I readily allowed. He got well, and it was supposed she got well also. The intercourse was continued between them for many months after, without any mischief received on his side, or any suspicion of remaining disease on hers. At last this connexion was broken off ; and she formed another attachment. She no sooner formed this new attachment than she gave her new lover a gonorrhœa ; she now flew to me for a cure, and declared that she had no connexion but with the two gentlemen before mentioned, and therefore that the present disease must be the same for which I had attended her formerly. Her second lover was not a patient of mine: but I gave her medicines, which she very much neglected to take. Her lover continued his connexion, as the first had done, for several months after he had got well, without any further infection from her. But, unfortunately, her first lover returned about a twelvemonth after; and thinking himself secure, as she lived in peace with the present, renewed his acquaintance with her, and but once; the consequence, however, was a gonorrhœa.

Had the woman the gonorrhœa all this time? And what was the reason why those gentlemen did not catch the disease, except after that the acquaintance had been interrupted for some time? Was it the effect of habit, by which the parts lost their susceptibility of that irritation?

The case of a young woman from the Magdalen Hospital is a striking proof of this, as far as circumstances can prove a fact. She was received into that house, and continued the usual time, which is two years. The moment she came out she was picked up by one who was waiting for her with a post-chaise to carry her off immediately. She gave him a gonorrhœa.

This opinion of parts being so habituated to this irritation as hardly to be affected by it is strengthened by observing that in the gonorrhœa the violent symptoms shall often cease, and the disease shall still continue, spinning itself out to an amazing length, with no other symptoms than a discharge; yet that discharge shall be venereal. This I have frequently seen; and the following is an abstract of a singular case of this kind.

A gentleman had connexion with a woman of the town, and received a venereal gonorrhœa in the beginning of April 1780. He at first could hardly believe it to be venereal, as he had kept the woman in the country, where she had scarcely ever been out of his sight; but the violent pain in making water, great running, chordee, and swelled testicle convinced him that it was venereal. When the cure was going on tolerably well, and he had got the better of one swelled testicle, the other began to swell; however, all the symptoms gradually disappeared, except the chordee, hardness of the epididymis, and a small gleet which was slimy. On the 12th of June he went into the country: while he was in the country the chordee went off, and the hardness of the epididymis entirely disappeared; but still a slimy gleet remained, although but trifling.

September the first, he married a young lady, and endeavouring to enter the vagina, he found great difficulty, which brought on a return of the chordee, and an increased discharge. On the 10th, she began to complain of heat and pain, and of a difficulty and frequency in making water; and when she made water there was forced out some matter;

she had also a dull heavy pain, and a sense of weight at the bottom of her belly and round her hips, with great soreness of the parts when she sat. These symptoms had been preceded by an itching about the orifice of the vagina.

By taking a mercurial pill, and rubbing the parts with mercurial ointment, in about eight days the violence of the symptoms abated. They were now allowed to cohabit; but whenever they came together the pain which she suffered was excessive. The parts were washed with a solution of corrosive sublimate and sugar of lead, and anointed with mercurial ointment, which applications being continued for some time, the soreness went off. He was treated medically, and afterwards all was well.

Here was a venereal gonorrhœa contracted about the beginning of April; all the symptoms had disappeared by the first of June, and there only remained some of the consequences, such as chordee, hardness of the epididymis, and a discharge of a little slimy mucus, which could only be observed in the morning. In a short time the chordee and hardness in the epididymis had entirely gone off, and merely the small discharge of mucus, which appeared only in the morning, remained; yet three months after he communicated the disease to his wife.

I was consulted in the following case by the surgeon who attended. July 13th, 1783, a person had connexion with a woman of the town; the 30th, that is, seventeen days after, a gonorrhœa came on, which was violent. He took mercurial pills and gentle purges. In twelve days the violent symptoms abated, and about the 4th of September the discharge was stopped. On the 9th it began to appear again, but only lasted a few days; and would come and go in this way sometimes every two days, often six or seven days. On the 28th of September he had connexion with his wife, while he had a small discharge. The 9th of October he had connexion again; and three days after she complained of heat in making water, with a discharge and other symptoms of gonorrhœa, which were violent. About the latter end of October her complaints were almost removed, some only of the symptoms appearing and disappearing till January 1784, when he had connexion with her to try whether she could give it him, viz. three months after the second connexion; and in fourteen days after this he had all the symptoms of a gonorrhœa. April 29, he was not perfectly well, having a discharge, with a pain in the perinæum; and she also had a discharge. If this last attack, in January 1784, in him was a gonorrhœa, then of course she must have had it; and also of course he must have lost his in the intermediate time, between the 9th of October 1783 and January 1784; for if he had it also then, it could not have produced any effect upon him.

It was impossible to say whether they had now the infection or not, for any trials upon themselves would prove but little, except one of them only had it so as to infect the other; but if both had it, no alteration could take place in either, as it could not be ascertained whether they had the disease or not; and as there were suspicious symptoms in both, when joined with all the circumstances, I agreed with the attending surgeon, that it was most prudent to treat them as if actually affected with a gonorrhœa.

If it is true, as is asserted in the Voyage round the World, that the venereal disease was carried to Otaheite, it shows that it can be long retained after all ideas of its existence have ceased; and when it is retained for such a length of time it is most probably in the form of gonorrhœa*.

In like manner, a venereal bubo, if it could be kept a considerable time between the point of suppuration and resolution, would become indolent from habit, continue in that point of suspension, and remain perhaps almost incurable.   Such, I think, I have seen.

§. 4. Of the Venereal Gonorrhœa.

In treating of the seat, extent, and symptoms of gonorrhœa, I shall begin with such particulars as are constant or most frequent, and take them as much as possible in the order they become less so; for there is a considerable variety in different gonorrhœas.

§. 5. Of the Seat of the Disease in both Sexes.

The seat of this disease, in both sexes, is commonly the parts of generation.   In men it is generally the urethra, though it sometimes takes place on the inside of the prepuce and surface of the glans.   In women it is the vagina, urethra, labia, clitoris, or nymphæ.

The disease has its seat in these parts from the manner in which it is caught.   But if we were to consider the surface of contact simply in men, we should naturally suppose that the glans penis†, or the orifice of the urethra, would be the first, or indeed the only parts affected; yet most commonly they are not, for though there are cases where the glans is affected, and where the disease goes no further, I believe it seldom attacks the orifice of the urethra without passing some way along that

---

* Vide page 143.

† Inserted: "inner surface of the prepuce near to the glans."—*Home.*

canal. How far it ever can be said to affect the prepuce only I am not quite certain, although I believe it sometimes happens; for I have seen inflammation there, as well with as without a discharge from the ure-thra, which appeared to me to be venereal. I have seen in such cases the inflammation extending into the loose cellular membrane of the prepuce, and producing a phimosis; and this inflammation I suspect to be of the erysipelatous kind.

When the disease attacks the glans and other external parts, as, for instance, the prepuce*, it is principally about the root of that body and the beginning of the prepuce, the parts where the cuticle is thin-nest, and of course where the poison most readily affects the cutis; but sometimes it extends over all the glans, and also the whole external surface of the prepuce. It produces there a soreness or tenderness, with a secretion of thinnish matter, commonly without either excori-ation or ulceration. I am not certain, however, that it does not some-times excoriate those parts, for I once saw a case where almost the whole cuticle was separated from the glans. The patient assured me that it was venereal, and, from the particular circumstances which he related, I had no reason to think his opinion ill founded. He never had had any such complaint from connexion with women before that time. Per-haps the disease begins oftener on those parts than is commonly ima-gined, but being defended by a cuticle, they are but little susceptible of this kind of irritation; and this may be the reason why a permanent effect is not produced, and why it is often so slight as not to be observed. When the glans or prepuce, or both, suffer the venereal inflammation, it often rests there, and goes no further, not being attended with a dis-charge of matter, nor with pain in the urethra. This the following case illustrates.

A young gentleman from Ireland slept with a woman at Bristol, and a fortnight afterwards he had intercourse with another woman in London, which last happened to be on a Monday, and on the Tuesday, or the day following, he observed a discharge from the end of his penis when co-vered with the prepuce. On the Saturday following he applied to me. Upon examination, I found that the running came from the inside of the prepuce, near to the glans; and the corona glandis, as also that part of the prepuce which is behind it, appeared to be in a tender and exco-riated state, and covered with matter. He told me he had once had a gonorrhœa before, and upon being asked if it was in the same place, he said it was. Not being certain how far this might be venereal, I made the following inquiry: whether he had been subject to such excoriations

---

* Inserted: "I believe it is principally in those patients whose glans is commonly covered with the prepuce, and—".—*Home.*

before he had visited women ? And his answer was, that he never had; and that he had not this complaint always after coition, but only twice, as has been above mentioned, which, being uncommon, inclined him to suppose the effect to be venereal.

I suspect that when the prepuce swells in a gonorrhœa of the urethra, producing a phimosis, which is often the case, it arises from the same disease having affected its inside, and that not being sufficient to produce ulceration, it goes no further. It seems probable that this inflammation is of the erysipelatous kind, a circumstance very necessary to be known in the cure.

The urethra is the part in which this form of the venereal disease is most frequent; and although the inflammation attending the disease in this part has many of the common symptoms of inflammation, yet it can hardly be called inflammatory when moderate, at least it does not constantly produce all the effects of common inflammation, though there is a tendency towards it. The parts seldom have all the characteristic symptoms; for there is no throbbing sensation; there is but little pain, except from the irritation of the urine and distention of the parts; the inflammation seldom goes deeper than the surface, and we have there-. fore rarely any tumefaction or thickening of the parts. It should rather seem to be an error loci on the surface of the urethra, like a bloodshot eye.

The secretion of pus with so little inflammation is perhaps owing to these parts being naturally in a state of secretion; therefore the transition from a healthy to a diseased secretion is more easily produced. It sometimes happens, however, that the parts do inflame considerably, and the inflammation goes deep into the cellular, or rather reticular, membrane of the corpus spongiosum urethræ, especially near the glans. Sometimes it extends further along the corpus spongiosum urethræ, producing tumefaction, that is, an extravasation of the coagulable lymph, which is the common cause of chordee. It may be observed in general, that in most cases when suppuration is produced there is a decrease of inflammation. The inflammation in the reticular membrane of the surrounding parts would appear not to be always confined to the adhesive stage, for in those parts we have sometimes suppurations, especially in the perinæum, which suppurations I suspect to be in the glands, as will be taken notice of hereafter.

The gonorrhœa does not always attack an urethra otherwise sound; nor does it always attack an urethra the relative parts of which are always sound. Thus we find people contracting this disease while they are affected with strictures, a swelled prostate gland, as also diseased testicles, or such testicles as very readily run into disease, by which the malady becomes more complicated, and requires more attention in the method of cure. Sometimes such diseases are relieved by the gonorrhœa, at other times increased.

§. 6. Of the most common Symptoms, and the Order of their Appearance.

Although the irritation must always begin first, yet it is not certain which of the symptoms, in consequence of that irritation, will first appear, for any one may appear singly without the others, though this is rarely the case. The first symptom, when carefully attended to, is generally an itching at the orifice of the urethra, sometimes extending over the whole glans*; a little fulness of the lips of the urethra: the effects of inflammation are next observable, and soon after a running appears; the itching changes into pain, more particularly at the time of voiding the urine; there is often no pain till some time after the appearance of the discharge, and other symptoms; and in many gonorrhœas there is hardly any pain at all, even when the discharge is very considerable; at other times the pain, or rather a great degree of soreness, will come on long before any discharge appears†.

There is generally at this time a greater fulness in the penis, and more especially in the glans, although it is not near so full as when erected, being rather in a state of half-erection. Besides this fulness, the glans has a kind of transparency, especially near the beginning of the urethra, where the skin is distended, being smooth and red, resembling a ripe cherry, this is owing to the reticular membrane, at this time loaded with a quantity of extravasated serum, and the vessels filled with blood. Near the beginning of the urethra there is in many cases an evident excoriation, which is marked by the termination of the cuticle all around. The surface of the glans also is often in a half-excoriated state, which gives it a degree of tenderness, and there oozes out from it a kind of matter, as has been before observed‡. The canal of the urethra becomes narrower, which is known by the stream of the urine being smaller than common. This proceeds from the fulness of

---

* These symptoms are most carefully observed by those who are under apprehensions of having the disease, and therefore are attentive to every little sensation about those parts.

† Added: "and extend a little way down the canal. I have known these sensations to be felt half way down the urethra."—Home.

‡ Added: "but this is more evident in those whose glans penis is commonly covered by the prepuce, for when denuded the cuticle becomes thicker, and is less easily irritated."—Home.

the penis in general, and from the internal membrane of the urethra being swollen by the inflammation, and also from its being in a spasmodic state. Besides these changes, the fear of the patient whilst voiding his urine assists in diminishing the stream of urine. The stream, as it flows from the urethra, is generally much scattered and broken as soon as it leaves the passage, which is owing to the internal canal having become irregular, and is not peculiar to a venereal gonorrhœa, but common to every disease of the urethra that alters the exact and natural figure of the canal, even although the irregularity is very far back. This we find in many diseased prostate glands*.

There is frequently some degree of hæmorrhage from the urethra. This I suppose arises from the distention of the vessels, more especially when there is a chordee, or a tendency to one.

There are often small swellings observable along the lower surface of the penis in the course of the urethra. These, I suspect, are the glands of the urethra so enlarged as to be plainly felt on the outside. They inflame so much in some cases as to suppurate, and, according to the laws of ulceration, the matter is brought to the skin, forming one, two, or more abscesses, along the under surface of the urethra; and some of these breaking internally, form what are called internal ulcers. I have observed in several cases a tumour on the under side of the penis, where the urethra is, which would swell at times very considerably, even to the size of a small flattened nut, inflame, and then, a gush of matter flowing from the urethra, would almost immediately subside. The discharge has continued for some time, gradually diminishing till it has entirely gone off, and the tumour has been almost wholly reduced; yet after some months it has swelled in the same manner again, and terminated in the same way. How far these tumours, and the matter they discharge, are really venereal when they appear first, may be doubtful; and it is difficult to determine this, for the patients in general have recourse to medicine immediately; but in their subsequent attacks they are certainly not venereal, for they cure themselves.

I have suspected these tumours to be the ducts or lacunæ of the glands of the urethra, distended with mucus, from the mouth of the duct being closed, in a manner similar to what happens to the duct leading from the lachrymal sac to the nose: and in consequence of the distention of the ducts or lacunæ, inflammation and suppuration come on, and ulcera-

---

* Added: "In some instances the first symptoms are unusual sensations in the penis, especially while making water, which come on a few days after receiving the infection, attended with constitutional irritability, sensations in the testicles, neck of the bladder, and anus; these continue for about ten days, when a discharge comes on, and they disappear."—*Home.*

tion takes place, which opens a way into the urethra; but this opening soon closes up and occasions a return. Cowper's glands have been
suspected to inflame, and hardness and swelling have been felt externally very much in the situation of them, which, coming to suppuration,
have produced considerable abscesses in the perinæum. These tumours
break either internally or externally, and sometimes in both ways, making a new passage for the urine, called fistulæ in perinæo.

A soreness is often felt by the patient all along the under side of the
penis, owing to the inflamed state of the urethra. This soreness often
extends as far as the anus, and gives great pain, principally in erections;
yet it is different from a chordee, the penis remaining straight.

Erections are frequent in most gonorrhœas. These, arising from the
irritation at the time, often approach to a priapism, especially when
there is the above-mentioned soreness, or when there is a chordee.

Priapisms often threaten mortification in men; and I have seen an
instance of it in a dog. The erection never subsided, and the glans penis
could not be covered by the prepuce, from the swelling of the bulb. The
penis mortified and dropped off; the bone in it was denuded, and an
exfoliation followed. As opium is of great service in priapism, there is
reason to suppose the complaint is of a spasmodic nature.

§. 7. *Of the Discharge.*

The natural slimy discharge from the glands of the urethra is first
changed from a fine transparent ropy secretion to a watery, whitish fluid;
and the natural exhaling fluid of the urethra, which is intended for moist-
ening its surface, and which appears to be of the same kind with that
which lubricates cavities in general, becomes less transparent; and both
these secretions becoming gradually thicker, assume more and more the
qualities of common pus. In some cases of gonorrhœa, the glands that
produce the slime which is secreted in consequence of lascivious ideas,
are certainly not affected; for I have seen cases, when, after the passages had been cleared of the venereal matter by making water, the pure
slime has flowed out of the end of the penis on such occasions. When
this matter is more in quantity than what lubricates the urethra, it is
forced out of the orifice by the peristaltic action of that canal, and appears
externally*.

---

* That the urethra has considerable powers of action is evident in a vast number of
instances; and that action is principally from behind forwards. We find that a bougie
may be worked out by the action of the urethra. This action, I believe, is often inverted, as in spasmodic stranguries.

The matter of gonorrhœa often changes its colour and consistence, which is owing to the disposition of the parts which form it; sometimes from a white to a yellow, and often to a greenish colour. These changes depend on the increase or decrease of the inflammation, and not on the poisonous quality of the matter itself; for any irritation on these parts, equal to that produced in a gonorrhœa, will produce the same appearances; and the changes in the colour of the matter are chiefly observable after it has been discharged upon a cloth and become dry. The appearance upon the cloth is of various hues: in the middle the matter is thicker or more in quantity, and it is therefore generally of a deeper colour; the circumference is paler, because the watery or serous part of the matter has spread further; and at the outer edge of all it is darkest: this last appearance is owing to its being only water with a little slime, in which some of the tinge is suspended, which when dry gives a transparency to the part that takes off from the white colour of the linen. It is very probable that there is a small extravasation of red blood in all the cases where the matter deviates from the common colour, and to this the different tinges seem to be owing. As this matter arises from a specific inflammation, it has a greater tendency to putrefaction than common matter from a healthy sore, and has often a smell seemingly peculiar to itself.

As it should appear that there is hardly a sufficient surface of the urethra inflamed to give the quantity of matter that is often produced, especially when we consider that the inflammation does in common go no further than two or three inches from the external orifice, it is natural to suppose that the discharge is produced from other parts, the office of which is to form mucus for natural purposes, and which are therefore more capable of producing a great quantity upon slight irritations, which hardly rise to inflammation. These parts, I have observed, are the glands of the urethra. In many cases where the glands have not been after death so much swelled as to be felt externally, and where I have had an opportunity of examining the urethra of those who have had this complaint upon them, I have always been able to discover that the ducts or lacunæ leading from them have been loaded with matter, and more visible than in the natural state. I have observed too that the formation of the matter is not confined to these glands entirely; for the inner surface of the urethra is commonly in such a state as not to suffer the urine to pass without considerable pain, and therefore most probably this internal membrane is also affected in such a manner as to secrete a matter.

This discharge, in common cases, should seem not to arise much further back in the urethra than where the pain is felt, although it is commonly believed that it comes from the whole of the canal, and even from Cowper's glands and the prostate, and even what are called the vesiculæ seminales*. But the truth of this I very much doubt. My reason for supposing that it comes only from the surface where the pain is, are the following. If the matter arose from the whole surface of the urethra and from the glands near the bladder, there would certainly be many other symptoms than do actually occur : for instance, if all the parts of the urethra beyond the bulb, or even in the bulb, were affected so as to secrete matter, that matter would be gradually squeezed into the bulb as the semen is, and from thence it would be thrown out by jerks; for we know that nothing can be in the bulbous part of the urethra without stimulating it to action, especially when in a state of irritation and inflammation. In such a state we find that even a drop of urine is not allowed to rest there ; and also if an injection of warm water only is thrown into the urethra as far as the bulb, the musculi acceleratores are uneasy till they act, and throw it out. Hence it is natural to suppose, that if the membranous and bulbous part of the urethra, with the vesiculæ seminales, prostate, and Cowper's glands, assisted in forming the matter, whenever it collected in the bulb it would probably be immediately thrown forwards by the muscles above mentioned, and we should be sensible of it every moment of the day. But such symptoms are seldom observed. Sometimes indeed a spasmodic contraction of these muscles occurs, which may probably arise from this cause, though it is more frequently felt immediately after the urine is discharged.

When the inflammation is violent, it often happens that some of the vessels of the urethra burst, and a discharge of blood ensues, which is in greater quantity at the close of voiding urine. This, however, happens at other times, and generally gives temporary ease. Sometimes this blood is in small quantity, and only gives the matter a tinge; as I observed when treating of the colour of the discharge. The erections of the penis often stretch the part so much as to become a cause of an extravasation of blood. This extravasation generally increases the soreness at the time of emptying the bladder, and in such a state of parts the urethra is usually sore when pressed; yet the bleeding diminishes the inflammation, and often gives ease.

---

* Those bags are certainly not reservoirs for the semen. The difference between the contents of them and the semen gave me the first suspicion of this; and from several experiments on the human body, as also a comparative view of them in other animals, I have been able to prove that they are not.

§. 8. *Of the Chordee.*

The chordee appears to be inflammatory in some cases, and spasmodic in others. We shall treat first of the inflammatory chordee.

When the inflammation is not confined merely to the surface of the urethra and its glands, but goes deeper and affects the reticular membrane, it produces in it an extravasation of coagulable lymph, as in the adhesive inflammation, which uniting the cells together, destroys the power of distention of the corpus spongiosum urethræ, and makes it unequal in this respect to the corpora cavernosa penis, and therefore a curvature takes place in the time of erection, which is called a chordee. The curvature is generally in the lower part of the penis, arising from the cells of the corpus spongiosum urethræ having their sides united by adhesions*. Besides this effect of inflammation, when the chordee is violent, the inner membrane is, I suppose, so much upon the stretch, as to be in some degree torn, which frequently causes a profuse bleeding from the urethra, that often relieves the patient, and even sometimes proves the cure. As chordee arises from a greater degree of inflammation than common, it is an effect which may, and often does, remain when all infection is gone, being merely a consequence of the adhesive inflammation.

§. 9. *Of the Manner in which the Inflammation attacks the Urethra.*

In what manner the disease extends itself to the urethra is a question not yet absolutely determined. I suspect that it is communicated or creeps along from the glans to the urethra, or at least from the beginning or lips of the urethra to its inner surface ; because it is impossible to conceive that any of the venereal matter from the woman can get into the canal during coition, although the contrary is commonly asserted. It is impossible, at least, that it can get so far as the common seat of the disease, or into those parts of the urethra where it very often exists, that is, through the whole length of the canal. The following case amounts almost to a proof of this opinion.

A gentleman, on whose veracity I have an entire confidence, when in Germany, where he had not lain with a woman for many weeks, sat in a necessary-house some time. Upon arising, he found something that seemed to give the glans penis a little sharp pull, and he found a small

---

* The preceding sentence omitted.—*Home.*

bit of the plaster of the necessary-house sticking to it. He paid no further attention to it at that time than merely to remove what stuck to his penis; but five or six days after, he observed the symptoms of a clap, which proved a pretty severe one. The only way of accounting for this is, that some person who had a clap had been there before him, and had left some venereal matter upon this place, and that the penis had remained in contact with it a sufficient time for the matter to dry.

When the disease attacks the urethra it seldom extends further than an inch and a half, or two inches at most, within the orifice, which distance appears to be truly specific, and what I have called the specific extent of the inflammation*.

As the cause of a gonorrhœa is commonly an inflammation, it is accompanied with pain and the formation of matter. In such a state neither the sensations of the patient nor the actions of the parts themselves are confined to the real seat of the disease. In consequence of the neighbouring parts sympathising, a variety of symptoms are produced, many of which do not exceed what might arise from an irritable state. An uneasiness partaking of soreness and pain, and a kind of weariness, are everywhere felt about the pelvis; the scrotum, testicles, perinæum, and hips become disagreeably sensible to the patient, and the testicles often require being suspended; and so irritable are they indeed in such cases, that the least accident or even exercise, which would have no such effect at another time, will make them swell. The glands of the groin are often affected sympathetically, and even swell a little, but do not come to suppuration. When they inflame from the absorption of matter, they in general suppurate. I have seen cases where the irritation has extended so far as to affect with real pain the thighs, the buttocks, and the abdominal muscles, so that the patient has been obliged to lie quiet in a horizontal position. The pain has at times been very acute, and the parts have been very sore to the touch; they have even swelled, but the swelling has not been of the inflammatory kind; for notwithstanding a visible fulness, the parts have been rather soft. I knew one gentleman who never had a gonorrhœa but that he was immediately seized universally with rheumatic pains: this had happened to him several times. The blood at such times is generally free from the inflammatory appearance, and therefore we may suppose that the constitution is but little affected.

* It is to be here remarked, that specific diseases, among which I shall reckon such as arise from morbid poisons, have their specific distance or extent as one of their properties; but this can only take place where the constitution is not susceptible of erysipelas, or any other uncommon mode of action; for where there is an erysipelatous disposition no bounds are set to the inflammation.

When the gonorrhœa (exclusive of the affections arising from sympathy) is not more violent than I have described, it may be called common or simple venereal gonorrhœa; but if the patient is very susceptible of such irritation, or of any other mode of action which may accompany the venereal, then the symptoms are in proportion more violent. In such circumstances we sometimes find the irritation and inflammation exceed the specific distance, and extend through the whole of the urethra. There is often also a considerable degree of pain in the perinæum; and a frequent though not a constant symptom is a spasmodic contraction of the acceleratores urinæ, which is always attended with contractions of the erectores muscles. Whether these spasms arise from a secretion of matter, which being collected in the bulbous part of the urethra produces uneasiness, and excites contractions in order to its own expulsion, like the last drops of urine, I have not been able to determine. I have seen such spasms in the time of making water, from the urine irritating the parts in its passage through the urethra, and throwing the musculi acceleratores into contractions, so that the water has come by jerks. This kind of inflammation sometimes is considerable, goes deep into the cellular membrane, and produces tumefaction without any other effect*. In other cases it goes on to suppuration, often becoming one of the causes of fistulæ in perinæo. I have sometimes, as I have already observed, suspected Cowper's glands to be the seat of such suppurations; for I have observed externally circumscribed swellings in the situation of those glands. The small glands likewise of the bulbous part of the urethra may be affected in a similar manner; and the irritation is often extended even to the bladder itself†.

When the bladder is affected it becomes more susceptible of every kind of irritation, so that very disagreeable symptoms are often produced: it will not allow of the usual distention, and therefore the patient cannot retain his water the ordinary time; and the moment the desire of making water takes place, he is obliged instantly to make it, with violent pain in the bladder, and still more in the glans penis, exactly similar to what happens in a fit of the stone. If the bladder be not allowed to discharge its contents immediately, the pain becomes almost intolerable; and even when the water is evacuated, there remains for some time a considerable pain both in the bladder and glans, because the very contraction of the muscular coat of the bladder becomes a cause of pain.

* Added: " There is often a pain in the urethra after making water, in the same part in which it is usually felt while the water passes; this I believe to be the effect of the contraction of the internal membranes, which lasts for some time after the action has ceased."—*Home.*

† Added: " This happens more commonly towards the going off of the gonorrhœa." —*Home.*

The ureters, and even the kidneys, sometimes sympathise, when the bladder is either very much inflamed, or under a considerable degree of irritation; however, this but rarely happens. I have even reason to suspect that the irritation may be communicated to the peritonæum by means of the vas deferens. This suspicion receives some confirmation from the following history. A gentleman had a gonorrhœa, which was treated in the antiphlogistic way. The discharge being in some degree stopped, a tension came upon the lower part of the belly on the right side, just above Poupart's ligament, but rather nearer to the ilium. There was hardness and soreness to the touch, which soreness spread over the whole belly, producing rigors every third day, with a low pulse, which to me indicated a peritonæal inflammation, arising, in my opinion, from the vas deferens of that side being affected in its course through the belly and pelvis.

When the inflammation, or perhaps only the irritation, runs along the whole surface of the urethra, attacks the bladder, and even extends to the ureters and the kidneys, so as to cause a disagreeable sensation in all these parts, the disease is generally very violent, and I suspect is something of the erysipelatous kind; at least it shows an irritable sympathising habit.

This disease sometimes produces very uncommon symptoms. A gentleman had a gonorrhœa; and when the inflammatory symptoms were abating, the urethra lost both the involuntary and voluntary powers of retaining the urine. His water came away involuntarily, nor could he stop it. I advised him to do nothing, and to wait for some time, as probably the method of cure might be more disagreeable than the disease itself, although it was very troublesome to him when in company. The complaint gradually lessened, and in time went entirely off.

§. 10. *Of the Swelled Testicle.*

A very common symptom attending a gonorrhœa is a swelling of the testicle. This I believe, like the affection of the bladder, and many of the symptoms mentioned before, is only sympathetical, and not to be reckoned venereal, because the same symptoms follow every kind of irritation on the urethra, whether produced by strictures, injections, or bougies. It may be observed here, that those symptoms are not similar to the actions arising from the application of the true venereal matter, whether by absorption or otherwise, for they seldom or never suppurate; and when suppuration happens, the matter produced is not venereal.

The testicles seem, as it were, in many cases, rather to be acting for the urethra than for themselves, which is an idea applicable to all sympathies. Thus the swelling and inflammation appear suddenly, and as suddenly disappear, or in a few minutes go from one testicle to the other; the affection depending upon the state of the urethra, and not at all upon the part itself. A part, however, of the testicle, the epididymis, assumes all the characters of inflammation, remaining swelled even for a considerable time after the inflammation has subsided.

The first appearance of swelling in the testicle is generally a soft pulpy fulness of the body of the testicle, which is tender to the touch; this increases to a hard swelling, accompanied with considerable pain. The hardest part is generally the epididymis, and principally that portion of it which is at the lower end of the testicle, as may be distinctly felt. The hardness and swelling, however, often run the whole length of that body, and form a knob at the upper part. The spermatic chord is likewise often affected, and more especially the vas deferens, which is thickened and sore to the touch. The veins of the testicle sometimes become varicose. I have seen such a state of veins accompany a swelling of the testicle in two instances. A pain in the small of the back generally attends inflammations of the testicle of all kinds, with a sense of weakness of the loins and pelvis. The bowels generally sympathise with most complaints of the testicle; in some by cholicy pains, in others by an uncommon sensation both in the stomach and intestines. Sickness is a common symptom, and even vomiting; the powers of digestion by this means are impaired, and a disposition for the accumulation of air takes place, which is often very troublesome. Here we have from the testicles a chain of sympathies, as we had in consequence of the irritation running along the whole urinary passages: first the testicle is affected from the urethra; then the spermatic chord, the loins, intestines, stomach; and from thence in some measure the whole body.

In a case of swelled testicle, I have known the buttocks swell; but the swelling was not of the inflammatory kind, and in making water pain was felt in that part. Whether this symptom arose from the swelling of the testicle, or from the same common cause, that is, the gonorrhœa, is not easily determined, although the latter supposition is the most probable.

It has been asserted, but without proof, that in cases of swelled testicles in consequence of a gonorrhœa, it is not the testicle that swells, but the epididymis. The truth is, it is both the one and the other. Any man that is accustomed to distinguish between a swelling of the whole testicle, and that of the epididymis only, will immediately be sensible that in the hernia humoralis the whole testicle is swelled. The testicle assumes the same shape that it does from other causes, where we know, from being obliged to remove it, that the whole has swelled. The pain is in every part of the testicle. I have seen such swellings suppurate on the fore part, and have known several instances of adhesions between the tunica albuginea and vaginalis, from such causes. This has only been discovered after death, or in the operation for a partial hydrocele. Such changes could not have taken place if the body of the testicle had not been in a state of inflammation. This inflammation of the testicle most probably arises from its sympathising with the urethra, and in many cases it would appear to arise from what is understood by a translation of the irritation from the urethra to the testicle. Thus a swelling of the testicle coming on shall remove the pain in making water, and suspend the discharge, which shall not return till the swelling of the testicle begin to subside; or the irritation in the urethra first ceasing shall produce a swelling of the testicle, which shall continue till the pain and discharge return, thus rendering it doubtful which is the cause and which the effect. I have nevertheless known cases where the testicle has swelled and yet the discharge has become more violent; nay, I have seen instances where a swelling has come on after the discharge has ceased, yet the discharge has returned with violence, and remained as long as the swelling of the testicle. Sometimes the epididymis only is affected, sometimes the vas deferens, and at other times only the spermatic chord, producing varicose veins. No reason can be assigned why one of these parts is affected more than another, and indeed the immediate cause in all is as yet unknown; for although an action in the urethra is the remote cause, yet it is still impossible to say whether it be the cessation of that action that is the cause of the swelling in the testicle, or the swelling in the testicle the cause of the cessation. It is described as arising from an irritation taking place in the mouths of the vasa deferentia. Were this the cause, it ought in general to affect both testicles at the same time: but I have seen this complaint happen as often where the inflammation has gone no further back in the urethra than about an inch and a half or two inches, as where it has extended further; and the circumstance of the swelling shifting suddenly from one testicle to the other shows it to arise from some other principle in the animal œconomy.

A strangury often attends such cases of sympathy, and more frequently when the running stops, than when it is continued along with the swelling of the testicle. Indeed any sudden stoppage of the discharge gives a tendency to a strangury*.

* Added: " When the testicle is swelled, blood comes away with the semen; this may either be thrown out in the act of secretion, or come from the blood-vessels of the urethra in the act of emission."—*Home*.

As singular a circumstance as any respecting the swelling of the testicle is that it does not always come on when the inflammation in the urethra is at the height. I think it oftener happens when the irritation in the urethra is going off, and sometimes even after it has entirely ceased, and when the patient conceives himself to be quite well.

I may be allowed to remark, that swellings in the testicle in consequence of venereal irritation in the urethra subject it to a suspicion that every swelling of this part is venereal; but from what I have said of its nature when it arises from a venereal cause, which was, that it is owing to sympathy only, and from what I shall now say, that it is never affected with the venereal disease, either local or constitutional, as far as my observation goes, it is to be inferred that such suspicions are always ill founded. This, perhaps, is an inference to which few will subscribe[a].

I have known the gout produce a swelling in the testicle of the inflammatory kind, and therefore similar to the sympathetic swelling from a venereal cause, having many of its characters. Injuries done to the testicle produce swellings; but they are different from those above mentioned, being more permanent, having the disease or cause in the part itself. Cancers and the scrofula produce swellings of the testicle; but these are generally slow in their progress, and not at all similar to those arising from an irritation in the urethra.

§. 11. *Of the Swellings of the Glands from Sympathy.*

Since our knowledge of the manner in which substances get into the circulation, and our having learned that many substances, especially poisons, in their course to the circulation, irritate the absorbent glands to inflammation and tumefaction, we might naturally suppose such swellings, accompanying complaints in the urethra attended with a discharge, to be owing to the absorption of that matter, and therefore, if it be a venereal discharge, that they must also be venereal. But we must not be too hasty in drawing this conclusion, for we know that the glands will sometimes swell from an irritation at the origin of the lymphatics, where no absorption could possibly have taken place. They often swell and become painful upon the commencement of inflammation, before any suppuration has taken place, and subside upon the coming on of suppuration, because when the suppuration begins, the

---

[a] [This assertion is contradicted by experience. There is an affection of the testicle which occurs so often in combination with venereal symptoms that it must be allowed to be a constitutional effect of the virus. It will be described hereafter among the secondary symptoms of lues venerea.]

inflammation abates. I have known a prick in the finger with a clean sewing-needle produce a red streak all up the fore arm, pain along the inside of the biceps muscle, a swelling of the lymphatic gland above the inner condyle of the humerus, and also of the glands of the arm-pit, immediately followed by sickness and a rigor, all which, however, have soon gone off. As it should therefore appear that the absorbent system is capable of being affected as well by irritation as by the absorption of matter, in all diseases of this system arising from local injuries attended with matter, one must always have these two causes in view, and endeavour, if possible, to distinguish from which the present affection proceeds. For in those arising from an irritated surface in consequence of poison, especially the venereal, it is of considerable consequence to be able to say from which of the two it arises, since it sometimes happens, although but seldom, that the glands of the groin are affected in a common gonorrhœa with the appearance of beginning buboes, but which I suspect to be similar to the swelling of the testicle, that is, merely sympathetic. The pain they give is but very trifling, when compared to that of the true venereal swellings arising from the absorption of matter, and they seldom suppurate. However, there are swellings of these glands from actual absorption of matter in gonorrhœa, and which consequently are truly venereal ; and as it is possible to have such, they are always to be suspected. As they have sometimes arisen upon a cessation of the irritation in the urethra, similar to the swelling of the testicle, it has been supposed that the matter was driven, as it were, into them by unskilful treatment. From our acquaintance with the absorbing system we know that the matter can go that way ; but we also know that we have no method of driving it that way ; and if we had, there is no reason why more should not be formed in the urethra. This therefore does not account for the cessation of secretion of matter in that part.

It is difficult to say what is the nature of those sympathetic diseases. They are not venereal, for they subside by the common treatment of inflammation. without the use of mercury : and I have known an instance of a swelled testicle from a venereal gonorrhœa that suppurated, and was treated by my advice as a common suppuration, and healed without a grain of mercury being given. Neither can they be called truly inflammatory, having rarely any of the true characters of inflammation, such as thickening of the parts, symptomatic fever, or sizy blood, except in swellings of the testicle and glands. The swelling of the testicle has several peculiarities attending it ; it is often very quick in its increase, and not being of the true inflammatory disposition, it requires less time for the removal of the inflammation ; but even where it ap-

pears to have more of the true inflammatory action, we find that the removal of the inflammation and tumefaction takes place more rapidly than
when proceeding from other causes. A swelled testicle in consequence
of the radical cure of the hydrocele does not subside after inflammation
is gone, in as many weeks, as the swelled testicle in consequence of its
sympathy with other parts, does in days; and probably the reason of
this is, that it arises from sympathy, for an inflammation arising from
real disease in a part, or from an external injury, as in the hydrocele,
must always last either till the disease be removed, or the injury repaired;
but that from sympathy will vary as the cause varies, which may happen very quickly, for we find a testicle swell in a few minutes, and in as
little time subside; and also the swelling move suddenly from one testicle to the other. These sympathies are often peculiar to constitutions,
and even to temporary constitutions, in so much as to be in some degree epidemic, for there is often such an influence in the atmosphere as
predisposes the body to this kind of irritation, and bodies so predisposed
require only the immediate cause to produce the effect.

§. 12. *Of the Diseases of the Lymphatics in a Gonorrhœa.*

Another symptom, which sometimes takes place in gonorrhœa, is a
hard chord leading from the prepuce along the back of the penis, and
often directing its course to one of the groins, and affecting the glands.
There is most commonly a swelling in the prepuce at the part where
the chord takes its rise. This happens sometimes when there is an excoriation and discharge from the prepuce or glans, which may be called
a venereal gonorrhœa of these parts. Both the swelling in the groin,
and the hard chord, we have reason to suppose arise from the absorption of pus, and therefore that they are the first steps towards a lues
venerea; but as that form of the disease seldom happens from a gonorrhœa, I shall not take any further notice of it in this place. However,
I may remark, that from this observation of the lues venerea being seldom produced from a gonorrhœa, it should appear that a whole surface,
or one only inflamed, does not readily admit of the absorption of the
venereal poison; and therefore, although the venereal matter lies for
many weeks in the passage, and over the whole glans, it seldom happens that any absorption takes place*. I have seen a case where blood

* Added: "As a further proof that these chords often arise from an inflammatory
excoriation and tumefaction of the prepuce, a gentleman had a chancre on the right
side, at the root of the prepuce, close to the penis, besides which there was an excoriation of the penis everywhere, with a thickening of that part. Although the chancre

has been discharged from the urethra, and the above-mentioned symptoms have come on. I at first suspected that the absorption had taken place where the vessel gave way; but as this symptom rarely happens, even where there has been a considerable discharge of blood, I am inclined to think that wounds are also bad absorbing surfaces, especially when I consider that few morbid poisons are absorbed from wounds.

§. 13. *Short recapitulation of the Varieties in the Symptoms.*

From what has been advanced above, it must appear that the variety of symptoms in a gonorrhœa, and the difference of them in different cases, are almost endless. I shall now recapitulate a few of the most material or common varieties. The discharge often appears without any pain, and the coming on of the pain is not at any stated time after the appearance of the discharge. There is often no pain at all, although the discharge be considerable in quantity, and of a bad appearance. The pain often goes off, while the discharge continues, and will sometimes return again. An itching in some cases is felt for a considerable time, which sometimes is succeeded by pain, though in many cases it continues to the end of the disease. On the other hand, the pain is often troublesome, and considerable even when the discharge is trifling, or none at all. In general, the inflammation in the urethra does not extend beyond an inch or two from the orifice; sometimes it runs all along the urethra to the bladder, and even to the kidneys; and in some cases spreads into the substance of the urethra, producing a chordee. The glands of the urethra inflame, and often suppurate; and I suspect that Cowper's glands sometimes do the same. The neighbouring parts sympathise, as the glands of the groin, the testicle, the loins, and pubes, with the upper parts of the thighs and abdominal muscles. Sometimes the disease appears soon after the application of the poison, as in a few hours, at other times not till after six weeks. It is often not possible to determine whether it is venereal, or only an accidental discharge arising from some unknown cause.

It may not be improper to mention here, that I have seen a chancre on the prepuce produce a pain in the urethra in making water, which most probably depended upon a sympathy similar to that by which the application of venereal matter to the glans produces a discharge from the urethra, as was observed above. If the application of venereal mat-

was on the right side, and the excoriation principally on the left, yet there was a hard chord along the left side of the penis, leading to an enlarged gland in the groin."— *Home.*

ter to the glans can produce a discharge from the urethra, it is possible that any acrid matter, though not venereal, may have a similar effect. The discharge from the vagina, in cases of what is called fluor albus, is sometimes extremely irritating, in so much as to excoriate the labia and thighs ; and the following history shows that it may sometimes produce effects similar to venereal matter.

Mr. and Mrs. —— have been married these twenty years and up-wards. She has for many years past been at times troubled with the fluor albus. When he has connexion with her at such times, it has ge-nerally, although not always, produced an excoriation of the glans and prepuce, and a considerable discharge from the urethra, attended with a slight pain. These symptoms commonly take a considerable time before they go off, whether treated as a gonorrhœa or as a weakness. Is this a new poison ? And does it go no further because the connexion takes place only between two? What would be the consequence if she were to have connexion with other men, and these with other women ? Such cases, as far as I have seen, have only been in form of a go-norrhœa. They have not produced sores in the parts ; nor, as far as I know, do they ever produce constitutional diseases.

CHAPTER II.

OF THE GONORRHŒA IN WOMEN.

THE venereal disease in the form of a gonorrhœa in women is not so complicated as in men ; the parts affected are more simple, and fewer in number. But it is not so easily known in them as it is in men, be-cause the parts commonly affected in women are very subject to a disease resembling the gonorrhœa, called *fluor albus* ; and the distinguishing marks, if there are any, have not yet been completely ascertained. A discharge simply from these parts in women is less a proof of the exist-ence of the venereal infection than even a discharge without pain in men ; therefore in general little or no attention is paid to it by the patient herself, and we often find the venereal virus formed in those parts without any increase of the natural discharge. The kind of mat-ter gives us no assistance in distinguishing the two diseases, for it often happens that the discharge in the fluor albus puts on all the appearances of the venereal matter; and an increase of the discharge is no better mark by which we can distinguish the one from the other. Pain, or any peculiarity in the sensations of the parts, is not a necessary attendant upon this complaint in women, therefore not to be looked for as a distinguishing symptom.

The appearance of the parts often gives us but little information, for I have frequently examined the parts of those who confessed all the symptoms, such as increase of discharge, pain in making water, soreness in walking, or when they were touched; yet I could see no difference between these and sound parts. I know of no other way of judging in cases where there are no symptoms sensible to the person herself, or where the patient has a mind to deny having any uncommon symptoms, but from the circumstances preceding the discharge, such as her having been connected with men supposed to be unsound, or her being able to give it to others, which last circumstance, being derived from the testimony of another person, is not always to be trusted to, for very obvious reasons. Thus a woman may have this species of the venereal disease without knowing it herself, or without the surgeon being able to discover it, even on inspection. It may appear very strange, that a disease which is so violent and well marked in men should be so obscure in women; but when we consider that this poison generally produces symptoms according to the nature of the parts affected by it, it becomes an easy matter to account in some measure for this difference.

When we attend to the manner in which this disease is contracted by women, it is evident that it must principally attack the vagina, a part that is not endowed with much sensation, or action of any kind. While it is confined to the vagina it may be compared to the same disease on the glans penis in men. In many cases, however, it extends much further, and becomes the cause of disagreeable feelings, producing a considerable soreness in all the parts formed for sensation, such as the inside of the labia, nymphæ, clitoris, carunculæ myrtiformes, the orifice of the meatus urinarius, and often affecting that canal in its whole length. Those parts are so sore in some cases as not to bear being touched; the person can hardly walk; the urine gives pain in its passage through the urethra, and when it washes the above-mentioned parts, which can hardly be avoided. Such symptoms are not much increased at one time more than another, excepting at the time of making water, and then principally in those who have the urethra affected, for as these parts are less exposed to circumstances of change, the increased irritation arising from such change of parts must necessarily in this sex be less. But in men the urethra, which is the part most commonly affected, has great sensibility, is capable of violent inflammation, is often distended with a stimulating fluid, and the body of the penis, urethra, and glans, stretching the passage with erections, always produce an increase of the symptoms, especially of the pain.

But as this disease frequently attacks parts more sensible than the vagina, and which are more susceptible of inflammation, as has been observed, under such circumstances women have nearly the same symptoms as men; a fulness about the parts, almost like an inflamed tonsil, a discharge from the urethra, violent pain in making water, and great uneasiness in sitting, from pressure on those parts.

The bladder sometimes sympathises, producing the same symptoms as in men, and it is probable that the irritation may be communicated even to the kidneys. It has been asserted that the ovaria are sometimes affected in a similar manner to the testicles in men. I have never seen a case of this kind, and I should very much doubt the possibility of its existence; for we have no instance, in other diseases, of the ovaria sympathising with those parts, or at least producing such symptoms as would enable us to determine that they did. That there do, however, uncommon symptoms now and then occur, should appear from the following case.

A lady had all the symptoms of a venereal gonorrhœa, such as a discharge, pain and frequency in making water, or rather a continued inclination to void it, and a heaviness approaching to pain about the hips and loins. The uncommon symptom in this case was great flatulency in the stomach and bowels; this last symptom was most probably a sympathy with the uterus. There may possibly be sympathies therefore with the ovaria.

The inflammation frequently goes deeper than the surface of the parts; often running along the ducts of the glands, and affecting the glands themselves, so as to produce hard swellings under the surface of the inside of the labia, which sometimes suppurate, forming small abscesses, opening near the orifice of the vagina. These are similar to the inflammations and suppurations of the glands in the urethra in men. The different surfaces or parts which the disease attacks, make no distinction in the disease itself. It is immaterial whether it is a large or small surface: in one case the parts are more susceptible of this irritation than in another; but the method of cure may be more complicated.

It sometimes happens that the venereal matter from the vagina runs down the perinæum to the anus, producing a gonorrhœa or chancres there.

How far the gonorrhœa in women is capable of wearing itself out, as in men, I cannot absolutely determine; but am much inclined to believe that it may, for I have known many women who have got rid of a violent gonorrhœa without having used any means to cure it; and indeed the great variety of methods of cure employed in such cases, all of which cannot possibly do good, though the patients get well, seems to confirm this opinion. One circumstance, which appears as curious as any, is the seeming continuance of the disease in the vagina for years; at least we have reason to believe this, as far as the testimony of patients can be relied on; and this long continuance of it, without wearing itself out as it does sometimes in men, is probably owing to its being less violent in the vagina*.

* A case is here added:

" The following account of a lady having all the symptoms of gonorrhœa immediately after connexion, shows how early in some cases the disease is produced; it was sent to me from Bath for my opinion upon it, drawn up by her medical attendant.

" A lady of a delicate habit of body, great sensibility of mind, and extreme irritability of the whole nervous system, in general had enjoyed good health until her present illness, which began in the following manner. The morning after her marriage she complained of great soreness and swelling of the pudenda, attended with a good deal of pain, and difficulty in making water; this was considered as the natural consequence of her connexion, and she continued her journey in a post-chaise, though in much pain, the whole day. The following morning her complaints were much increased, and a considerable discharge came on from the parts. In this situation she came to Bath a few days after, when I was desired to see her. I found her in an agony of distress, her husband having informed her, that, from circumstances attending himself, he was apprehensive her complaints might prove venereal. Upon questioning him, I found that for some months he had had a running from the urethra attended with heat of urine; that he had been under the care of a surgeon in the country, who had assured him his disease was not venereal; that, confiding in this assurance, he had married, not doubting that he was perfectly well, except a trifling gleet which remained still: he further stated, that in having connexion with his wife, from the natural tightness of the parts he had not been able to penetrate; that in the attempt she complained of much pain, and some blood was discharged: upon examining his shirt, some discharge was observed upon it, and he still was troubled with heat of urine. I was at first inclined to hope that (as women are not so easily infected with the venereal poison as men) all these complaints might be the consequences of a first connexion, followed by a long and rapid journey in a post-chaise; I therefore ordered an opening mixture, and desired the parts might be fomented with a decoction of poppy-heads in milk and water, and a soft poultice of bread and milk applied. Finding no advantage from the use of these means, I examined the state of the parts affected, and found there was a considerable discharge of matter, principally from the urethra, the orifice of which was much swelled and inflamed, as well as the ducts of the glands on each side the urethra: there did not appear to be any discharge from the vagina; the hymen still appeared unbroken, and very firm and fleshy; the lacunæ from Cowper's glands on each side were very much inflamed; and there was a hard tumour on one side of the hymen, which afterwards suppurated. There was no appearance of disease anywhere about the labia or nymphæ. It was treated as venereal, and she went through a course of mercury, which was persisted in for some time: the abscess above mentioned burst; her mouth grew a little tender; her complaints were so much mended, that there was no doubt of a speedy and happy termination of her disorder, when she was seized with a most violent diar-

§. 1. *Of the Proofs of a Woman having this Disease.*

It may be asked, what proof there is of a woman having a gonorrhœa when she is not sensible of having any one symptom of the disease,
and none appears to the surgeon on examination. In such a case, the
only thing we can depend upon is the testimony of those whom we look
upon as men of veracity. Such men have asserted that they have been
affected by a woman in the situation above described, having had no
connexion for some months with any other woman. From this evidence
it is reasonable to suppose that the disease has been caught from such
women; and it should seem to put it beyond a doubt when the same

rhœa, which was with the utmost difficulty restrained. Mercurials of every kind were
then left off; the former symptoms grew more troublesome; the heat of urine increased,
and extended to the bladder, as appeared by the continuance of the pain for an hour or
two after she had made water. She was now desired to rub about a drachm of mercurial ointment upon the thighs, labia, and inside of the pudenda. About this time
another abscess formed, in nearly the same situation with the former, which was opened
with a lancet; this gave her much relief; the heat of urine went off in a great measure,
but the discharge from the urethra still continued as much as before: she continued
the mercurial frictions with great freedom during the healing of the abscess, insomuch
that her mouth was greatly affected; she then left off the ointment for a little time, and
soon after, the orifice of the urethra swelled and inflamed very much, the discharge
greatly increased in quantity, and there was likewise a discharge of matter from the
vagina; an injection of crude mercury rubbed down with mucilage of gum arabic till
it was extinguished, and mixed with water, was ordered to be used twice or thrice a
day; she had all along taken the almond emulsion with gum arabic for her constant
drink, and this was continued in large quantities; she also again resumed the use of
the ointment as before, by which her mouth was at times made exceedingly sore.
" The disease had now continued nearly five months; the catamenia regularly appeared ever since her first complaint; at the last return of them she was free from pain,
and the discharge as little as it had been at any time during her illness, and she continued free from uneasiness during that period, but soon after its cessation the heat of
urine again returned in a most violent degree, and continued for an hour or two, with
unabating violence; the orifice of the urethra again swelled as much as before. The
discharge from the vagina at present is much the same, to which is superadded a shooting pain in almost every direction of that passage and the parts adjacent, which frequently recurs during the day. I can feel no swelling of any other part within the
reach of my finger; nor does the pressure give pain in any direction. Being now fully
persuaded that the venereal virus must be fully subdued, all mercurials are left off, and
she uses only an injection of opium and thin starch, keeping the bowels open with a
little castor oil now and then. Every fresh return of the ardor urinæ has been accompanied with a train of most distressing nervous symptoms, hysterics, and extreme de-
jection of spirits, and the pain is generally most violent in the night, though she drinks
an astonishing quantity of diluting liquors with gum arabic, pulvis tragacanth., comp.,
&c., and has frequently taken opiates, from which she has certainly received relief; but
as they always increase her nervous symptoms, she is greatly overcome by their use."
—Home.

woman gives the disease in this way to more than one man. The case of the woman giving the disease to two men alternately at an interval of twelve months each time*, which gives a space of at least two years for the continuance of the disease, proves that its communication is almost the only criterion of its presence. The case too of the young woman at the Magdalen Hospital† confirms the same opinion. Yet all this does not amount to an absolute proof; for a sound woman may have had a connexion with a man who had a gonorrhœa, or a man with chancres, and soon after, that is perhaps within forty-eight hours, she may have admitted the embraces of a sound man. In such a case it is very possible that he may receive the infection from that matter which was lodged in the vagina by the unsound man, and yet the woman may not catch the disease, for the matter may be washed away before it irritates the vagina; and this woman may be suspected of having a gonorrhœa, and apparently with great justice. A repetition of these circumstances may be the cause of many women appearing to have the disease for years, without really having it. Again, I have seen a bubo come on at a time when the patient was not sensible of any disorder till that appeared. This, one would think, is an absolute proof that there may be a gonorrhœa, and the patient not be conscious of it. But even this is not altogether without fallacy; for there may have been an absorption of venereal matter deposited in the vagina by some infected man, which may not have produced any irritation in that part‡.

CHAPTER III.

OF THE EFFECTS OF THE GONORRHŒA ON THE CONSTITUTION IN BOTH SEXES.

THE disease I have been describing, both in men and women, is local, and generally confined to the part affected; yet it sometimes happens that the whole constitution is more or less affected by it. Thus we find, before there is any appearance of matter from the parts, that some patients complain of slight rigors: these are most considerable when the

---

* See p. 165.   † See p. 166.
‡ The last three sentences omitted.—*Home.*

suppuration is late in taking place. A remarkable instance of this happened in a gentleman who had the infection twice* The first time he assured me that it was six weeks between the time it was possible for him to have contracted the disease, and its appearance; and that for a considerable part of that time he had often been indisposed with slight rigors, attended with a little fever and restlessness, for which he could assign no cause, nor was he relieved by the usual remedies prescribed in such cases. A violent gonorrhœa came on, and these symptoms went off, which appeared to me to explain the case. The second time it was a month from the time of infection before the gonorrhœa appeared, and for some weeks of that time he was subject to a similar indisposition, which went off as before when the running came on. Here it would appear that we have something of a suppurative fever, which perhaps often happens in this disease; but the inflammation being small, and the fever therefore inconsiderable, it is commonly little noticed by the patient. The above gentleman, not suspecting any such complaint in the first attack, had connexion with his wife as usual, and was afraid, when the disease appeared, that he might have given it to her; but she never complained, which is a strong circumstance in confirmation of the principle laid down above, that it cannot be communicated but by matter.

These constitutional sympathies from local specific diseases are the same, from whatever cause they proceed: they are the sympathetic effects of irritation or of violence. And it is probable that all remote sympathies are, at least in this respect, similar; for if they were similar to their cause, it is most probable that they would produce in the constitution the same kind of disease that gave rise to them.

CHAPTER IV.

OF THE CURE OF THE GONORRHŒA.

FROM the idea which I have endeavoured to give of the venereal disease in general, namely, that, in whatever form it appears, it always arises from the same cause, it might be supposed that, since we have a spe-

---

* The case is mentioned before, p. 165.

cific for some of the forms of the disease, this specific should be a certain cure for every one; and therefore that it must be no difficult task
to cure the disease when in the form of inflammation and suppuration
upon the secreting surfaces of any of the ducts or outlets of the body.
But from experience we find the gonorrhœa the most variable in its symptoms while under a cure, and the most uncertain with respect to its
cure, of any of the forms of this disease; many cases terminating in a
week, while others continue for months, under the same treatment.

The only curative object is, to destroy the disposition and specific
mode of action in the solids of the parts; and as that is changed, the
poisonous quality of the matter produced will also be destroyed. This
effects the cure of the disease, but not always of the consequences.

I have already observed that this form of the disease is not capable
of being continued beyond a certain time in any constitution; and that
in cases where it is violent, or lasts long, it is owing to the parts being
very susceptible of such irritation, and readily retaining it. As we have
no specific medicine for the gonorrhœa, it is fortunate that time alone
will effect a cure: it is therefore very reasonable to suppose that every
such inflammation ceases of itself: yet although this appears to be nearly
the truth, it is worthy of consideration whether medicine can be of any
service in this form of the disease. I am inclined to believe it is very
seldom of any kind of use, perhaps not once in ten cases: but even this
would be of some consequence, if we could distinguish the cases where
it is of service from those where it is not. Upon the idea that every
gonorrhœa cures itself, I gave certain patients pills of bread, which were
taken with great regularity. The patients always got well; but some
of them, I believe, not so soon as they would have done, had the artificial methods of cure been employed.

The methods of cure hitherto recommended, and still followed by different people of the profession, are of two kinds. They consist either
of internal remedies or local applications. But in whichsoever of these
two ways this disease is to be treated, we are always to pay more attention to the nature of the constitution, or to any attending disease in the
parts themselves, or parts connected with them, than to the disease itself.

The nature of the constitution is principally to be learned from the
local effects; for the local effects of this poison are so different in different people as to require great variety of treatment; but this has been
too little attended to, every one endeavouring to attack the immediate
symptoms, as if he had a specific for a gonorrhœa.

The first thing to be considered is the nature of the inflammation,
whether violent or mild, whether common or irritable. Yet even when

this is ascertained, we have not in all cases the cure in our power; for
I have already observed that some people are very susceptible of this
irritation, who are, as it were, insensible to others; and, on the contrary, many are easily affected by common inflammation, who are insensible to this. These last are rather uncommon dispositions, and the
cure being always easy they demand little attention. When the symptoms are violent, but of the common inflammatory kind, which is to
be collected from the attending circumstances, particularly the extent
of the inflammation not exceeding the specific distance, the local mode
of cure may be either irritating or soothing. Irritating applications in
the present case may be attended with less danger than in the irritable
inflammation*, and may alter the specific action; but to produce this
effect it must be greater than the irritation from the original injury.
The parts will afterwards recover of themselves, as from any other common inflammation. After all, however, I believe the soothing plan is
the best at the beginning. If the inflammation be great, and of the irritable kind, no violence is to be used in the cure (for it will only increase
the symptoms), unless we know that the great degree of inflammation
arises entirely from a susceptibility of this irritation, and that there is
no general irritability in the constitution, which seldom can be ascertained. In cases where the symptoms run high, nothing should be done
that may tend to stop the discharge, either by internal or external means;
for nothing would be gained thereby, as we may stop the discharge, and
not put an end to the inflammation. The constitution is to be altered,
if possible, by remedies adapted to each disposition, with a view to alter
the actions of the parts arising from such dispositions, and reduce the
disease to its simple form. If the constitution cannot be altered, nothing
is to be done but to allow the action to wear itself out.

When the inflammation has considerably abated, and the disease only
remains in a mild form, its cure may be attempted either by internal remedies or local applications. If a local cure be attempted, violence is
still to be avoided, because it may bring back the irritation. At this
period gentle astringents may be applied with a prospect of success; or,
if the disease has begun mildly, and there are no signs of an inflamma-

* It is very difficult to give clear ideas of distinctions in disease, when they are not
marked by something permanent as to time, space, &c. I have used the term "irritable inflammation," because I think this kind of inflammation takes place more in weak
irritable habits than in others: it appears to be guided by no law that I am acquainted
with. It may be called an ill-formed inflammation, as not going through the usual
process to a natural termination, but continuing with little variation; and if such inflammation were to take place in the cellular membrane, it would rather produce an
œdematous swelling than such as arises from the extravasation of coagulable lymph,
which takes place in what I would call the true inflammation.

tory disposition either of the common kind or the irritable, in order to get rid of the specific mode of action quickly, an irritating injection may be used, which will increase the symptoms for a time, but when it is left off they will often abate or wholly disappear. In such a state of parts, astringents may be used; for the only thing to be done is to procure a cessation of the discharge, which is now the principal symptom.*

In those cases where the itching, pain, and other uncommon sensations are felt for some time before the discharge appears, I should be inclined to recommend the quieting or soothing plan instead of the irritating, with a view to bring on the discharge, as that effect is a step towards a resolution of the irritation; but how far it would really be the proper plan I cannot absolutely say, not having had experience enough in such cases. One thing, however, I think I may assert from reasoning, that to use astringents would be bad practice, as they would rather tend to prevent the discharge from taking place, which might prolong the inflammation and protract the cure. In cases of stricture, or in cases of diseased testicles, I believe, astringents should not be used; for we find in either case, while the discharge lasts, both complaints are relieved; therefore in such cases we should proceed with more caution than when all the parts are otherwise sound. If we had a specific for venereal gonorrhœa, it would still be a question whether this specific could cure the irritation before the full action had taken place.

§. 1. *Of the different Modes of Practice.—Evacuants,— Astringents.*

The internal remedies commonly recommended in a gonorrhœa may be divided into evacuants and astringents. The evacuants are principally of the purgative or diuretic kind, and these not confined to any particular medicines; for every practitioner supposes that he is in possession of the best. Some use mercurial evacuants, while others carefully avoid mercury in every form. The neutral salts have been given, from the idea of their being cooling. Some of the profession have kept principally to diuretics, perhaps with two views, as evacuants acting upon the urinary passages mechanically, to wash off the venereal matter, or as specifics for the latter purpose : nitre has been given with this view; besides, it has been supposed to lessen inflammation; but its

---

* Added: " It is very common when the discharge is stopped by an injection, even of a mild kind, to have an uneasy sensation in the perinæum, and continued on to the bladder, producing frequency in making water, and on the return of the discharge these sensations immediately cease."—*Home.*

virtues in this way I very much doubt. Under these different modes
of treatment the patients always get well, and the cures are ascribed by
each practitioner to his own method of treatment.

To keep the body open in most cases, even when the patient is in
other respects in health, must no doubt be proper; but what idea can
we form of an irritation, produced all along the intestinal canal, curing
a specific inflammation in the urethra? Yet there are cases where a
brisk purge has been of service, and even in some has performed a cure.
But I suspect that in such cases the disease has been continued by habit
only, and that this practice would not have succeeded in the beginning.
A gentleman had a gonorrhœa, all the symptoms of which continued for
two months, and by taking at once ten grains of calomel, which purged
him most violently, he was almost immediately cured. The calomel
could not have acted specifically, but by a kind of derivation : that is,
an irritation produced in one part cured one that subsisted in another.
But, even if it should be granted that in some constitutions purges have
the power of making the solids less susceptible of this irritation, it cannot be supposed they will have this effect in every case ; in some constitutions they might debilitate, increase irritability, and of course increase the symptoms. These contrary effects must take place in different constitutions in which a medicine has no specific action. On the
supposition of the cure being promoted by an evacuation from the blood,
what service can purging out some of the blood in form of a secretion
from one part do to an inflammation of another part? On such a supposition, would not a sweat, or an increase of saliva by chewing tobacco,
or stimulating the nose by snuff, all tend equally to cure a gonorrhœa?
But humours having been considered as the universal cause of every
disease, especially those in which pus is formed or a discharge produced,
and purging having been supposed to be the cure for humours, purgatives were of course made use of in this disease : and as the patients have
always been cured, the practice became generally established.

Those who recommended mercury in this form of the disease, did it
most probably from the opinion that this medicine was a specific for the
venereal disease in all its forms. On this supposition, we can see some
reason for their practice, as it would be absorbed from the intestines,
circulate through the inflamed vessels of the urethra, and thereby destroy the venereal irritation. Here we can only suppose it to act by its
specific virtue; but I doubt very much of mercury having any specific
virtue in this species of the disease, for I find that it is as soon cured
without mercury as with it ; and where this medicine is only used as a
purge, or purged off the next day, and therefore allowed to act merely.
upon the bowels, I cannot conceive that it could have any more effect

upon the venereal inflammation in the urethra than an irritation in the
bowels arising from any other purgative. So little effect indeed has this
medicine upon a gonorrhœa, that I have known a gonorrhœa take place
while under a course of mercury sufficient for the cure of a chancre.
Whether the gonorrhœa arose from the same infection that produced
the chancre I cannot say; nor can it be easily determined in such cases.
Men have also been known to contract a gonorrhœa when loaded with
mercury for the cure of a lues venerea; the gonorrhœa, nevertheless,
has been as difficult of cure as in ordinary cases.

A gentleman committed himself to my care, on the 27th of June, for
the cure of two chancres and a bubo. I dispersed the bubo; but as he
disliked the unction, I was obliged to substitute mercurius calcinatus
daily instead of it, giving two grains in the evening and one in the morning. About the middle of July his mouth became sore, and the mercury was left off; we began its use again in a week, and he appeared
to be quite well of his venereal complaints. I, however, continued the
use of mercury, keeping his mouth sore; and on the 16th of August,
while in this state, he had a connexion with a woman, both on that and
the following evening, and in five days after a gonorrhœa appeared, and
proved to be very violent.*

The same general observations may be made with regard to the effects
of diuretics, considered as evacuants.

It is possible that specific medicines taken into the constitution (if
we had such), and passing off by urine, might act upon the urethra in
their passage through it. The balsams and turpentines pass off in this
way, and become specifics for many irritations in the urinary passages;
but how far medicines which have the power of affecting particular parts
when sound, or when under diseases peculiar to those parts, have also
the powers of affecting a specific irritation in these parts, I know not;
but do not believe they have any considerable powers in this way. It
is possible, however, that they may remove any attending irritation,
although not the specific one. Diuretics have, nevertheless, their advantages, for if they produce a greater quantity of water they do good;
but I believe this had better be effected by simple water, or water joined
with such things as will encourage the patient to drink a good deal, as
tea, syrup of capillaire, orgeate, and the like.

Astringents, although often given, yet have always been condemned
by those who have called themselves the judicious and regular practitioners; because, according to them, there is something to be carried

---

* Added: " Another gentleman, while under a course of mercury for the cure of
chancres, had connexion with a woman before he left off the use of mercury, and in
two days a gonorrhœa made its appearance."—*Home.*

off, and if that is not carried off a lues venerea is to be the consequence.
This reasoning is not just; and therefore the question to be considered
is, do they or do they not assist us in the cure of the gonorrhœa? I
believe they do not, in any case, lessen the venereal inflammation; but
certainly they often lessen the discharge. As that effect, however, does
not constitute a cure, it is not necessary to produce it.

I can conceive that a combination of astringents, especially the specific astringents of those parts, as the balsams, with any other medicine
which may be thought to be of service, may help to lessen the discharge
in proportion as the inflammation abates; and this I have often seen, as
will be explained more at length hereafter.

§.2. Of local Applications—different kinds of Injections: irritating, sedative, emollient, astringent.

Local applications may be either internal to the urethra, external to
the penis, or both; all of which will in many cases be necessary. The
internal, applied to the urethra, should seem the most likely to cure this
species of disease, by coming immediately in contact with the diseased
parts; for if they have any power of action, whatever that be, it must
be in opposition to the venereal irritation. Therefore we might suppose that most irritations that are not venereal would tend to a cure;
but certainly this is not universally the case. If, on the contrary, the
applications are such as quiet irritation, they must also be of service.

Local applications to the urethra may be either in a solid or fluid
form, each of which has its advantages and disadvantages. A fluid is
only a temporary application, and that of very short duration, and is
similar to the washing of a sore, which is, I believe, in most cases unnecessary; for I imagine that matter from any sore whatever is always
such as cannot stimulate that sore into any action. It can be of no
consequence, therefore, whether the matter is allowed to lie upon it or
not; but it being removed, the medicines are allowed to come in contact with the inflamed surface. I apprehend it is only in this way
that the removal of it can be of service. The solid applications may
remain a long time, and are similar to the dressings in the case of a
wound. When the parts are not so much inflamed as to prevent the
use of them, they would appear to have an advantage over the fluid applications by continuance; but they in general irritate immediately, in consequence of their solidity alone. These applications must be in the form
of a bougie; but I should be inclined to suppose that the less use that
is made of bougies, when these parts are in an inflamed state, the bet-

ter, although I cannot say that I ever saw any bad effects from them in any case, when applied with caution.

Fluid applications to the inside of the urethra are commonly called injections, and, like the internal remedies, are without number; every practitioner thinking, or wishing to make the world think, that his own is the best. But, as every venereal inflammation is frequently removed under the use of injections of various kinds (which was observed with respect to internal medicines), have we not here a strong corroborating circumstance in favour of an opinion, that every such complaint will in time cure itself? I think, however, it appears from practice, that an injection will often have almost an immediate effect upon the symptoms, and that, therefore, they must have some powers; and yet the kind of injection which would have the greatest specific powers I believe is not yet known: if an injection has no specific powers, it must be very uncertain in its effects, and can only be of service as far as it may be adapted to a peculiarity of constitution or parts. As injections are only temporary applications, it becomes necessary to use them often, especially in cases where they are found to be of service; they should therefore be applied as often as convenient, perhaps every hour, or even oftener; but this must be regulated in some measure by the kind of injection, for if it be irritating it will not be proper to use it so often, as it may be productive of bad consequences.

Many injections immediately, or at least soon after the application, remove the symptoms, and prevent the formation of matter, which has given rise to the notion of their shutting up the disease, and driving it into the constitution; but this supposed mode of producing a constitutional complaint is the reverse of what really happens, for I have already endeavoured to prove that matter is the only substance in which the poison is contained, and that the formation of the poison is inseparable from the formation of matter; therefore if we can prevent the one, the other cannot take place, and of course there can be no room for absorption; so that there can neither be any power of infecting the constitution in the same person, nor of communicating the infection to others.[*]

When the discharge is an effect of present inflammation it may be stopped by injections, though the inflammation still continue in some degree, and may afterwards be removed without the discharge ever reappearing. But I believe that by this practice little is gained, for the effect of the inflammation is not the disease which we wish to remove. However, we find that the same method which stops the discharge also removes the inflammation, although not always, and only I believe when the inflammation is slight.

---

[*] Vide, p. 140, what was said of the method of contracting the lues venerea.

I shall divide injections, according to their particular effects upon the urethra, into four kinds,—the irritating, sedative, emollient, and astringent. The specific, I believe, is not yet discovered, although a mercurial injection, in some form or other, is by most people supposed to be possessed of such a power, and of course this mineral makes part of many of the injections now in use.

Irritating injections, of whatever kind, I suspect in this disease act upon the same principle; that is, by producing an irritation of another kind, which ought to be greater than the venereal, by which means the venereal is destroyed and lost, and the disease is cured, although the pain and discharge may still be kept up by the injection. Those effects, however, will soon go off when the injection is laid inside, because they arise only from its irritating qualities. In this way bougies, as well as many injections, may be supposed to form a cure; and although they increase the symptoms for the time, they never can increase the disease itself, any more than the same injection which would produce the same symptoms, if applied to the urethra of a sound man, can communicate the disease. Most of the irritating injections have an astringent effect, and prove simply astringents when mild, their irritating quality depending chiefly upon their strength.

As irritating injections do not agree with all inflammations arising from the venereal poison*, it may be asked, In what cases are the irritating injections to be used with advantage? This I have not been able to determine absolutely; but I think irritating injections should never be used where there is already much inflammation, especially in constitutions which cannot bear a great deal of irritation, as a previous knowledge of the disease in the same person sometimes teaches us; nor should they be used where the irritation has spread beyond the specific distance; nor where the testicles are tender; nor where, upon the discharge ceasing quickly, they have become sore; nor where the perinæum is very susceptible of inflammation, and especially if it formerly has suppurated; nor where there is a tendency in the bladder to irritation, which is known from the patient having had for some time a frequency in making water. In such cases I have not succeeded with them; they not only do no good, but they often do harm, for I have seen them make the inflammation spread further in the urethra†; and I think I have had reason to suspect that they have been the cause of abscesses in perinæo. But in cases that are mild, and in constitutions that are not irritable, injections often succeed, and remove the disease

* For I have already remarked, that the inflammation varies according to the constitution.

† It is, however, to be remarked, that this symptom is not always to be attributed to the injection, for it often happens when none has been used.

almost immediately. The practice, however, ought to be attempted with caution, and not, perhaps, till milder methods have failed. Two grains of corrosive sublimate, dissolved in eight ounces of distilled water, are nearly as good an injection as any of the kind. But an injection of only half this strength may be used where it is not intended to attempt a cure so quickly. If, however, the injection, even in that proportion, gives considerable pain in its application, or if it occasions a great increase of pain in making water, it should be diluted.

Sedative injections will always be of service in cases where the inflammation is considerable, not by lessening the disease itself, but by lessening the diseased action, which always allows the natural actions of the part more readily to take place. They are likewise very useful in relieving the painful feelings of the patient. Perhaps the best sedative we have is opium, as well when given by the mouth or anus, as when applied to the part affected in the form of an injection. But even opium will not agree, or act as a sedative, in all constitutions or parts. On the contrary, it has often opposite effects, producing great irritability. Lead may be reckoned a sedative, so far as it abates inflammation, while at the same time it may act as a gentle astringent. Fourteen grains of saccharum saturni, in eight ounces of distilled water, make a good sedative astringent injection.

The drinking freely of diluting liquors may, perhaps, be considered as having a sedative effect, as it in part removes some of the causes of irritation, rendering the urine less stimulating, either to the bladder, when the irritation is there, or to the urethra in its passage through it; and it is possible that diluting may lessen the susceptibility of irritation. The vegetable mucilages of certain seeds and plants, and the emollient gums, are recommended; but I suspect that this practice is founded on a mechanical notion, and that none of them are of much service. I believe the advantage arises chiefly from the quantity of water that is drunk, and that if the water be joined with anything, spirits excepted, that can induce the patient to drink freely, the purpose is fully answered. I have, however, been informed by some patients, that they have thought that when the liquids they drank have been impregnated with mucilaginous substances, they have had less uneasiness in making water.

Emollient injections are the properest applications where the inflammation is very great. They are most probably useful by first simply washing away the matter, and then leaving a soft application to the part, in which way I can conceive them to be of singular service, by lessening the irritating effects of the urine. Indeed practice proves this, for we often find that a solution of gum arabic, milk and water, or sweet oil, will lessen the pain and other symptoms, when the more active injections have done nothing, or have seemed to have done harm.

It very often happens that the irritation is so great at the orifice of the urethra that the point of the syringe cannot be suffered to enter. When this is the case, nothing should be done in the way of injection till the inflammation abate. Emollients may likewise be used externally, in form of fomentation.

The astringent injections can only act by lessening the discharge. They can have no specific effect upon the inflammation; but, as they must affect the actions of the living powers, it is possible they may alter the venereal disposition. They should only be used towards the latter end of the disease, when it has become mild, and the parts begin to itch. But this should be according to circumstances, and, if the disease begins mildly, they may be used at the very beginning, for by gradually lessening the discharge, without increasing the inflammation, we complete the cure, and prevent a continuation of the discharge called a gleet. Injections of this kind very probably stimulate in such a way as to make the vessels of the part contract, and probably hinder the act of secretion. We can hardly suppose that they act chemically by coagulating the juices. They will have an irritating quality if used strong, which in some measure destroys their astringency, or rather makes the parts act contrary to what they would do from the application of a simple astringent. Thus, they often increase the discharge instead of lessening it; by which means the disease also may be cured, in the same way as by irritating injections, that is, by altering the disposition of the inflammation. When more mild they often stop the discharge, without, however, in all cases, hastening the cure; for the inflammation may still continue even longer than it otherwise would have done if the tendency to secretion had not been stopped. I have already observed, that a surface that discharges has assumed the complete action of the disease, which is one step towards a cure or termination. However, it sometimes happens that an astringent injection will cure a slight irritation in a very few days. My experience has not taught me that one astringent is much better than another.

The astringent gums, as dragon's blood, the balsams, and the turpentines, dissolved in water; the juices of many vegetables, as oak bark, Peruvian bark, tormentil root; and perhaps all the metallic salts, as green, blue, and white vitriols, the salts of mercury, and also alum, probably all act much in the same way, although we may assert that they do not always act equally well in every gonorrhœa, for on our changing the injection we sometimes succeed after several others have been tried in vain.

The external applications are generally poultices and fomentations, but they can be of little service, except when the external parts, such as the prepuce, glans, and orifice of the urethra, are in some degree inflamed; the last, indeed, is almost always more or less affected.

When the glands of the urethra are so much swelled so as to be felt externally, the application of mercurial ointment to the part may be proper; but most probably this will be of more service after the inflammation has subsided. Indeed, mercurial ointment is often applied to all the external surfaces of those parts when in a state of inflammation, with an emollient poultice over it. I am not perfectly satisfied of the utility of this practice.

CHAPTER V.

OF THE CURE OF GONORRHŒA IN WOMEN.

In women the cure of the gonorrhœa is nearly the same as in men; but the disease itself is milder, and the secondary symptoms less numerous in women. This arises from there not being so many parts to be affected, and from those parts not being either of so great extent, or so liable to inflammation. Hence the cure becomes more simple.

When the disease is in the vagina only it is easily cured. Injections are the best means that can be used, and, after the use of them, it may be proper to anoint the parts, as far up as possible, with mercurial ointment*, and also to wash the external parts often with the injection.

If the inflammation has attacked the urethra, injections there cannot be so conveniently used, as it is almost impossible for the patient to throw an injection into that canal.

The injections recommended in the cure of men are equally serviceable here; but they may be made doubly strong, as the parts of women are not nearly so irritable as the common seat of this disease in men.

If what I have said of the disease in women be just, we must see that it will be a difficult thing to say, with any degree of certainty, when the

---

* How far mercurial ointment assists in the cure I have not been able to determine; the use of it arises more from a kind of practical analogy than real experience in such cases.

patient is well, because, whenever the symptoms have ceased, the surgeon and the patient will naturally suppose the cure to be complete; but a new trial of those parts may prove the contrary, or in cases where the disease has never affected the urethra, but only the vagina, and still more where no symptoms have ever been observed, it will be more difficult to fix the date of the cure; but general experience must direct the practitioner.

When the inflammation runs along the ducts of the glands, whether those of the mouth of the vagina, or urethra, or affects the glands themselves, the same method is to be followed; in particular, the mercurial ointment is to be freely applied to the parts. If the inflammation on the mouths of the ducts is so great as to shut them up, the duct and glands will suppurate, and form abscesses; in such cases it will be necessary to open them, or enlarge the opening already formed, and dress the abscess as a chancre or bubo.

In the case of a simple running the constitutional treatment will be taken notice of hereafter; but if any suppuration follow, the constitution is to be treated as in chancres or buboes, for most probably absorption will take place, and its effects must be guarded against.

CHAPTER VI.

OF THE TREATMENT OF THE CONSTITUTION IN THE CURE OF THE GONORRHŒA.

In the cure of the gonorrhœa the constitution is in some cases to be as much attended to as the parts affected, if not more; but in general this is not necessary. The knowledge of the constitution is to be obtained in a great measure from the local symptoms, and as far as the constitutional treatment can be made similar to the local, they should correspond.

We find in many strong plethoric constitutions, where both the powers and actions are great, that the symptoms are violent. These constitutions have generally a strong tendency to fever of the inflammatory kind; and probably the most distinguishing mark of such a constitution is that of the symptoms not extending beyond the specific

distance. Many medicines which might be of service in another constitution will often prove hurtful here, in so much as to increase the very
symptoms which they were meant to relieve. I have seen even opiate
clysters, though they relieved at first, yet in the end produce or increase
fever, and by that means increase all the symptoms. I have seen the
balsam capivi, given in such cases, increase the inflammatory symptoms,
probably by stopping the discharge in part, which appears to be salutary. The treatment of such a constitution, when affected with this
disease, consists chiefly in evacuations, the best of which are bleeding
and gentle purging. To live sparingly, and above all to use little exercise, is necessary; for although such a treatment does not lessen the
venereal irritation, yet it lessens the violence of the inflammation, and
allows the parts to relieve themselves. In this kind of constitution,
therefore, the disease is in the end soonest cured, as there is not a tendency to a continued inflammation.

In the weak and irritable constitution the symptoms are frequently
very violent, arising from great action in the parts, and often extend
beyond the specific distance, the inflammation running along the urethra, and even affecting the bladder. Instead of evacuations, which
would rather aggravate the symptoms than relieve them, the constitution should be strengthened, and thus it will be less susceptible of irritation in general.

I have seen patients, whose constitutions were such that they were
never sure of twenty-four hours' health, where the inflammation has
been both considerable and extensive. I have seen evacuations tried,
and the symptoms increased; but as soon as the bark was given freely
they have become almost immediately mild, and without using any
other medicine the patients have soon recovered. The medicine here
acted upon the constitution, destroyed the irritability, gave the parts a
true and healthy sense of the venereal irritation, and brought the inflammation to that state in which it ought to be in a healthy subject,
whereby the constitution was enabled to cure itself.

So capricious sometimes is this form of the disease in its cure, that
the accession of an accidental fever has stopped the discharge, the pain
in making water has ceased, and the gonorrhœa has finally terminated
with the fever. In others I have seen all the symptoms of the gonorrhœa cease on the accession of a fever, and return when the fever has
been subdued. In some I have seen a gonorrhœa begin mildly, but a
severe fever coming on, and continuing for several days, has greatly increased the symptoms, and on the fever going off the gonorrhœa has
also gone off. Although a fever does not always cure a gonorrhœa, yet,
as it possibly may, nothing should be done while the fever lasts; and if

it continues after the fever is gone, it is then to be treated according to the symptoms.*

Unfortunately, there are cases where no known method lessens the symptoms; evacuations have produced no abatement; the strengthening plan has been as unsuccessful; sedatives and emollients have procured no relief; and time alone has performed the cure. In such cases the soothing plan, I believe, is the best, till we know more of the disease. Astringents should not be used, their action upon the inflamed parts being uncertain, for they often do not lessen the inflammation or the pain, although they may perhaps lessen the discharge. The turpentines, especially the balsam capivi and Canada balsam, lessen the disposition of the parts to form matter, which effect has always a salutary appearance; but as they have not at the same time the power of lessening the inflammation, they can be of little service.

Besides the various effects arising from the difference of constitution in the gonorrhœa, we find that it is considerably affected by the patient's way of life during the inflammatory state, and also by other diseases attacking the constitution at the same time. But this is common to all other diseases, for whenever we have a local disease (in which light I have considered a gonorrhœa) it is always affected by whatever affects the constitution. Most things that hurry, or increase the circulation, aggravate the symptoms, such as violent exercise, drinking too much of strong liquors, eating strong indigestible food, some kinds of which act specifically on these parts, thereby increasing the symptoms more than by simply heating the body, such as peppers, spices, and spirits.

From what has been said in general, it must appear that a gonorrhœa is to be cured in the same way as every other inflammation; and it must also appear that all the methods used are only to be considered as correctors of irritation in general, and of disordered circulation. In cases that have begun mildly, where the inflammation has been but slight, or in those cases where the violent symptoms above taken notice of have subsided, such medicines as have a tendency to lessen the discharge may be given, along with the local remedies before mentioned. The turpentines, I believe, are the most efficacious. Cantharides, the salts of some metals, such as of copper, zinc, and lead, and also some earths, as alum, are strongly recommended as astringents when given internally.

Whatever methods are used for the cure, locally or constitutionally,

---

* Added: "A gentleman, while using an injection for a gonorrhœa, was seized with a vomiting and purging, which brought on a fit of the piles; they bled profusely: as soon as he recovered from these attacks he found that all the symptoms of gonorrhœa had gone away."—*Home.*

it is always necessary to have in view the possibility of some of the matter being absorbed, and afterwards appearing in the form of a lues venerea, to prevent which I should be inclined to give small doses of mercury internally. At what time this mercurial course should begin is not easily ascertained; but if the observation be just, that a disposition once formed is not to be cured by mercury, but that mercury has the power of preventing a disposition from forming, as was formerly explained, we should begin early, and continue it to the end of the disease, till the formation of venereal matter ceases, and even for some time after. The mercurial ointment may be used where mercury disagrees with the stomach and intestines.

This practice appears to be more necessary if the discharge has continued a considerable time, and especially if the treatment has been simply by evacuants, for in the former case there is a greater time for absorption, and in the latter we may suppose a greater call for it, such medicines having no effect in carrying off the virus.

To prevent a lues venerea being produced from absorption, a grain of mercurius calcinatus taken every night, or one at night and another in the morning, may be sufficient; but should be continued in proportion to the duration of the disease.

The success of this practice in any particular case can never be ascertained, because it is impossible to say when matter has been absorbed, except in cases of buboes; and where it is not known to be absorbed, it is impossible to say that there would have been a lues venerea if mercury had not been given, as very few are infected from a gonorrhœa, although they have taken no mercury. It is, however, safest to give mercury, as we may reasonably suppose it will often prevent a lues venerea, as it does when given during the cure of a chancre or bubo, where we know, from experience, that without it the lues venerea would certainly take place.[a]

---

[a] [The principles which the author has laid down for the treatment of gonorrhœa, though generally correct, yet require some modification. In one or two instances he seems to have been misled by opinions, which are at the least very questionable.

It is pretty well established, that a course of mercury is neither necessary nor useful in a gonorrhœa: it has no peculiar influence on the course of the disorder, and it is an error to suppose that it is necessary for the sake of preventing secondary symptoms; and this is equally true, notwithstanding the occurrence of suppuration in the glands of the urethra, or in the groin, or of breach of surface from any other cause. At the same time mercury is not particularly hurtful, except it be given in such doses, and for such a length of time, as would materially depress the general tone, render the urine alkaline, or induce universal irritability of the system.

From the opinion, "that no matter of whatever kind can produce any effect on the part that forms it" (see p. 164), the author has been led to disregard altogether the

CHAPTER VII.

OF THE TREATMENT OF OCCASIONAL SYMPTOMS OF THE GONORRHŒA.

As the following symptoms are only occasional consequences of a venereal gonorrhœa, being the effects of an irritation on the urethra, and therefore not venereal, they are to be treated in the same manner as if they had arisen from any other cause.

---

discharge of gonorrhœa, and to conclude, that in no degree, and under no circumstances, is the inflammation increased by its stimulus, or relieved by arresting it. This doctrine, however, seems scarcely consistent with experience. It is difficult to understand the effects of astringents in the early periods of the disorder, except on the supposition, that by arresting the discharge they relieve the urethra from the stimulus of the virus, and thus take away the very cause of the inflammation. Again, the distinction between venereal gonorrhœas, and simple purulent discharges which are not derived from infection, is to be found less in the severity of the symptoms than in their obstinacy. The urethra is often attacked with inflammation as violent as that of a gonorrhœa, in cases where there has been no possibility of infection. The discharge may be as copious, and exactly similar both in colour and appearance. But in these cases the inflammatory symptoms will in a few days spontaneously subside, and the discharge will diminish with it; whereas the inflammation and discharge of a gonorrhœa, shall, under similar circumstances, continue for weeks, or even months, without any visible abatement. Whence this difference, unless that in simple cases the cause is temporary, and hence the inflammation which it has excited soon exhausts itself; in gonorrhœas a poison is generated, which acts as a perpetual stimulus, and constantly renews the excitement which originally gave rise to the disorder?

It does not appear that the plan on which a gonorrhœa should be treated differs from that which should be adopted in other inflammations of the urethra. But it must be remembered, that inflammation of mucous membranes generally, of Schneider's membrane for instance, or the inner membrane of the bladder, does not require, and is not benefited by much reduction; and that, if the constitution be rendered irritable from weakness, these inflammations often become aggravated and obstinate. This rule, which is generally applicable to mucous membranes, is more especially important in all inflammations of the bladder and urethra, perhaps because depletion tends to change the state of the urinary secretion, and to render it alkaline and irritating.

The duration and severity of a gonorrhœa depend much on the part of the urethra which is attacked by it. There is great variety in this respect. In most cases the inflammation is confined to the neighbourhood of the glans; but in many it involves also the membranous portion, as may be shown, not only by the symptoms during life, but also by dissections after death. If the disease is limited to the last three inches of the urethra, it is seldom very violent or tedious; if it extends to the bulb and parts adjacent, the symptoms are most obstinate and distressing. Except in very rare instances, the disease commences at the glans. If it affects the membranous portion, it is by the

§. 1. *Of the Bleeding from the Urethra.*

It has been already observed, that when the inflammation is violent, or spreads along the urethra, there is frequently a discharge of blood from the vessels of that part. In such bleeding, the balsam capivi,

---

progressive extension of the inflammation which gradually creeps up the urethra. This extension seldom occurs until the complaint has existed for a fortnight or longer, and, if the cure can be effected within that time, may almost certainly be avoided.

The true principles on which the treatment should be conducted will naturally follow from these considerations.

If the patient be seen on the first access of the disorder, when the discharge has only just appeared, and is small in quantity, before the orifice of the urethra has become turgid, and the passage has become sensible to the stimulus of the urine, the disease may often be entirely arrested by astringent injections, or by internal medicines, which have the property of acting as astringents on the urethra, such as the balsam of copaiba, or cubebs. But such a result can only be obtained when the inflammatory symptoms have scarcely commenced, and are in the slightest possible degree. After the expiration of twenty-four hours it is often too late, and generally so at the end of forty-eight hours. When active inflammation is present, the stoppage of the discharge can seldom be effected completely, and scarcely ever permanently. It may be greatly diminished; but this diminution rather aggravates than relieves the inflammation, as it lessens a secretion which has the effect of unloading the distended vessels, and the continuance of the inflammation will in a short time inevitably reproduce the discharge as profusely as before. It is to be observed, that it is necessary for the success of this plan that the discharge should be entirely stopped. If a single drop remains, it will go on to cause inflammation, and the disease will hold its ordinary course.

Should the malady be in such a state as to render this mode of treatment hopeless, it will be necessary to allow it to run its natural course. A period will arrive when the urethra will become accustomed to the virus, and the inflammation will then spontaneously subside. In the mean time the surgeon must endeavour to moderate its violence, by the removal of all stimulants which can be avoided. The chief stimulants are the urine and the discharge. The urine must be rendered mild, by neutralising its acidity, and by copious dilution; and the discharge must be moderated by astringent medicines, given in such doses as will only slightly check the increase of the secretion, without occasioning any immediate or sensible diminution in its quantity. Everything should be avoided which would determine to the parts affected. The diet should be light, and rather sparing, and no violent exercise should be taken; but there is no advantage in rigid abstinence or absolute rest, or in any restrictions which would interfere with the general health, or materially lower the general tone.

However, should the inflammation extend to the parts surrounding the urethra itself, or, as Mr. Hunter expresses it, beyond the specific distance, this rule will not always apply. If there is tenderness and swelling of the perinæum, or inflammation of the neck of the bladder, a horizontal posture and a careful regimen may be necessary. Yet even here it is better that blood should be abstracted locally and not generally, and that the diet should not be much reduced below the usual standard of health.

When the inflammatory symptoms have nearly subsided; when the ardor urinæ and chordee have disappeared, when the orifice of the urethra has lost its red and turgid aspect, and the discharge is less profuse and less purulent, astringents may again be given in full doses, and will generally complete the cure.]

given internally, has been of service; and it may be supposed that all the turpentines will be equally useful. I have not found any good effects from astringent injections, and in some cases have suspected that they have been the cause of this complaint. They always go off in the usual time of the cure of the gonorrhœa.

§. 2. *Of preventing Painful Erections.*

Opium, given internally, appears to have great effects in preventing painful erections in many cases. Twenty drops of tinctura thebaica, taken at bedtime, have procured ease for a whole night. The cicuta likewise seems to have some powers in this way.

§. 3. *Of the Treatment of the Chordee.*

In the beginning of this complaint bleeding from the arm is often of service; but it is more immediately useful to take away blood from the part itself by leeches, for we often find by a vessel giving way in the urethra, and a considerable hemorrhage ensuing, that the patient is greatly relieved. Relief will often be obtained by exposing the penis to the steam of hot water. Poultices likewise have beneficial effects, and both fomentations and poultices will often be assisted in removing inflammation by the addition of camphor. Opium, given internally, is of singular service, and if it be joined with camphor the effect will be still greater; but opium in such cases acts rather by lessening the pain than by removing the inflammation, though by preventing erections it may be said to obviate the immediate cause of the complaint.

When the chordee continues after all other symptoms are gone, little or nothing, in the way of evacuation, seems to be necessary, the inflammation being subdued, and a consequence of it only remaining, which will cease gradually by the absorption of the extravasated coagulable lymph. Therefore bleeding in this case can be of no use. Mercurial ointment applied to the parts will promote the absorption of the extravasated coagulable lymph, for experience has shown that mercury has considerable powers in exciting absorption. The friction itself also will be of use. In one case considerable benefit seemed to result from giving the cicuta, after the common methods of cure had been tried. Electricity may be

---

a [Bleeding from the urethra in gonorrhœa is beneficial, and should very seldom be repressed. If, however, the quantity which is lost is very excessive, and it becomes necessary to check it, the application of cold, in the form of a bladder filled with ice, to the perinæum will be found by much the most effectual remedy.]

of service. This symptom is indeed often longer in going off than either the running or pain; but no bad consequences arise from it. Its declension is gradual and uniform, as happens in most consequences of inflammation.

In relieving the chordee, or the remains of it, which appear to arise from spasm, I have known the bark of great service. Evacuations, whether from the part or from the constitution, generally do harm.

§. 4. Of the Treatment of the Suppuration of the Glands of the Urethra.

Suppurations in the glands of the urethra are to be treated as chancres. Therefore mercury ought to be given, as will be explained hereafter.

Should a suppuration take place in Cowper's glands, it demands more attention. The abscess must be opened freely and early, as the matter, if confined, may make its way either into the scrotum or urethra, whence would arise bad consequences. Here also mercury must be given, and perhaps as freely as in a bubo. In short, the treatment should be the same as in a venereal ulcer; and in this respect it will differ from the treatment of those abscesses which arise in consequence of stricture.[a]

§. 5. Of the Treatment of the Affection of the Bladder from Gonorrhœa.

When the disease extends as far as the bladder, it produces a most troublesome complaint, from which, however, bad consequences seldom arise. But I suspect that it sometimes has laid the groundwork of future irritation in that part, which has proved very troublesome and even dangerous.

Opiate clysters, if nothing in the constitution forbid the use of them, procure considerable temporary relief. The warm bath is of service, although not always; and bleeding freely, if the patient is of a full habit, often does good. Leeches also, applied to the perinæum, have good effects. But in many constitutions bleeding will rather do harm; and we should be cautious in making use of this evacuation, for it has

[a] [Experience does not confirm this doctrine. Suppurations in the glands of the urethra are not very uncommon in gonorrhœa, yet they heal readily without the use of mercury; nor are they ever followed by secondary symptoms.]

been already observed that many of these cases are rather from sympathy than inflammation. As this affection of the bladder often continues for a considerable time, producing other sympathies in the neighbouring parts, and is not in the least mitigated by the methods commonly used, I would recommend the following trials to be made use of in such cases. An opiate plaster to be applied to the pubes, or the small of the back, where the nerves of the bladder take their origin; a small blister on the perinæum, which is of service in irritations of the bladder arising from other causes.

§. 6. *Of the Treatment of the Swelled Testicle.*

When the testicle sympathises either with the urethra or bladder, and is inflamed, rest is the best remedy. The horizontal position of the body is the easiest, as such a position is the best for a free circulation. If the patient cannot submit to a horizontal position, it is absolutely necessary to have the testicle well suspended. Indeed the patient will be happy in having recourse to that expedient as soon as he is acquainted with the ease which it affords.

In this complaint, perhaps, no particular method of cure can be laid down. It is to be treated as inflammation in general, by bleeding and purging, if the constitution requires them, and by fomentation and poultices. Bleeding with leeches has often been of service. This we cannot well account for, as the vessels of the scrotum have but little connexion with those of the testicle.

As I do not look upon the swelling of the testicle to be venereal, mercurials, in my opinion, can be of no service in these cases while the inflammation continues; but they are useful when that is gone and the induration only remains.[a]

Vomits have been recommended in such cases, and are sometimes of service. I have known a vomit remove the swelling almost instantaneously. The effects of the vomit most probably arise from the sympathy between the stomach and the testicle. Opiates are of service, as they are in most irritations of those parts. When such swellings suppurate, which they seldom do, they require only to be treated as common suppurations, and mercury need not be given.

---

a [Though mercurials are not required for the sake of counteracting the venereal virus, yet experience shows that calomel is of the greatest service, even in the acute stage of inflammation of the testicle. It is probable that it acts here, as in many other cases of adhesive inflammation, by controuling the capillary circulation of the inflamed part. It should always be combined with purgatives, and generally with local bleeding.]

In the history of this disease I observed, and indeed it has been observed by most writers, that when a swelling comes upon the testicle in consequence of a gonorrhœa the running ceases, or when the running ceases the testicle swells; but which is the cause, or which is the effect, has not yet been ascertained. It has been also observed that when the running returns, the testicle then shows the first symptoms of recovery; so that the testicle having lost its sympathising action, the action is restored to the urethra. And here also it has not yet been ascertained which is the cause or which is the effect; but, from a supposition that the cessation of the discharge in the urethra is the cause of the swelling, it has been attributed to the mode of treatment of that irritation, and by some to injections.

It has been advised by many, and attempted by some, to procure a return of the running; but the methods used have hardly been founded upon any sound principle. Mr. Bromfield appears to have been the first who recommended a treatment suitable to this theory, which was to irritate the urethra to suppuration again, by introducing bougies. I have not seen that benefit that could have been wished, or that the first idea might induce us to expect, from this practice. Some have gone further, by recommending the introduction of venereal matter into the urethra; but this appears to be only conceit, and is founded upon a supposition that such swellings arise only from venereal irritations. But I have already observed that they are produced by other causes.

It is generally a long time before the swelling of the testicle entirely subsides, although it does so more quickly at first than swellings of this part arising from other causes. Before it becomes less, it generally becomes softer, commonly on the anterior surface; and by degrees the whole becomes perhaps softer than natural, and then it diminishes. It is still much longer (sometimes even years) before the epididymis returns to its natural state; sometimes it is never reduced to its natural size and softness. However, this is of no great consequence, as no inconvenience results from a continuance of the hardness simply; though sometimes, perhaps, such testicles are rendered totally useless. I never had an opportunity of examining the testicle of one that was known to have this complaint; but have examined testicles where the epididymis has had the same external feel, and where the canal of the vas deferens has been obliterated. But this I suspect too, seldom happens, for there are people who have both testicles swelled, and, notwithstanding, discharge their semen as before.[a]

_____

a [The hardness which is left after inflammation of the testicle does not appear in most instances to interfere with its functions. The obliteration of the vas deferens is not a frequent occurrence: and the induration which often remains in the epididymis,

It is in this stage of the complaint that resolvents may be of service, such as mercurial friction joined with camphor. Likewise we may usefully apply fumigations with aromatic herbs, in order to stimulate the absorbents to take up the superfluous matter. Electricity has been in some cases of singular service.

§.7. Of the decline and termination of the symptoms of Gonorrhœa.

The decline of the disease is generally known by an abatement of some or all of the above-mentioned symptoms. The pain in the part becomes less, or terminates in an itching similar to what is felt in the beginning of many gonorrhœas, and at last entirely goes off. The sense of weariness about the loins, hips, testicles and scrotum is no longer felt; and the transparent cherry-like appearance of the glans penis gradually disappears. These are the most certain signs of an abatement of the disease.

The running becomes less; or, if it does not diminish, becomes first whiter, then of a paler colour, and gradually acquires a more slimy and ropy consistence, which has always been considered as the most certain sign of an approaching cure. When the running becomes more slimy, it is then changed from matter to the natural fluid which lubricates the passage, and also to that fluid which appears to be preparatory to coition. But it is often very inconstant in its appearances, arising frequently from different modes of living, exercise, or other causes.

It often happens that all the symptoms shall totally disappear, and the patients shall think themselves cured, and yet the same symptoms shall come upon them anew, commonly indeed milder than at first; though in some cases as violent, or even more violent; and this takes place sometimes at a considerable distance of time. I have known the symptoms return a month after every appearance of the disease has been removed. However, in such cases, they seldom last long. How far this second attack is to be looked upon as truly venereal has not as yet been ascertained. Nothing can prove it absolutely to be venereal but the circumstance of having given it to a sound person. What may be

---

is usually from deposition in the cellular membrane which connects its convolutions, or mere thickening of the membranes which invest it. And though it is not uncommon that some of the vasa efferentia should be totally obstructed, and converted into solid cords: yet unless the whole of these vessels should be thus changed, such an occurrence is of little consequence; as those which still remain pervious will be sufficient to carry the semen as before into the vas deferens.]

the case with those in whom it has returned soon after the going off of the symptoms, I will not pretend to say; but I should very much suspect that, where the patient has continued well for a month, a return cannot be venereal. This is only conjecture: and if we were to reason upon it we might easily reason ourselves into a belief of its being venereal; for if the parts can fall back again into one mode of action, that of inflammation and suppuration, there can be no reason why they should not fall back again into the specific mode of action. However, as the common effect of irritation is suppuration, and as the specific suppuration requires a peculiar irritation, it is easier to conceive that the parts may fall into the common mode of action than into both. It is possible, however, that in such cases the venereal action may be only suspended, similar to what happens between the contamination and complete appearance of the disease.

In women, returns of the symptoms are more frequent than in men, particularly of the discharge; which being similar to the fluor albus, and frequently taken for that disease, gives less suspicion, although they are perhaps equally virulent as those in men.

The distinction between a gonorrhœa and a gleet is not yet ascertained: for the inflammation subsiding, the pain going off, and the matter altering are no proofs that the poison is destroyed. It is no more necessary that there should be a continuance of the inflammation to produce the specific poison than that there should be a continuance of the inflammation to produce the gleet, as will appear evident from two cases before related*.

The first of these cases shows that the inflammation is not necessary to the existence of the venereal poison; and, on the contrary, the inflammation may exist after the matter discharged has ceased to be venereal. I have known cases where the inflammation and discharge have continued for twelve months, and with considerable violence: in the mean time a free intercourse with women has not communicated the disease. However, this is not an absolute proof that there is no virus in the discharge.

* Vide pages 166 and 167.

CHAPTER VIII.

OBSERVATIONS ON THE SYMPTOMS WHICH OFTEN REMAIN AFTER THE DISEASE IS SUBDUED.

It often happens, after the virus is destroyed and the venereal inflammation removed, that some one, two, or more of the symptoms shall continue, and perhaps prove more obstinate than the original disease itself. Some of these symptoms shall continue through life, and even new ones shall sometimes arise as soon as the first have subsided. All these symptoms are commonly imputed by the patients themselves, and what is still worse, by some of the profession, to the original disease having been ill treated. But certainly, so far as we are yet acquainted with the disease and method of cure, this is not true; for the methods of treatment, though numerous, may be said to be very similar; and we shall find these symptoms not to be consequences of any one mode of treatment, but that they happen indiscriminately after them all. Yet I can conceive that many constitutions and particular parts often require one mode of treatment in preference to another, and probably require modes that we are not as yet acquainted with; but if these peculiarities of constitution or of parts are not yet known, which must often be the case, the practitioner is not to be rashly accused of ignorance.

In the Introduction, I observed that the venereal disease is capable of calling into action such susceptibilities as are remarkably strong, and peculiar to certain constitutions and countries; and that, as the scrofula is predominant in this country, some of the effects of gonorrhœa may partake of a scrofulous nature.

The symptoms which continue after the virus is gone do not owe their continuance to the specific qualities of the virus, but to its effects upon the parts, such as inflammation and its consequences; for the same degree of inflammation, arising from any other cause, would leave most of the same effects. But I suspect that the continuance of the discharge called a gleet is an exception to this; for we find that it is often cured by the same mode of action which would produce the other symptoms, that is, inflammation; and we find in general that a discharge brought on by violence of no specific kind does not last longer than the violence, even although the cause has been continued for some time, as is often the case during the use of bougies.

The first of the continued symptoms may be reckoned the remains of the disagreeable sensations excited by the original disease.

The second, the discharge called a gleet.

The third, the chordee.

The fourth, the irritable state of the bladder.

The fifth, the increase and hardness of the epididymis.

§. 1. Of the remains of the disagreeable Sensations excited by the original Disease.

The disagreeable sensations which continue in the urethra and glans occur most frequently when the bladder has sympathised with the urethra during the disease; for then there are often the remains of the old shooting pains in the glans, or on its surface, which take their rise from the bladder. These, however, commonly go off, seldom being the fore-runners of any bad symptoms, and therefore are not to be considered as part of the disease, but merely a consequence; yet they are often very troublesome and teazing to the patient, keeping his mind in doubt whether he is cured or not, which makes him frequently become the dupe of ignorant or designing men.

As these remaining sensations vary considerably in their nature, per-haps no one method of treatment will always be proper. I have known a bougie, introduced a few times, take off entirely the disagreeable sen-sation in the urethra; and I have known it do no good. Gentle irri-tating injections, used occasionally, will often alleviate in some degree those complaints. A grain of corrosive sublimate to eight ounces of water makes a good injection for this purpose; but all such applica-tions are in general no more than palliatives.

I have known the use of hemlock relieve the symptoms very much, and in some cases entirely cure them; while in many others it has not had the least effect.

A blister applied to the perinæum will entirely cure some of the re-maining symptoms, even when they extend towards the bladder, as will be explained hereafter: indeed it appears to have more effect than any other remedy. A blister to the small of the back will also give relief, but not so effectually as when applied to the perinæum.

The following cases are remarkable instances of this. A Portuguese gentleman, about twenty-five years of age, had contracted a venereal gonorrhœa, of which he was cured; but two years after, many of the symptoms still continued, and even with considerable violence. The symptoms were the following: a frequency in making water, and when the inclination came on he could not retain it a moment; a straining, and pain in the bladder after voiding it; a constant pain in the region of the bladder; a shooting pain in the urethra, which extended often to the anus; strange sensations in the perinæum; a sense of weariness in the testicles; and if he at any time pressed his thighs close together the pain or sensation in the perinæum was excited. It was supposed at Lisbon that he had the stone, and he came over to London for a cure of that disease. He was examined, but no stone was found. He was ordered to wash the external parts every morning with cold water, which he did for a fortnight, but found no benefit. I was consulted, and informed of all the above-mentioned circumstances. As a staff had been passed, there could be no stricture; however, I thought it was possible there might be a diseased prostate gland, and therefore examined him by the anus, but found that gland of its natural size and firmness. As there was no visible alteration of structure anywhere to be found, I looked upon the disease as only a wrong action of the parts, and therefore ordered a blister to be applied to the perinæum, which being kept open only a few days all the symptoms were entirely removed. He retained his water as usual; all the disagreeable sensations went off; and the blistered part was allowed to heal. About a fortnight after, he got a fresh venereal gonorrhœa, which alarmed him very much, as he was afraid it might bring back all his former symptoms, which however did not return, and he was soon cured of the gonorrhœa. He staid in London some time after, without any relapse.

Another case was that of a gentleman's servant in the country. He had, from a venereal cause, a disagreeable sensation whenever he made water, also a running, and some degree of chordee; which symptoms he had laboured under for a considerable time. He had gone through a course of mercury, which lasted two months, on a supposition that the venereal virus had not been destroyed; but without benefit. He had after that been bled, used powders of gum arabic and tragacanth, and taken calomel in small doses, with no better success. He then had recourse to injections and bougies of all kinds, but with no better success. On the ground of the symptoms not being venereal, but only wrong actions of the parts, a blister was applied upon the perinæum, repeated and kept open six days, upon which the symptoms totally disappeared, and had not recurred a twelvemonth afterwards.

This practice is not only of service where there has been a preceding gonorrhœa, but I have found it remove, almost immediately, suppressions of urine from other causes, when the turpentines and opium, both by the mouth and anus, had proved ineffectual, and when the catheter had been necessarily introduced twice a day to draw off the water. But of this more fully hereafter.

Electricity has been found to be of service in some cases, and therefore may be tried either in the first instance, or when other means have failed.

§. 2. Of a Gleet.

Whatever method has been had recourse to in the cure of the venereal inflammation, whether injections have been used, or internal medicines, (mercurials, purgatives, or astringents,) it often happens that the formation of pus shall continue, and prove more tedious and difficult of cure than the original disease. For, as I have already observed, the venereal inflammation is of such a nature as to go off of itself, or to wear itself out; or, in other words, it is such an action of the living powers as can subsist only for a certain time. But this is not the case with a gleet, which seems to take its rise from a habit of action which the parts have contracted, and as they have no disposition to lay aside this action, it of course is continued; for we find in those gonorrhœas which last long, and are tedious in their cure, that this habit is more rooted than in those which go off soon.

This disease, however, has not always the disposition to continue, for it often appears to stop of itself, even after every method has been ineffectually used. It is most probable that this arises from some accidental changes in the constitution, not at all depending upon the nature of the disease itself.

I have suspected that there was something scrofulous in some gleets. We find frequently that a derangement of the natural actions of a part will be the cause of that part falling into some new disease to which there may be a strong tendency in the constitution. We find that a cold falling on the eyes produces a scrofulous weakness in those parts, with a considerable discharge. There are often scrofulous swellings in the tonsils, from the same cause.

This opinion of the nature of some gleets is strengthened by the methods of cure; for we find that the sea-bath cures more gleets than the common cold bath, or any other mode of bathing. I have never yet tried the internal use of those medicines which are generally given in the scrofula; but I have found sea-water, diluted and used as an injection, cure some gleets; though it is not always effectual.

A gleet is generally understood to arise from a weakness: this certainly gives us no idea of the disease, and indeed there is none which can be annexed to the expression. By mechanical weakness is understood the inability to perform some action or sustain some force. By animal weakness the same is understood. But when the expression is applied to the animal's performing an uncommon or an additional action, I do not perfectly understand it.

Upon this idea of weakness depended in a great measure the usual method of cure; but we shall find that the treatment founded on this idea is so far from answering in all cases that it often does harm, and that a contrary practice is successful.

A gleet differs from a gonorrhœa: first, in this, that though a consequence of it, it is perfectly innocent with respect to infection; secondly, when it is a true gleet it is generally different in some of the constituent parts of the discharge, which consists of globular bodies, floating or wrapt in a slimy mucus instead of a serum. But the urethra is so circumstanced as easily to fall back into the formation of pus; and this commonly happens upon the least increase of exercise, eating or drinking indigestible food, or anything which increases the circulation or heats the patient. The virus, however, I believe, does not return; but of this I am not certain, for there are cases that make it very doubtful, as was before observed.

I am inclined to suspect that a gleet arises from the surface of the urethra only, and not from the glands: for I have observed in several instances that when the passage has just been cleared, either by the discharge of urine or by the use of an injection, a lascivious idea has caused the natural slime to flow very pure, which I do suppose would not have happened if the parts secreting the liquor had assisted in forming the gleet*.

A gleet is supposed to be an attendant upon what we call a relaxed constitution; but I can hardly say that I have observed this to be the case: at least I have seen instances where I should have expected such a termination of a gonorrhœa, if this had been a general cause, but did not find it; and I have seen it in strong constitutions, at least in appearance, in every other respect. Gleets do not in all cases arise from preceding gonorrhœas, but sometimes from other diseases of the urethra. A stricture in the urethra is, I believe, almost always attended with a gleet. It sometimes arises also from a disease in the prostate gland.

When a gleet does not arise from any evident cause, nor can be supposed to be a return of a former gleet in consequence of a gonorrhœa, a

* Added: " A gentleman has a gleet, occasionally attended with pain in making water: it is brought on by sitting in a post-chaise, if he sits on the cushion, but not if he sits on a hard seat; it never comes on after riding on horseback, but he believes that riding upon a padded saddle would produce it."—*Home.*

stricture or diseased prostate gland is to be suspected; and inquiry should be made into the circumstances of making water, whether the stream is smaller than common, whether there be any difficulty in voiding it, and whether the calls to make it are frequent. If there should be such symptoms, a bougie, of a size rather less than common, ought to be used, which, if there is a stricture, will stop when it reaches it; and if it passes on to the bladder with tolerable ease, the disease is probably in the prostate gland, which should be next examined. But more fully of both these complaints hereafter.[a]

§.3. Of the Cure of Gleets—constitutionally—locally.

As this discharge has no specific quality, but depends upon the constitution of the patient or nature of the parts themselves, there can be no certain or fixed method of cure; and as it is very difficult to find out the true nature of different constitutions or of parts, it becomes equally difficult to prescribe with certainty the medicines that will best suit this disease; for so great is the variety in constitutions, that what in one case proves a cure will in another aggravate the complaint.

There are two ways of attempting the cure of this complaint : constitutionally, or locally.

Medicines, taken into the constitution with a view to the cure of gleet, may be supposed to act in three ways : as specifics[†], strengtheners, and astringents.

† It may be necessary to remark here, that by specific I do not mean a specific for the disease, but only such medicines as act specifically on the parts concerned, as the turpentines, cantharides, &c.

---

a [A gleet may arise from any source of irritation in any part of the urinary passages, or even in the neighbourhood. Hæmorrhoids are a frequent cause, and, in children, worms in the intestines. In like manner it may be occasioned by a calculus, or by other disease in the bladder or kidneys, and still more commonly, as the author has stated, by stricture in the urethra. But perhaps the most common cause, if we except stricture, is some derangement in the secretion of the urine, by which that fluid is rendered too acid or alkaline, and is converted into a perpetual source of irritation, occasioning various derangements of the urinary organs, and none, at least in those who have suffered from gonorrhœa, more frequently than gleet.

The cure of a gleet depends chiefly on the discovery, and the removal of the causes which excite it. While these continue, the effect of any remedies which are calculated to act directly on the discharge is generally inadequate, and at the best temporary. When the source of irritation, whatever it may be, is taken away, there is seldom much difficulty in repressing the excessive secretion from the urethra.

The same remark applies to leucorrhœa in women. This is very generally kept up by some uterine derangement, as amenorrhœa, or irritability of the os uteri. While this derangement subsists, no remedies are effectual: but if it is first corrected by appropriate treatment, the discharge may usually be arrested, without great difficulty, by a little perseverance in the use of the commonest astringents.]

The specific power of internal medicines upon those parts is not very great; however, we find that some of them, such as the balsams, turpentines, and cantharides, are of use, especially in slight cases. I think I have been able to ascertain this fact, that when the balsams, turpentines, or cantharides, are of service, they are almost immediately so; therefore if upon trial they are not found to lessen, or totally remove the gleet in five or six days, I have never continued them longer. And even where they have either lessened or totally removed the gleet in that time, it will often recur upon leaving them off, and therefore they should be continued for some time after the symptoms have disappeared. I have known cases where the gleet has disappeared immediately upon the use of the balsam capivi, and recurred upon the omission of it; and I have also seen where that medicine has kept it off for more than a month, and yet it has recurred immediately upon laying it aside, and stopped again as quickly when the patient has returned to it. In such cases the other methods of cure should be tried. The balsams may either be given alone, or mixed with other substances, so as to make them less disagreeable*.

The general strengtheners of the habit need only be given when the parts act merely as parts of that habit. The whole being disposed to act properly, these parts are also disposed to act in the same way. By general strengtheners are here meant, the cold bath, the sea bath, the bark, and steel. Astringents, taken into the constitution, have no great powers; and if they had, they might be very improper, as anything that could act with powers in the constitution equal to what would be necessary here, might very much affect many natural operations in the animal œconomy. The astringent gums and salt of steel are commonly given.

The second mode of cure is by local applications. These may be divided into four, which are, specifics, astringents, irritating medicines, and such as act by derivation.

The specifics, applied locally, we may reasonably suppose, will have greater effects than when given internally, because they may be applied stronger than can safely be thrown into the circulation. Of this, I think, I have had experience.

The astringents commonly used are the decoction of the bark, white vitriol, alum, and preparations of lead. The aqua vitriolica cœrulea of the London Dispensatory, diluted with eight times its quantity of water, makes a very good astringent injection. The same observations that I made on the specifics are applicable to the astringents; I believe that

---

* Added: "I believe that the balsam of capivi cures a gleet more permanently than injections, its action being specifically upon the parts."—*Home*.

they act nearly in the same manner, and have the same effect. What their mode of action is it is difficult to say.

When either of these methods has been used, and has had the desired effect, it should be continued for a considerable time after the symptoms have disappeared; and the time must be in proportion to the duration of the complaint, or the frequency of its returns. If it has been of long standing, we may be sure that the disposition to such a complaint is strong; and if it has returned frequently, upon the least increase of circulation, we may expect the same thing to happen again. Therefore, to correct the bad habit, it is necessary to continue the medicines a considerable time.

Irritating applications are either injections or bougies, simple, or medicated with irritating medicines. Violent exercise may be considered as having the same effect. Such applications should never be used till the other methods have been fully tried and found unsuccessful. They differ from the foregoing by producing at first a greater discharge than that which they are intended to cure; and the increased discharge may or may not continue as long as the application is used. It becomes, therefore, necessary to inquire how long they are to be used to produce a cure of the gleet. That time will generally be in proportion to the violence used, and the nature of the parts which form the matter, and according to the disposition being strong or weak, joined to its duration, and the greater or less irritability of the parts. If the parts are either weak or irritable, or both, an irritating injection should not be used; if strong, and not irritable, it may be used with safety. In this last case, if it is an injection that stimulates very considerably, perhaps it may be sufficient to use it twice or thrice a day. I knew a gentleman who threw into the urethra, for a gleet of two years' standing, Goulard's extract of lead, undiluted, which produced a most violent inflammation; but when the inflammation went off, the gleet was cured. Two grains of corrosive sublimate to eight ounces of water are a very good irritating injection.

If it is a gleet of long standing, it may require a week or more to remove it, even with an irritating injection; and if the injection is less irritating, so as to give but little pain, and to increase the discharge in a small degree, it may require a fortnight. But one precaution is very necessary respecting the use of irritating injections; it should be first known, if possible, that they will do no harm. To know this may be difficult in many cases; but the nature of the parts is to be ascertained as nearly as possible; that is, whether they had ever been hurt before by such treatment; whether they are so susceptible of irritation as that

the irritation may be expected to run along the urethra and produce
symptoms in the bladder, for in such cases irritating applications do not
answer, but, on the contrary, often produce worse disorders than those
they were meant to cure.

Bougies may be classed with the irritating applications, and in many
cases they act very violently as such. They appear to be more efficacious than injections, but they require longer time to produce their full
effect. A simple, or unmedicated bougie, is, in general, sufficient for
the cure of a gleet, and requires a month or six weeks' application before the cure can be depended upon. If bougies are made to stimulate
otherwise than as extraneous bodies, then a shorter time will generally
be sufficient. Probably the best mode of medicating them would be by
mixing a little turpentine, or a little camphor with the composition, so
as to act specifically on the parts ; but great care should be taken not
to irritate too much.

The size of the bougie should be smaller than the common, and need
only be five or six inches long, as it seldom happens that a greater extent of the urethra has the disposition to gleet; but no harm will arise
from passing a bougie of the common length through the whole extent
of the urethra.

In the cure of a gleet, attempted by means of the bougie, we have no
certain rules to direct us when it should be left off, as the discharge
will often continue as long as the bougie is used. If, upon leaving off
the bougie, after the use of it for several weeks, the running ceases,
then we may hope there is a cure performed ; but if it should not be in
the least diminished, it is more than probable that bougies will not effect a cure, and therefore it is hardly necessary to have recourse to
them again. Yet, if the gleet is in part diminished, it will be right to
begin again, and probably it may be proper to increase the irritating
quality of the bougie, in order to suit it to the diminished irritability of
the parts.

The fourth mode of cure is by sympathy, or by producing an irritation in another part of the body, which shall destroy the mode of action
in the urethra.

I knew a case of obstinate gleet attended with very disagreeable sensations in the urethra, especially at the time of making water, removed
entirely by two chancres appearing upon the glans. The patient had
taken all the medicines commonly recommended, and had applied the
bougie without effect.

A gentleman informed me that he had cured two persons of gleets
by applying a blister to the under side of the urethra ; and I have known

several old gleets, after having baffled all common attempts, cured by electricity. All these different methods of cure alter the disposition of the part.

In whatever way the cure is attempted, rest or quietness in most cases is of great consequence; for, as I have observed, exercise is often a cause, not only of its continuance, but of its increase and return. But this idea is not to be too rigidly adhered to, especially in cases which have been treated unsuccessfully, as I have known some that have got immediately well by riding on horseback after long disuse of that exercise.

Regularity and moderation in diet should be particularly attended to; for irregularities of this kind either hinder the cure or bring on a return of the disease.

Intercourse with women often causes a return, or increase of gleet, and in such cases it gives suspicion of a fresh infection; but the difference between this and a fresh infection is, that here the return will follow the connexion so close as to be almost immediate, and that circumstance, joined with the other symptoms, will in general ascertain the nature of the discharge.

The cure of the gleet in women is nearly the same as in men, except in the use of what I have called specifics to the parts, for as the gleet in women is principally from the vagina, I believe that this part is not more affected by the turpentines than other parts are; but as the vagina is less irritable than the urethra in men, the astringents which are applied to it may be considerably stronger. Neither can we use the bougie in cases of gleet in the vagina; and when the gleet is only from the urethra, I imagine it is hardly ever attended to in women.

§. 4. *Of the Remaining Chordee.*

This symptom, I have already observed, often remains after every mark of the true virus is removed, and may or may not be attendant on any of the other continuing symptoms.

Mercurial ointment applied to the part may be of service, and if joined with camphor, its powers will be increased. I have known electricity cure a chordee of long standing. If it is the spasmodic chordee that remains, bark should be given.

§. 5. *Of the continuance of the Irritation of the Bladder.*

The irritation of the bladder sometimes continues after every other symptom has ceased, and it may be an attendant upon all, or any of the other continuing symptoms; it seldom lasts with the same violence, although it is often very troublesome. When this irritation is kept up with the same violence, the bladder itself may be suspected of being diseased; or it may arise from its connexion with other parts, such as the urethra, or prostate gland; for a stricture in the urethra coming on will prove the cause of its continuance, and a disease in the prostate gland will do the same.

Neither of these diseases will probably follow the gonorrhœa so closely as to keep up this irritation, though perhaps they may have been taking place prior to the gonorrhœa, and so contribute to its increase and continuance, which may probably be ascertained by a history of the patient preceding the present complaint; however, before the bladder itself is attempted to be cured, a bougie should be passed, and if no stricture is found, then the prostate gland should be examined, as shall be described.

When the disease is in the bladder only, I think the pain is principally at the close of making water, and for a little while after. The cure of this symptom consists in opiate clysters, cicuta, bark, sea-bathing, and I should be inclined to recommend the application of a blister to the perinæum in men. How far opiate clysters can affect the bladder in women as they do in men, I am not certain.

§. 6. *Of the remaining Hardness of the Epididymis.*

This symptom I have observed remains long after every other symptom is removed, and may continue even for life; but seldom or ever any bad consequences happen from it if the vas deferens is not rendered impervious, and not even then if it is only in one testicle, the other being equal to all the purposes of generation. As this is the case, we must at once see that no certain method of resolution is yet known. The application of the steam of hot water with camphor may be tried, especially in such cases as are not disposed to be permanent; and the scrotum may be rubbed with mercurial ointment, joined with camphor. But in most cases this practice will prove too tedious, or rather too inefficacious to be long persisted in.

PART III.

CHAPTER I.

OF DISEASES SUPPOSED TO ARISE IN CONSEQUENCE OF VENEREAL INFLAMMATION IN THE URETHRA OF MEN.

THE gonorrhœa produces, or at least is supposed to produce, besides those disorders already mentioned, many others which are totally different from the original disease. How far they do all or any of them arise in consequence of this disease, is not clear; but as they are diseases of the urethra, and are both numerous and important, I mean to treat fully of them in this place. If any of these diseases arise from a gonorrhœa, they are most probably not the consequences of any specific quality in the venereal poison, but are such as might be produced by any common inflammation in those parts, as was observed of the *continued symptoms*.

In this investigation we shall find some of the complaints arising out of each other, so that there is frequently a series of them. Thus a stricture of the urethra produces an irritable bladder, a frequent desire to make water, increased strength of the bladder, a dilatation of the urethra between the bladder and stricture, ulceration, fistulæ in perinæo, dilatation of the ureters and enlargement of the pelvis of the kidneys, besides other complaints that are sympathetic, such as swellings of the testicle, and of the glands in the groin. I shall treat of the diseases of those parts in the order in which they most commonly arise.

It may be observed that most of these diseases, especially the diminution of distensibility in the bladder, attack men advanced beyond the middle age, although many, if not all of them, are at times found in younger subjects, and the circumstance of their appearing at this period arises probably in some degree from a long habit of an unnatural mode of life producing many diseases, such as gout; for certainly such complaints do not so frequently take place among the more uncivilized nations.

The most frequent disease in the urethra is an obstruction to the passage of the urine; it happens both in young and old, although most frequently in the latter. Before I begin to treat of this subject, I shall, for the better understanding of the whole, make some observations on the uses of this passage in its natural state.

It may first be observed, that the urethra in man is employed for two purposes. On this occasion I may be allowed to make the following general remark, that nature has not been able to apply any one part to two uses with advantage, as might be illustrated in many instances in different animals. The animals whose legs are contrived both for swimming and walking, are not good at either, as seals, otters, ducks, and geese. The animals also whose legs are intended both for walking and flying, are but badly formed for either, as the bat. The same observations are applicable to fish, for the flying fish neither swims nor flies well; and whenever parts intended for such double functions are diseased, both are performed imperfectly. This is immediately applicable to the urethra, for it is intended as a canal or passage both for the urine and the semen. The urine requires the simplest of all canals, and of no greater length than the distance from the bladder to the external surface, as we find the urethra in women, birds, the amphibia, and fish; but the passage for the semen in the quadruped requires to be a complicated canal, and of a length capable of conveying the semen to the female, provided with many additional and necessary parts, as the corpus spongiosum urethræ, musculi acceleratores, Cowper's glands, prostate gland, and vesiculæ seminales. As all these parts are to serve the purposes of generation, and as the diseases of this canal are principally seated in them, we at once see how much the urinary organs must suffer from a connexion with parts so numerous and so liable to disease; and what adds to the evil is, that the actions of the urinary organs are constant, and absolutely necessary for the well-being of the machine, whereas the evacuation of the semen takes place only during a certain portion of life, is then only occasional, and never essentially necessary to the existence of the individual. The force of this observation is at once seen by making the comparison between the inconveniences that attend the expulsion of the urine in the male, and in the female.

The canal of the urethra is liable to such diseases as are capable of preventing in some degree the passage of the urine through it; and in some of these diseases the passage at last becomes completely obstructed. In all cases there is a diminution of the size of the canal, but in different ways. There are five modes of obstruction, four of which are diseases of the passage itself, the fifth is a consequence of the diseases of other parts. Three of the former are a lessening of the diameter of the passage; the fourth an excrescence in the passage; the fifth arises from the sides being compressed, which may be done either by exterior contiguous swellings, or by a swelling of the prostate gland.

§. 1. *Of Strictures.*

The three first I shall now consider, of which the first is the true permanent stricture arising from an alteration in the structure of a part of the urethra. The second is a mixed case, composed of a permanent stricture and spasm. The third is the true spasmodic stricture. Most obstructions to the passage of the urine, if not all, are attended with nearly the same symptoms, so that there are hardly sufficient marks for distinguishing the different causes. Few take notice of the first symptoms of a stricture till they have either become violent, or have been the cause of other inconveniences. For instance, a patient shall have a considerable stricture without observing that he does not make water freely; he shall even have, in consequence of a stricture, a tendency to inflammation, and suppuration in the perinæum, and not feel any obstruction to the passage of his urine, nor suspect that he has any other complaint than the inflammation in the perinæum. In all of these obstructions the stream of water becomes small, and that in proportion to the obstruction; but this symptom, though probably it is the first, is not always observed by the patient. In some the water is voided only in drops, and then it cannot escape notice; in others the stream of urine is forked or scattered: under such circumstances, the passage should be examined with a bougie; and if one of a common size passes with tolerable ease, the fifth cause of obstruction is to be suspected, which will most probably be found to be a swelled prostate gland, for any other cause that can produce a compression of the sides of the urethra sufficient to obstruct the urine, will be known to the patient, such as a tumour forming anywhere along the canal, or an inflammation along its sides. If, therefore, neither of these is known to exist, the prostate gland should be examined, as will be described hereafter.

The spasmodic obstruction will commonly explain itself when the symptoms are well investigated, for the obstruction arising from this cause will not be permanent. These obstructions, but more particularly that from a permanent stricture, are generally attended with a discharge of matter, or a gleet. This is often considered by the patient as the whole disease, and he applies to the surgeon for the cure of a gleet. The surgeon often perseveres in attempting the cure of this disease; but, no success attending him, at last other symptoms are observed, and a stricture is suspected, either by the surgeon or patient. In diseases of this passage, and also of the prostate gland and bladder, there is commonly an uneasiness about the perinæum, anus, and lower part of the abdomen, and the patient can hardly cross his legs without pain.

CHAPTER II.

OF THE PERMANENT STRICTURE.

In the permanent stricture* the patient seldom complains till he can hardly procure a passage for the urine ; and frequently has a considerable degree of strangury, and even other symptoms that happen in stone and gravel, which are therefore too frequently supposed to be the causes of the complaint. The disease generally occupies no great length of the passage ; at least, in most of the cases that I have seen, it extended no further in breadth than if the part had been surrounded with a piece of packthread, and in many it had a good deal of that appearance. I have, however, seen the urethra irregularly contracted for above an inch in length, owing to its coats or internal membrane being irregularly thickened, and forming a winding canal.

A stricture does not arise in all cases from an equal contraction of the urethra all round, but in some from a contraction of one side, which probably has given the idea of its having arisen from an ulcer on that side. This contraction of one side only throws the passage to the opposite side, which often renders it difficult to pass the bougie. The contracted part is whiter than any other part of the urethra, and is harder in its consistence. In some few cases there are more strictures than one. I have seen half a dozen in one urethra, some of which were more contracted than others ; and indeed many urethras that have a stricture have small tightnesses in other parts of them. This we learn from successive resistance felt in passing the bougie.

Every part of the urethra is not equally subject to strictures, for there appears to be one part which is much more liable to them than the whole of the urethra besides, that is, about the bulbous part. We find them, however, sometimes on this side of the bulb, but very seldom be-

* Vide Plate IX, fig. 1.

yond it. I never saw a stricture in that part of the urethra which passes through the prostate gland ; and the bulb, besides being the most frequent seat of this disease, has likewise strictures formed there of the worst kind. They are generally slow in forming, it being often several years from their being perceived before they become very troublesome.

The same stricture is not at all times equally bad, for we find that in warm weather it is not nearly so troublesome as in cold. These changes are often very quick. A cold day, even an hour of cold weather, shall produce a change in them; and the same stricture is almost always worse in winter than in summer. However, this observation is not free from exceptions ; I knew one case that was always worse in the summer. There are other circumstances besides cold that make a stricture worse. A gentleman who had an ague always found the stricture increased during the fit. It is also increased by drinking, violent exercise, and by the retention of urine after an inclination to void it has been felt. This last cause is often so great as to produce a total stoppage for a time. It is sometimes rendered much worse by a small calculus passing from the bladder, of the formation of which this stricture was probably the cause. The calculus not passing, will produce a total stoppage of urine, the cause of which can hardly be known at the time, and if known it could not be remedied without an operation*.

It is impossible to say what is the cause of that alteration in the structure of the urethra which diminishes the canal: it has been ascribed to the effects of the venereal disease, and often to the method of cure. But I doubt very much if it commonly, or even ever, arises from these causes ; yet as most men have had venereal complaints some time or other, it is natural to ascribe the stricture to them, and therefore it may be very difficult to refute this opinion. Many reasons, however, can be given why we should suppose that it is not commonly a consequence of a venereal inflammation. Strictures are common to most passages in the human body; they are often to be found in the œsophagus; in the intestines, especially the rectum ; in the anus ; in the prepuce, producing phimosis ; in the lachrymal duct, producing the disease called fistula lachrymalis, where no disease had previously existed. They sometimes happen in the urethra where no venereal complaint has ever been. I have seen an instance of this kind in a young man of nineteen, who had had the complaint for eight years, and which therefore began when he was only eleven years of age. It was treated at first as stone or gravel. He was of a scrofulous habit, the lips thick, the eyes sore, a thickened cornea of one eye, and the general habit weak.

* Vide Plate XII.

This stricture was in the usual place, about the membranous part of the urethra.　I have seen an instance of a stricture in the urethra of a boy of four years, and a fistula in perinæo in consequence of it.　They are as common to those who have had the gonorrhœa slightly as those who have had it violently.

I knew a young gentleman who had a very bad stricture.　He had had several gonorrhœas, but they were so slight that they seldom lasted a week, nor in any of them did the pain extend beyond the frænum ; but the stricture was about the membranous part.　Cases of this kind occur every day.　They are never found to come on during the venereal inflammation, nor for some time after the infection is gone.　There have been thirty, and sometimes forty, years between the cure of a gonorrhœa and the beginning of a stricture, the health being all that time perfectly good.　If they arose in consequence of the venereal inflammation, we might expect to find them of some extent, because the venereal inflammation extends some way ; and we should also expect to find them most frequent in that part of the urethra which is most commonly the seat of the venereal disease.　But I remarked before, that they are not so frequent there as they are in other parts of the urethra.

It is supposed by many that strictures arise from the use of injections in the cure of the gonorrhœa ; but this opinion appears to be founded in prejudice, for I have seen as many strictures after gonorrhœas that have been cured without injections as after those cured with them.

Such modes of accounting for strictures give no explanation of those where there has been no previous gonorrhœa, or where the gonorrhœa has not been cured by injections ; and indeed if we consider the mode of cure of strictures, we must see that an injection is a mild application to the urethra compared to a bougie ; yet a bougie has never been supposed or known to be the cause of a stricture.　Further, some have injected by mistake very irritating liquors, such as the undiluted extract of lead, and caustic alkali, without giving the least tendency towards a stricture, although they produced violent inflammation, and even sloughing of the internal membrane of the urethra.

By many they have been supposed to have arisen from the healing of ulcers in the urethra ; but as I never saw an ulcer in these parts, except in consequence of a stricture, and as I do not believe there ever is an ulcer in the case of a common gonorrhœa, I can hardly subscribe to that opinion[a].

---

[a] [Many well-authenticated facts disprove the common prejudice which attributes stricture invariably to gonorrhœa or to the use of injections.　But when the author goes so far as to question whether it ever arises from these causes, his opinion is contradicted both by reason and by experience.　It would appear that any irritation on

§. 1. *Of the Bougie.*

The bougie, with its application, is perhaps one of the greatest improvements in surgery which these last thirty or forty years have produced. When I compare the practice of the present day with what it was in the year 1750, I can scarcely be persuaded that I am treating the same disease. I remember when, about that time, I was attending the first hospitals in this city, the common bougies were either a piece of lead*, or a small wax candle; and although the present bougie was known then, yet a due preference was not given to it, or its particular merit understood, as we may see from the publications of that time.

Daran was the first who improved the bougie and brought it into general use. He wrote professedly on the diseases for which it is a cure, and also of the manner of preparing it; but he has introduced so much absurdity in his descriptions of the diseases, the modes of treatment,

* When lead was used in place of bougies it has happened that a piece of the end has broken off in the bladder, which has been dissolved by injecting quicksilver. I at first suspected that quicksilver could not come in contact with lead while in water, so as to dissolve it; but upon making the experiment I found it succeeded.

---

the urethra, if sufficiently long continued, may give rise to stricture. It may be consequent on stone in the bladder, on disease of the prostate or disease of the bladder, on acid urine, on repeated attacks of strangury occasioned by the application of a series of blisters. But of all sources of irritation which can affect the urethra, the most common and the most severe is gonorrhœa, and hence a large proportion of cases of stricture follow so immediately on this disease as to be justly attributable to it. There are few cases of gonorrhœa in which the stream of urine is not diminished in size, from the existence of some degree of spasmodic contraction in the membranous portion of the canal. If the gonorrhœa lasts long, this spasm may become habitual, and terminate in stricture; and the likelihood of such a result is much increased if the inflammation is not confined to the extremity of the urethra, but extends to the bulb and neck of the bladder.

How far injections have a tendency to produce the same effect is more doubtful. When they are successfully used on the first appearance of the discharge, it is probable that, by cutting short the disorder, they rather prevent than promote stricture. But where injections fail, they unquestionably in many cases extend the sphere of the inflammation, and involve those parts of the urethra which are in the vicinity of the bulb, and are especially liable to this affection. Again, the discharge, as the author has elsewhere observed, relieves the spasm of a stricture. In cases where there exists already spasmodic contraction of the urethra, injections, by diminishing or arresting the discharge, will undoubtedly tend to increase the spasm and to render it permanent.

The old opinion was, that a stricture was the cicatrix of an ulcer which existed during a gonorrhœa. This notion the author justly repudiates. But he must not be understood to mean that ulceration may not sometimes arise from other causes, and leave behind it a stricture. When the urethra has been lacerated by external violence, as by a blow on the perinæum, stricture will usually follow, and will in most cases be of a kind which is peculiarly intractable and obstinate.]

and of the powers and composition of his bougies, as to create disgust. However, this absurdity has been much more effectual in introducing the bougie into universal use than all the real knowledge of that time, directed by good sense, could have been. Such extravagant recommendations of particular remedies are not at all times without their use. Inoculation would have still been practised with caution had it not been for the enthusiasm of the Suttons. Preparations of lead would not have been so universally applied if they had not been recommended by Goulard in the most extravagant terms; nor would the hemlock have come into such general use if its true merits only had been held forth. Improvements are often over-rated, but they come to their true value at last. Sutton has told us, that the cold regimen, in extreme, is infinitely better than the old method; but from general practice we have learned that moderation is best, which is all we yet know.

When Daran published his obsérvations on the bougie, every surgeon set to work to discover the composition, and each conceived that he had found it out, from the bougies he had made producing the effects described by Daran. It never occurred to them that any extraneous body, of the same shape and consistence, would do the same thing.

§. 2. Of the Treatment of the Permanent Stricture.

The cure of the permanent stricture is, I believe, to be accomplished only by local applications. Mercury has been given, upon the erroneous supposition of its being venereal, but without success. The cure is either a dilatation of the contracted part, or a destruction of it by ulceration, or escharotics. The dilatation is performed by the bougie, and this is seldom or never more than a temporary cure; for although the passage may be dilated sufficiently for the urine to pass, yet there is always the original tendency to contraction, which generally recurs sooner or later*. The ulcerative process is also effected by a bougie, and the destruction by escharotics is by means of caustics. It often

---

* In cases of stricture, when a patient applies for relief, it may often be proper to inquire into the history of the case previous to the passing of a bougie, especially to inquire if he ever used bougies before; if he has, then to inquire into the result; if they passed readily, or if they did not pass the stricture at all: if the first, then nothing further need be asked; but if the last, then to inquire if he or his surgeon observed that they were gaining ground with the bougie, viz., if the bougie went further in before it was left off than at first; if so, then to ask him how far. If they have visibly gained ground without getting through the stricture, I am afraid that the use of the bougie must not be pursued, because it is most probable that a new passage has been formed, which makes the passing of the bougie into the stricture impossible.

happens in strictures that the passage is so diminished as hardly to allow any water to pass, producing often a total stoppage; nor will a
bougie immediately pass; and if it can be made to pass, yet no water
follows it when withdrawn.   In such cases therefore we must have recourse to the means that afford a temporary relief, such as the warm
bath, which counteracts the effects of cold, and quiets any spasms that
may have taken place in the parts, and clysters with opium, which have
still more effect.   Producing an evacuation by stool often lessens the
spasm, for a spasmodic suppression of urine frequently arises from a
constipation, even where there is no stricture.

The cure by dilatation is, I imagine, principally mechanical when
performed by bougies, the powers of which are in general those of a
wedge.   However, the ultimate effect of them is not always so simple
as that of a wedge upon inanimate matter, for pressure produces action
of the animal powers, either to adapt the parts to their new position, or
to recede by ulceration, which gives us two very different effects of a
bougie, and of course two different intentions in applying them; one
to produce dilatation, the other ulceration, which last is not always so
readily affected.

It generally happens, as has been already observed, that the disease
has gone considerable lengths before application has been made for a
cure, and therefore the stricture has become considerable, in so much
that it is often with great difficulty that a small bougie can be made to
pass.   If the case is such as will readily admit the end of a small bougie
to pass, let it be ever so small, the cure is then in our power.   It often
happens, however, that the stricture is such as will resist the passing of
a small bougie at first, and even after repeated trials.   Yet it is necessary to persevere with the small bougie, for sometimes it happens that
the passage through the stricture is not in a line with the urethra itself,
which of course obstructs the bougie; such strictures, I suspect, are not
equally placed all round, so as to throw the small passage remaining into
the centre of the canal.

In many cases, where the stricture is very considerable, much trouble
is given by occasional spasms, which will either resist the bougie altogether, or only let a very small one pass, though at another time they
will admit one larger.   In such cases I have been able to get the point
of the bougie sometimes to enter, by rubbing the perinæum externally
with the finger of one hand while I pushed the bougie on with the other.
This, though it does not always succeed, yet is worth the trial.
Whether it alters the position of the stricture, so as to give entrance
to the point of the bougie, or by sympathy removes the spasm, I will
not absolutely determine, but I believe it rather acts by sympathy.   In

such cases of spasm in the stricture, I have often succeeded by letting the bougie remain a little while close to the stricture, and then pushing it on; this mode so often succeeds, that it should always be attempted when the bougie does not pass, or only passes occasionally. This will be mentioned more fully when we shall consider the spasmodic stricture.

The spasm may probably be taken off by dipping the glans penis into cold water, which succeeds sometimes in the common strangury; but this cannot be so easily done while a bougie is in the passage.

In cases of a permanent stricture, though the bougie does not at first pass, yet, after repeated trials, it will every now and then find its way, which helps to render a future trial more certain and easy. It, however, too often happens that the future success does not immediately depend upon passing the bougie once or twice, for it shall pass today and not tomorrow; and this uncertainty shall last for weeks, notwithstanding every trial we can make; yet I may observe, that in general its introduction becomes gradually less difficult, and therefore in no case should we despair of success. It is imagined by some that the best time for trial in these cases is just after making water, as the passage is supposed to be clear, and more in a straight line; but this is not confirmed by practice.

It is not an easy matter, in cases where the passage is very small, to know whether the bougie has entered the stricture or not, for such slender bougies as must generally be used at first bend so very easily, that the introducer is apt to think it is passing, while it is only bending. A surgeon, however, should in general first make himself acquainted with the situation of the stricture, by a common-sized bougie, and afterwards make use of a smaller one, and when he comes to the stricture, push gently, and for a little time only. If the bougie has passed further into the penis, he will know how far it has entered the stricture by taking off the pressure from the bougie, for if it recoil he may be sure that it has not passed, at least has not passed far, but only bent; for the natural elasticity of the bougie, and the direction of the passage having been altered by it, will force it back again. But if it remain fixed, and do not recoil, he may be sure that it has entered the stricture.

In using a very small bougie, however, these observations are not so applicable, for it may be bending, or bent, without being perceptible. It often happens that a bougie will enter only a little way, perhaps not more than one tenth of an inch, and then bend if the pressure be continued. To determine whether this be the case, it is necessary to withdraw the bougie and examine its end: if the end be blunted, we may be sure the bougie has not entered in the least; but if it be flattened for an eighth or tenth of an inch, or grooved, or have its outer waxy coat pushed up for that length; or if there be a circular impression made upon the bougie where the stricture is, or only a dent on one side, both of which last I suspect arise from spasm at the time, we may then be sure that it has passed as far as these appearances extend. It becomes then necessary to introduce another exactly of the same size, and in the same manner, and to let it remain as long as the patient can bear it, or convenience will allow; and by repeating this we may overcome the stricture. Sometimes we can judge of its having entered the stricture, by pulling it gently out; for if it stick a little at the first pull, we may be certain it has entered; but the appearance of the bougie itself will give the best information*. In such cases I have always directed my patient to preserve the bougie for my inspection, exactly in the same form it was when it was withdrawn. But when it passes with ease this nicety is not necessary.

The time that each bougie ought to remain in the passage must be determined by the feelings of the patient; for it should never give pain, if possible. To go beyond this point is to destroy the intention, to increase the very symptoms that are meant to be relieved, and to produce irritation, which for a time renders the further application of the bougie improper. While the bougie is passing, if the patient feel very acutely, it should not be left in the urethra above five or at most ten minutes, or not so long if it give great pain; and each time of application should be lengthened so gradually as to be insensible to the feelings of the patient and the irritability of the parts. I have known it days, nay, in many patients, weeks, before they could allow the bougie to remain in the passage ten or even five minutes, and yet in time they have been able to bear it for hours, and at last without any difficulty. The best time to let it remain in the passage is when the patient has least to do; or in the morning, while he is in bed, provided he can introduce it himself.

* It may be remarked that there are some lacunæ (vide plate IX, fig. 2.) near and also a little way from the glans penis, which often stop the bougie, and give at first the idea of a stricture. I have known them taken for such; and when the bougie stops so near to the glans this is to be suspected, and therefore we should vary the direction of the point of the bougie, bearing it against the under side of the urethra. When the bougie stops in one of those lacunæ, I think that the patient appears to have more pain than from a real stricture. The valvular part of the prostate gland formed by disease, (vide plate XIII.) very often obstructs the bougie, and is taken for a stricture by those who are not well acquainted with the different obstructions in this canal; and by those who are, it is a means of discovering disease in this part; and indeed in a natural state of parts I think I can ascertain when I come to this part with a bougie.

The bougie should be increased in size according to the facility with which the stricture dilates, and the ease with which the patient bears the dilatation. If the parts are very firm or very irritable, the increase of the size of the bougie should be slow, gradually stealing upon the parts, and allowing them to adapt their structure to the increased size. But if the sensibility of the parts will allow of it, the increase of the size of the bougie may be somewhat quicker, though never more quick than the patient can bear with ease. The increase should be continued till a bougie of the largest size passes freely ; nor should this be laid aside till after three weeks or a month, in order to habituate the dilated part to its new position, or to take off the habit of contracting from the part as much as possible. But, as was observed before, the permanency of this cure can seldom be depended upon.

Instead of proceeding with the caution recommended, it has been practised with success for a time to force a common-sized bougie through a stricture that only allowed a small one to pass.   This, I suppose, either tore the stricture or weakened it by stretching it suddenly so as to render it unable to recover its contractile power for a considerable time after. I have seen where this has produced good effects, and for a time removed the permanent stricture and prevented spasm. This is a practice, however, which I have never tried, having always preferred the mild treatment where I could pass a bougie.

I have known the passing of the bougie remove, almost immediately, a swelling of the testicle, which had arisen from the stricture ; therefore such a symptom should not prevent the use of the bougie.

In cases of strictures where the bougie is used, the patient is commonly in other respects well, and is with difficulty persuaded to restrain from his common habits, often making too free in eating, drinking, and exercise ; which are all in many cases pernicious, more especially where inflammation and suppuration have taken place.   It is, therefore, the duty of the surgeon to restrict the patient for some time within certain bounds, till he finds by trials what the parts are capable of bearing without producing inflammation.

§.3. Of the Cure of Stricture by Ulceration.

The cure of a stricture by means of ulceration is likewise effected by a bougie. This method may be employed both in cases where a bougie will and where it will not pass. In the first case there is not the same necessity for ulceration as in the second, because where a bougie will pass there is no immediate danger arising from the stricture, which may therefore be dilated, as has been already described. But if this method should be preferred to a slow dilatation, which allows the parts time to adapt themselves to their new position, the stricture may be destroyed by producing ulceration in the parts, especially if they are not irritable, but admit of considerable violence.

When this is intended, the bougie should be introduced as far into the stricture as possible, and the size of it increased as fast as the sensations of the patient can well bear. This will produce ulceration in the part pressed, which is a more lasting cure, because more of the stricture is destroyed than when the parts are simply dilated. I believe, however, there are few patients that will submit to this practice, and indeed few will be able to bear it; for I have seen it bring on violent spasms in the part, which have produced suppression of urine, and proved very troublesome. Therefore as there is no absolute necessity in such cases for pursuing this method, I do not recommend it as a general practice, although there have been cases in which it has succeeded. Where this method is to be practised, it might probably be right to accustom the passage to a bougie for some time before such violence is used.

If the smallest bougie which can possibly be made cannot be made to pass by some degree of force, dilatation becomes impracticable, and it is necessary that something else should be done for the relief of the patient; for the destruction of the stricture must be effected. In many cases it may be proper to attempt this by ulceration of the part; for we find from experience that a stricture may be removed by the simple pressure of a bougie. This effect must arise from the irritation of absorption being given to the diseased part, which, from the stricture not being an originally-formed part, nor having any power of resistance equal to the original one, is more susceptible of ulceration, and thereby is absorbed. The bougies, which are only to produce ulceration in consequence of their being applied to the stricture, need not be so small as in the former cases, as they are not intended to pass; and by being of a common size they will also be more certain in their application to the stricture. The force applied to a bougie in this case should not be great: for a stricture is the hardest part of the urethra; and if a bougie is applied with a considerable degree of pressure, and left in the passage, it sometimes happens that the end of it slips off the stricture before there is time for ulceration, and makes its way into the substance of the corpus spongiosum by the side of the stricture; and if the pressure be continued still longer, it will make a new passage beyond the stricture in the corpus spongiosum urethræ*. This more readily happens if the stricture be in the bend of the canal, as in such cases the bougie can hardly be applied exactly to it, not having the same curve. such mischief I have seen more than once; and sometimes the bougie has been pushed so far as to make its way into the rectum.

It often requires a considerable time before the whole is so far ulcerated as to admit the bougie, and this tires the patient and almost makes him despair of a cure. In this process great attention should be paid to the seeming progress of the cure; for if it appears to the surgeon that he is gaining ground by the bougie passing further in, and yet the patient does not make water better in the least, then he may be sure that he is forcing a new passage†.

When the stricture has so far yielded to these means as to admit a small bougie, the dilatation is to be made as in the former case where a bougie passed at first. Whenever a bougie of a tolerable size passes with ease, and the parts and patient have become accustomed to it, it is no longer necessary that the surgeon should continue to pass it: the patient may be allowed to introduce bougies himself; and when he can do it readily the business may be trusted to him, as he can make use of them at the most convenient times, so that they may be applied longer at a time and oftener, the surgeon only attending occasionally. This practice of the patient under a surgeon's eye, by which he is taught how to pass them, becomes more necessary, as strictures are diseases that commonly recur; and therefore no man, who has ever had a stricture, and is cured of it, should rely on the cure as lasting, but should be always prepared for a return; and should always have some bougies by him. He should not go a journey, even of a week, without them; and the number should be according to the time he is to be absent, or to the place whither he is going, for in many parts of the world he cannot be supplied with them. The bougies for such purpose should be of different sizes, as it is uncertain in what degree the disease may return.

Bougies, in all cases, from their shape and from the action of the parts, readily slip out, whereby the cure is retarded; but it is much worse when they pass into the bladder, which can only take place in cases where the stricture is in some measure overcome. The consequence of a bougie passing into the bladder must at once appear in its fullest force to every one: it subjects the patient in most cases to be

* Vide plate X.

† This makes it necessary in all cases of strictures where bougies will not pass to be very particular in our inquiries whether the patient has used bougies formerly, and whether there may not be reason to believe that they had taken a wrong direction.

cut as for the stone; and indeed if it is either not soon thrown out or cut out it becomes the basis of a stone. A young man was cut for a bougie only a fortnight after it had passed into the bladder, and it was almost wholly crusted over with calculous matter. Bougies have been known to be forced out of the bladder along with the water by the action of that viscus, and in several folds. It is probable that the bladder in a natural state has not power sufficient to perform such an action; but we shall show that in cases of strictures where the resistance to the passing of the water is very much increased, the strength of the bladder becomes proportionably greater. This happens principally in strictures of long standing.

Such accidents are often observed before the outer end of the bougie has got beyond the projecting part of the penis, but even then it is difficult of extraction. I have succeeded in some of these cases by fixing the bougie in the urethra some way below its end: for instance, in the perinæum, by pressing against it with one hand, and pushing back the penis upon the bougie with the other hand; then laying hold of the penis upon the bougie, removing the pressure below, and drawing the whole up; and, by performing these two motions alternately, I have been able to lay hold of the end of it. However, this does not always succeed; for when the bougie is either small, or becomes soft, it will not admit of the penis being pushed down upon it without bending; or if the thick end of the bougie has got beyond the moveable or projecting part of the penis, then this mode of treatment becomes impracticable. I have succeeded in these last cases with the forceps for extracting the stone out of the urethra; but if it has got into the bend of the urethra, this practice will also fail; and in such a state it would be most advisable to pass a catheter down to it, and cut upon that; and probably the above-mentioned forceps, introduced through the wound, might then lay hold of its end; or by cutting a little further, so as to expose some part of the bougie, it might be easily extracted, without the necessity of cutting into the bladder. This part of the operation, however, would be very difficult in a fat or lusty man.

To prevent the inconveniency of the bougie coming out or the mischief of its passing in, it is necessary to tie a soft cotton thread round that end of the bougie which is out of the urethra, and then round the root of the glans. This last part should be very loose, for an obvious reason; and the projecting part of the bougie should also be bent down upon the penis, which makes it both less troublesome and more secure.

§. 4. *Of the Application of a Caustic to Strictures.*

When a bougie can readily pass, there is no necessity for using any other method to remove the stricture; but there are too many cases where a bougie cannot be made to pass, or so seldom that it cannot be depended upon for a cure. This may arise from several causes. First, the stricture may be so tight as not to allow the smallest bougie to pass. Secondly, the orifice in the stricture may not be in a line with the urethra, which will make it uncertain, if not impossible, to pass a bougie. Thirdly, there may be no passage at all, it having been obliterated by disease, and the urine discharged by fistulæ in perinæo.

The first very rarely occurs : for if the passage in the stricture be in a line with the general canal, a small bougie will commonly pass; and although it may not readily do so upon every trial, it will be sufficient to make way for another bougie, which is all that is wanted.

The second case, where the canal is not in a line with the common passage, may arise from three causes. First, when the stricture is in the bend of the urethra, although the passage through it may be in the centre of the canal, yet as the bougie cannot have the exact curve, it will be very uncertain in its application. Secondly, from an irregularity in the formation of the stricture, which may throw the passage to one side, even in the straight part of the urethra; and thirdly, from ulceration having taken place, producing fistulæ in perinæo, which often make the canal irregular in its course.

The third case where the application of the caustic may be necessary is where there is no passage at all, which happens from ulceration and abscesses in the perinæum opening externally; and in the healing of them the passage is often closed up entirely. In all the above-mentioned cases I have succeeded with the caustic beyond expectation.

If the obstructions are anywhere between the membranous part of the urethra and the glans, where the canal is nearly straight, or can easily be made so by the introduction of a straight instrument, it becomes an easy matter to destroy them by caustic; but if beyond that, it becomes then more difficult. However, at the beginning of the bend of the urethra the obstruction may be so far removed as to admit of the passing of a bougie, or at least to procure a tolerably free passage for the urine. I have seen several cases where it was thought necessary to follow this practice; and it succeeded so well that after a few touches with the caustic the bougie could be passed, which is all that is wanted. The success in these cases was such as would incline me to have recourse to this practice very early; indeed whenever I could not pass a small bougie through the stricture. I look upon the caustic as a much safer method than using pressure with a bougie, for the reason before mentioned, that is, on account of the danger of making a new passage, without destroying in the least any part of the obstruction.

Most of the strictures which I have examined after death appeared to have been in the power of such treatment.   However, I have seen one or two cases where the contraction was of some length and irregular, which would have puzzled me if I had attempted the cure with the caustic; because I should have been apt to suspect that I was making a new passage by my gaining ground, and yet not relieving the patient by the removal of the symptoms.

I have often tried this practice in strictures where there were also fistulæ in the urethra, and where the water came through different passages.   Such cases were not the most favourable; yet I succeeded in the greater part of them, that is, I overcame the stricture and could pass a bougie freely.   I have seen several cases of fistulæ of these parts, where the natural passage was obliterated by the stricture, in which I have succeeded with the caustic, and the fistulous orifices have readily healed.

It does not happen always in cases of obstruction to the passage of the urine, that when the obstruction is removed by the caustic, and the water of course passes freely, a bougie will also pass.   This, I apprehend, arises from the caustic not having destroyed the stricture in a direct line with the urethra, so as to allow a bougie to catch the sound urethra beyond.   But this appears to me of little consequence, as it is as much in the power of the bougie to prevent a return at this part as if it had passed on to the bladder; for if the water flows readily it is certain that the caustic has gone beyond the stricture, although it may not be in the direct line, and that the only risk of a return of obstruction will be at the old stricture; but as a bougie can now pass beyond that part it does as much good as if it passed into the bladder; for I have known several cases where the bougie appeared to have the same effect as if it had passed on to the bladder.

The application of the caustic need not be longer than a minute, and it may be repeated every day, or every other day, allowing time for the slough to come off.   But there are other causes that may prevent the repetition of the caustic, besides waiting for the separation of the slough; for sometimes the use of it brings on irritation, inflammation, or spasm in the part, which frequently occasions a suppression of urine for a time, against which all the means used commonly on such occasions to procure relief must be employed, and we must wait till these symptoms are gone off.   If the patient can make water immediately after the application it will be proper, as it will wash away any caustic that may have been dissolved in the passage, which if left would irritate the parts. A little water injected into the urethra will answer the same purpose.

About the year 1752 I attended a chimney-sweeper labouring under a stricture. He was the first patient I ever had under this disease. Not finding that I gained any advantage after six months' trial with the bougie, I conceived that I might be able to destroy the stricture by escharotics*; and my first attempt was with red precipitate. I applied to the end of a bougie some salve, and then dipped it into red precipitate. This bougie I passed down to the stricture; but I found that it brought on considerable inflammation all along the inside of the passage, which I attributed to the precipitate being rubbed off in passing the bougie. I then introduced a silver cannula down to the stricture, and through this cannula passed the bougie with precipitate as before. Not finding, however, that the patient made water any better, and not as yet being able to pass the smallest bougie through the stricture, I suspected that the precipitate had not sufficient powers to destroy it. I therefore took a small piece of lunar caustic, and fastened it on the end of a wire with sealing-wax, and introduced it through the cannula to the stricture After having done this three times, at two days' interval, I found that the man voided his urine much more freely. Upon the application of the caustic a fourth time, my cannula went through the stricture†. A bougie was afterwards passed for some little time till he was perfectly well.

Having succeeded so well in this case, I was encouraged to apply my mind to the invention of some instrument better suited to the purpose than the before-mentioned, which I have in some degree effected, although it is not yet perfectly adapted to all the situations of stricture in the urethra. The caustic should be prevented from hurting any other part of the canal; which is best done by introducing it through a cannula to the stricture, making it protrude a little beyond the end of the cannula, by which it acts only upon the stricture. The caustic should be fixed in a small portcrayon. It is necessary to have a piece of silver of the length of the cannula, with a ring at one end, and a button at the other of the same diameter with the cannula, forming a kind of plug, which should project beyond the end of the cannula that enters the urethra, by which means it makes a rounded end; or the portcrayon may be formed with this button at the other end. The button being introduced into the cannula, it should be passed into the urethra, and when it reaches the stricture the silver plug should be withdrawn, and

---

* Having lately looked over some authors on this disease, I find that this is not a new idea.

† Wiseman had the same idea, but probably the clumsy way in which he attempted to put it in execution might be the reason why he seems not to have pursued it.

the portcrayon with the caustic introduced in its place; or, if the plug and portcrayon are on the same instrument, then it is only withdrawing the plug, and introducing the portcrayon with the caustic.   This plug, besides giving a smooth rounded edge to the cannula, answers another good purpose, by preventing the cannula from being filled with the mucus of the urethra as it passes along, which mucus would be collected in the end of it, dissolve the caustic too soon, and hinder its application to the stricture*.

If the stricture be in the bend of the urethra the cannula may be bent at the end also; but it becomes more difficult to introduce a piece of caustic through such a cannula, for the plug and portcrayon must also be bent at the end, which cannot be made to pass through the straight part of the cannula; but this I have in some measure obviated by having the cannula made flexible, except at the end where it is to take the curve †.

After the bougie can be made to pass, the case is to be treated as a common stricture, either by dilating it slowly, or by quickly increasing the size of the bougie, and thus continuing the ulceration.

There are sometimes more strictures than one; but it seldom happens that they are all equally strong.   One only becomes the object of our attention.   The smaller ones may, however, be sufficient to hinder the passing the cannula to that which is to be destroyed by the caustic. When that is the case, those small strictures are to be dilated with bougies, as in common, till they are sufficiently large to allow the cannula to pass‡ ᵃ.

---

* Vide Plate XI. fig. 1.   † Vide Plate XI. fig. 2 and 3.

‡ Added: " A. B., a soldier in the 16th regiment of light dragoons, had a stricture twenty years ago, and was in St. Thomas's Hospital: bougies were passed, and he got pretty well.   About eight years afterwards the stricture began to recur, and has been growing worse ever since, and for these two years past he has not been able to do his duty, the water only coming from him in drops.   In this state he applied to me. Finding the smallest bougie could not be made to pass, I desired that a full-sized one might be passed down to the stricture, and its end pressed against it, for as long a time and as often as he could bear with tolerable ease, and to continue this practice for some weeks.   This he did without any advantage.   Being now afraid of a total stoppage of urine without the common means of relief, and there being a sensation in the perinæum threatening inflammation, I resolved to use the caustic.   I applied it three times in the whole, at two days' interval; and after the last application, he told me he had made water much more freely and less frequently than before.   I introduced a bougie of the second or third size above the smallest, and it passed the stricture with great ease into the bladder.   I then ordered him to pass the bougie, and increase it gradually till he could use the largest, which he did; and he is now perfectly well."—*Home.*

ᵃ [Since the time when Mr. Hunter wrote, the use of caustic in the cure of stricture has been greatly extended, chiefly through the labours of Sir E. Home, whose valuable

CHAPTER III.

OF STRICTURES IN WOMEN.

OBSTRUCTIONS to the urine in women, I believe, generally arise from stricture, although not always; for I have known them produced by

---

work on strictures in the urethra and œsophagus should be consulted by all who wish to be acquainted with its various effects in detail.

The mode of applying the caustic has been greatly improved. The use of the cannula has been discarded, and an *armed* bougie has been substituted in its place; that is, a small piece of nitrate of silver has been let into a common bougie, in such a manner as to present only on the surface of the extremity, and to be encircled on all sides by the plaster of which the bougie is composed. This instrument can be applied with far greater accuracy than the cannula; the bougie can with ease be adapted to the curvature of the urethra, and the sides of the canal are protected from the action of the caustic. It appears that this contrivance was invented by Mr. Hunter himself, who employed it many years before his death in preference to that which he has detailed in this work.

When it is intended to apply the caustic, it is necessary in the first instance to pass down to the stricture a common bougie, of such a size as moderately to fill the passage, and composed of such soft materials as readily to receive the impression of the part against which it is pressed. By first introducing this bougie, and keeping it for the space of a minute pressed against the stricture, the surgeon obtains several advantages. The urethra is opened, and the subsequent passage of the armed bougie rendered more easy and rapid; the exact distance of the stricture from the orifice is ascertained; and such a cast is taken of the stricture as to show accurately its size and shape, and to ascertain what effect has been produced by previous applications of the caustic. This information is so necessary that without it the treatment by caustic could not be pursued. The destruction of the disease is frequently partial and irregular. The armed bougie, notwithstanding every precaution, is sometimes not applied accurately on the orifice, or the caustic is dissolved in the moisture of the passage, and runs down to the lower part of the urethra, leaving the upper part almost untouched. These deviations must be accurately ascertained, in order that they may be corrected in subsequent applications.

After this previous step, the armed bougie is to be introduced, the distance of the stricture having been first marked upon it. It should be of such a size as to fill the urethra, and should be pressed against the part for the space of a quarter of a minute or more. The time should be partly regulated by the sensations of the patient. As soon as a burning pain begins to be felt, it should be withdrawn. The use of the caustic should not be repeated oftener than every third or fourth day, since that interval must be allowed for the separation of the slough.

The effects of caustic on strictures have been found in practice to be somewhat different from those which were anticipated by its first proposers. Its first and great effect is the relief of spasm. The morbid irritability of the part is exhausted by the violence of the stimulus. When the contraction is merely spasmodic, it is in most instances entirely removed by one or two applications. All difficulty of voiding the urine then disappears, and a full-sized bougie can be passed readily into the bladder. When there

compression from some adjacent swelling, and they are common in uterogestation, as also in dropsical or scirrhous ovaria. But such causes are commonly known long before this effect is produced, by which the suppression is easily accounted for. It may also arise from excrescences as in men.

How far a stricture in the urethra of this sex is really a consequence of a venereal inflammation I am not certain; but I should suppose it is not, and for stronger reasons still than those which I gave in speaking of the cause of strictures in men; for I can say that none of the strictures that I have seen in women have arisen in consequence of this disease, at least I had no reason to believe that they did; and I have observed before that in most women who have the venereal disease in the form of a gonorrhœa, it seldom attacks the urethra. Therefore, if we find a stricture in a woman who has had the disease, we are not to im-

is a permanent stricture which is more or less affected with spasm, the spasm will be relieved as speedily, but the permanent contraction will remain. The stricture will not be removed, but its irritability will be lessened. The opening will be enlarged so as to admit a larger instrument than before, but it will not be dilated to the natural size of the urethra.

These effects are obtained by one or two applications of the caustic as perfectly as by a longer continuance of its use. The actual destruction of the stricture is a very slow process, and in old indurated strictures is scarcely attainable. The slough which is produced by the nitrate of silver is very superficial, and no material destruction can be effected without numerous repetitions of the remedy. In the mean time there is much danger of deviating from the true direction of the urethra, and the patient is subject to very serious accidents during the course.

Of these accidents the first is retention of urine, which is a very common consequence of caustic. It arises sometimes from the violence of the irritation, but at other times it appears to be derived from the obstruction which is given by the slough, which during the process of suppuration hangs like a fringe from the edge of the stricture, and where the opening is small seems to oppose a mechanical obstacle to the flow of the urine. Hæmorrhage is another effect which is of frequent occurrence, and often proceeds to a most formidable extent. This symptom however, though very alarming to the patient, is never fatal, and as it invariably facilitates the cure, it can scarcely be considered as undesirable. Again, caustic very frequently occasions rigors, especially in those who have previously suffered from them; and it is by no means rare that its use should be followed by the occurrence of an abscess in the perinæum.

Moreover, caustic has no advantage over bougies in respect to the permanent cure of the malady. Experience has fully proved that after a stricture has been removed by caustic, bougies are still necessary, and that unless they are occasionally passed it is almost certain to recur.

For these reasons the treatment by caustic has of late lost much of its former celebrity. Even those advantages which in some cases it unquestionably possesses have been insufficient to prevent it from falling more and more into disuse. Surgeons now generally prefer the treatment by bougies, which effects the same objects, sometimes indeed more slowly, but on the whole more certainly, and with less inconvenience and hazard.]

pute it to that, at least till we can ascertain the urethra was affected; and even then it will remain doubtful.

Strictures are not near so common in women as in men. This may be owing to the great difference in the length of the two canals; but more especially to the canal in women being more simple, and intended only for one purpose. The stricture in women does not produce such a variety of symptoms, or so much mischief, as in men, there not being so many parts to be affected.

§. 1. *Of the Cure of Strictures in Women.*

The cure of strictures in the urethra of women is similar to that in men; but it is rather more simple, from the simplicity of the parts. There is, however, an inconvenience attending the passing the bougie in women that does not occur in men, which is, that in most cases it must be passed for them, it being hardly possible for a woman to introduce a bougie herself. The confinement of the bougie is also more difficult; for although it can easily be prevented from going into the bladder by bending the outer end down upon the mouth of the vagina, yet it is very difficult to prevent it from slipping out. It will be necessary to have a bandage of the T kind passing down between the labia over the bend of the bougie.

It appears to me that the caustic would answer extremely well in such cases; and therefore I should prefer it to the bougie, both for convenience and efficacy.

§. 2. *Of the Gleet in consequence of a Stricture.*

I have already observed that it happens generally, if not always, that there is a gleet when there is a stricture in the urethra. This I suppose to arise from the irritation produced in the urethra beyond the stricture, by the urine in its passage distending this part too much, which distention is increased by the increased strength of the bladder. This symptom often leads us to the knowledge of a stricture, or at least gives a suspicion of such a disease; and when a stricture is known to be the cause, no attempts should be made to cure the gleet, for it is generally cured when the stricture is removed; but if it still remains, it may be cured in the manner recommended in the common gleet, as probably arising from a cause different from stricture.

CHAPTER IV.

OF STRICTURE ATTENDED WITH SPASMODIC AFFECTION.

THERE are very few strictures that are not more or less attended with spasms; but some much more than others, the spasm being in some cases more the disease than the stricture itself. But real strictures are attended with occasional contractions, which make the passing of the urine much more difficult at one time than another. In all the cases that I have seen of this kind, when not attended with spasms the disease is not formidable; but when the parts are in a spasmodic state the symptoms are as violent as in the simple stricture.

As this is a mixed case, it has all the characters both of the permanent and spasmodic stricture; for the urethra in such circumstances is in a state similar to what it is in the true spasmodic kind, being very irritable, giving great pain in the passing of the bougie, and often rejecting it altogether: as will be taken notice of when we shall treat of that disease.

Upon considering this subject, we should at first hardly be disposed to believe that the spasm in the urethra is in the strictured part, which can scarcely be supposed capable of contraction; and it might therefore naturally be referred to the sound part of the urethra, as being brought on by the waters not flowing freely. If this is a just mode of accounting for it, we must suppose that the contraction is behind the stricture, that being the only part dilated by the water; and such urethras being very irritable, that part may contract so as to stop the flowing of the water altogether. But some circumstances that occur in practice give reason to believe that such strictures have the power of contraction; for we find the bougie grasped by the stricture when allowed to remain some time, and the circumstance of the strictured parts refusing the bougie at times is also a proof of the same.

There is sometimes this singular circumstance attending these cases, that when there arises a gonorrhœa, or any other discharge of matter from the urethra, or an increase of an old gleet, the passage becomes free and allows the urine to pass as usual; but such relief is uncertain and only temporary, for whenever the discharge ceases the spasmodic affection returns. I think it is probable that it is only the spasm that is affected by the discharge, and not the real stricture. Two remarkable cases of this kind fell under my observation, which I shall now relate.

A gentleman had for a long time a complaint in the urethra, attended with a stricture, which was supposed to be originally from a venereal complaint. It was often attended with a discharge, which always produced a slight fever on its coming on; but while the discharge lasted the difficulty of making water was relieved, and that in proportion to the greatness of the discharge; and whenever he got a fresh gonorrhœa the same thing happened.

Another gentleman had a difficulty in making water, supposed to arise from a stricture. It was generally attended with such a running as is common to strictures; but when that discharge was much increased then the stricture was less in proportion. During this complaint he contracted two different infections, both of which relieved him of the stricture for the time.

As this is a mixed disease, it may be thought proper to treat it with a bougie for the real stricture, and for the other to use the method to be recommended hereafter for the cure of spasm.

It sometimes happens in these mixed kinds that a bougie does not immediately pass, but is rejected by the spasm; but by letting it lie in the urethra, almost close to the stricture, for ten, fifteen, or twenty minutes, you will often make it pass. This is as it were stealing upon it, and the water will often flow although the bougie is not attempted to be passed on. It is often relieved by gently irritating injections*.

CHAPTER V.

OF SOME CIRCUMSTANCES ATTENDING THE USE OF BOUGIES; THEIR FIGURE AND COMPOSITION.

In cases of strictures, where a bougie is used as a wedge, not as a stimulant, and where a stricture is so far overcome as to let a bougie pass on, the question is whether it may be better to pass the bougie through the whole length of the urethra, so that the end of it shall be in the

---

* Added: " A gonorrhœa or occasional gleet relieves the spasmodic state of a stricture upon the same principle as the passing a bougie a few inches down the urethra: the irritation near the glans penis takes off the spasm upon another part of the canal."
—*Home.*

bladder, or only to pass it through the stricture a little way, so that its end shall remain in the urethra. Nothing but experience can determine this question; and, perhaps, in such cases we seldom make a fair trial, generally pushing the bougie on to the bladder; though, if we observe the consequences of bougies not passing in those cases where they either cannot pass far beyond the stricture or not at all, we find no inconvenience arising from this circumstance, except when they are applied with too much force, so as to make a new passage. The common idea is that it will be more hurtful to allow the end of the bougie to lie in the urethra than in the bladder; but this seems to be more founded in theory than practice.

Some people have such a quantity of calculous matter in their urine, or so great a disposition in their urine to deposit its calculous matter, that it only requires the presence of an extraneous body in the bladder to become an immediate cause of stone; for I have observed in some that the end of a bougie cannot remain in the bladder a few hours without being covered with a crust of calculous matter. Such people I have generally advised to use as much exercise as all other circumstances will allow.

Bougies, when first introduced, often produce sickness, and sometimes even fainting. I have seen a patient become sick, the colour leave his face, a cold sweat come on, and at last a deliquium; but all these effects soon go off, and seldom return upon a second or third trial. They at first produce an irritation on the urethra, which gives pain in the time of making water, but goes off on repetition. They produce a secretion of pus in those cases where there was none, and generally increase the discharge where there is one previous to the application of them; but this effect gradually ceases.

It frequently happens that swellings in the lymphatic glands of the groin arise from the use of bougies, but I never saw them advance to suppuration. As in most of such cases there is a discharge of matter previous to the bougie being passed, they can hardly be owing to the absorption of matter, but must arise from sympathy.

When treating of the stricture I observed that it was often the cause of a swelling in one or both testicles; and further, that the passing of a bougie often removed that complaint. I may now observe that a very common consequence of the passing a bougie is a swelling of the testicle. This also arises from sympathy, and, like the swelling of the glands, is a common effect of all irritations of the urethra*.

It may not be improper here to add some observations on the figure

* Added: " A gentleman who has had a stricture for many years, which at times is attended with a great deal of spasm, but has never any irritation in the testicles, upon

and composition of bougies. They ought to be about two inches longer than the distance between the glans and the stricture, or more if they can pass freely, so as always to allow an inch to bend upon the glans, and another to pass beyond the stricture. The thickness should be according to the size of the stricture ; at first such as will pass with a small degree of tightness, and this should be gradually increased as the contracted part enlarges. But when the urethra has become of the natural size the bougie need not be further increased, but its use still continued, as has been observed.

With regard to the shape, they should not taper from end to end when very small, but should be nearly of an equal thickness till within an inch of their smallest end, after which they should taper to a point, forming a round wedge fitted to pass into the stricture; and this form gives them greater strength than when made to taper from one end to the other.

The consistence ought to vary according to the nature of the case and size of the bougie. If the stricture be near the glans, a stiff bougie may be used, and the whole may be made to taper gradually, because a short bougie will always have sufficient strength for any pressure that is necessary; but if the stricture be more deeply seated, as about the bulb, where the passage begins to take a curve, the bougie must be a little thicker in its body to support the necessary pressure. If the stricture be anywhere in the bend of the urethra, or near the bladder, the bougie should be very flexible (although this is contrary to our general position), because in this case it must bend in order to adapt itself to the curve of the passage, which it ought to do with ease: for when it bends with difficulty it does not make its pressure upon the stricture, but upon the back part of the urethra, and therefore does not enter so easily, which circumstance makes it more difficult to enter a stricture near the bladder than near the glans. In the composition of the bougie the consistence is the most material thing to be considered, the medical properties, as far as known, being of little consequence. The materials of which they are commonly made are wax, oil, and litharge. The litharge gives them smoothness, and takes off the adhesive quality which they would have if made of wax and oil only. A composition which answers well is three pints of oil of olives, one pound of beeswax, and a pound and a half of red lead, boiled together upon a slow fire for six hours.

my passing a bougie smeared with a stimulating oil for a few minutes to remove the spasm, an irritation and swelling of the left testicle came on. He afterwards caught a gonorrhœa, which entirely removed the spasm while it lasted, but also brought on a swelling of the testicle."—*Home.*

§. 1. *Of a new Passage formed by Bougies.*

The greatest evil arising from the improper use of the bougie, and the most dangerous, is where it makes a new passage*. I mentioned before that this generally rose from an attempt to produce ulceration by the application of the end of the bougie to the stricture in cases where a bougie could not pass; for in those cases where a bougie passes there can be no danger of such an effect.

This new passage is seldom carried so far as to produce either an increase of the present disease or a new one, although sometimes this happens; yet it prevents the cure of the original disease, for it renders both the application of the bougie and caustic to the stricture so uncertain that a continuance of either is dangerous, as it may increase the mischief and at last produce very bad consequences.

This new passage is generally along the side of the old one when in that part of the urethra which is on this side of the bend, and it is made in the spongy substance of the urethra; but when it is made at the beginning of the bend, it passes on in a straight line through the body of the urethra, about the beginning of the membranous part, and goes through the cellular substance of the perinæum towards the rectum. When the new passage is made between the glans and the bend of the urethra, it may take place on either side of the canal equally, in the spongy substance of the urethra; between the canal and the skin of the penis or scrotum; and it may be between the canal and the body of the penis. The situation of it will make some difference in the operation necessary for the cure of this complaint.

When a new passage is made I know of no other method of cure than to open the part externally; and the opening must be made in that part of the urethra which is most convenient for coming at the stricture, regard being had to the other external parts, such as the scrotum. If the stricture be before the scrotum the new passage will be there also, and therefore the operation must be made of course before that part; but if the stricture is opposite to the scrotum, the bottom of the new passage may also be opposite to this part; but if the new passage is of a considerable length, its bottom or termination may be in the beginning of the perinæum; and in either situation the operation must be begun behind the scrotum, or indeed may be made a little way into it. But if the stricture and new passage are in the perinæum, then the operation is to be performed there.

* Vide Plate X.

The method of performing this operation is as follows. Pass a staff, or any such instrument, into the urethra as far as it will go, which will probably be to the bottom of the new passage, and that we may be certain is beyond the stricture. Feel for the end of the instrument externally, and cut upon it, making the wound about an inch long if the disease be before the scrotum, and an inch and a half, or more, if in the perinæum. If the new passage be between the urethra and the body of the penis, then you will most probably get into the sound urethra before you come to the instrument or new passage; if so, it is not necessary to go further in order to get into the bladder, as we may be certain that this part of the urethra is behind the stricture. Having proceeded so far, take a probe, or some such instrument, and introduce it into the urethra, by the wound, and pass it towards the glans, which will be passing it forwards towards the stricture. If it meet with an obstruction there, we mav be certain it is the stricture, which is now to be got through, and which will afterwards be easily enlarged. To complete the operation, withdraw the probe, and introduce in the room of it a hollow cannula forwards to the stricture; then take another cannula and introduce it from the glans downwards till the two cannulas oppose each other, having the stricture between them, an assistant laying hold of the urethra on the outside, between the finger and thumb, just where the two cannulas meet, to keep them in their places; then through the upper cannula introduce a piercer, which will go through the stricture, and pass into the lower cannula; this done, withdraw the piercer, and introduce a bougie into the same cannula in the same way, being careful that it passes into the lower cannula; then withdraw the lower cannula, and the end of the bougie will appear in the wound; lay hold of the bougie there, and withdraw the upper cannula over the bougie, leaving the bougie in the urethra: now the lower end of the bougie is to be directed into the urethra leading on to the bladder, and pushed on to that viscus. It may be further necessary to lay the whole of the new passage open, that it may all heal up; for it is possible that this new passage may often receive the bougie, to be applied in future, which would be troublesome, and might prove an obstruction to the cure.

If the new passage be between the skin and the canal of the urethra, after cutting down to the instrument, you must go further on in search of the natural canal, and, when you have found it, introduce a probe into it towards the glans, to find the stricture; and when this is done go on with the operation as above described.

The bougie must be left in the passage, and as it may be found difficult afterwards to introduce another readily into the bladder, the longer the first is allowed to remain so much the more readily will the second pass.   I am not yet certain but that it would be better to push on the hollow cannula at first, and keep it there for some days, at least till the inflammation is over, and the parts have adapted themselves to that body, which will make a bougie pass more easily afterwards. The bougies must be gradually increased in size, and continued till the wound is healed up.

The first case of a new passage formed by a bougie which I ever saw was at the hospital of the third regiment of guards, about the year 1765. A young soldier had a stricture, for the cure of which he had bougies regularly passed for near half a year without any relief. The bougie had gone further than at first by two inches, and therefore seemed to have gained ground on the stricture.   This seemed to justify the continuance of the practice; but it being suspected that there was something more than was then understood, I was consulted, and without foreseeing what was really the case, I proposed that an opening should be made into the urethra where the obstruction was, and carried further back if necessary, in search of the sound urethra. This was accordingly done in the following manner: the grooved staff was first passed as far down as it could go, which was to the bottom of the new passage; the scrotum was pulled up upon the penis, when the end of the staff was prominent towards the skin a little way above the perinæum, and there an incision was made on the end of the staff about half an inch long; this disengaged the end of the staff, which was pushed out at the wound; then search was made for the other orifice which led to the bladder, on a supposition that that orifice was the stricture; but none being to be found, we tried to trace it by blowing with a blowpipe into the bottom and lower part of the wound; but no orifice could be observed. We then began to suspect that we were not in the urethra. To determine if we had been in the urethra, I began to dissect with care the parts at the bottom of the wound, and laid bare the musculi acceleratores. I then made an incision into the body of the urethra and came to the true canal, which was easily discovered. When this was done we passed a probe on to the bladder, then withdrew, turned, and passed it from this wound towards the glans penis, but found that it went not much more than two inches that way, and then stopped. This struck us with a new idea of the case, for we were now sure that the end of the staff had not been in the urethra, but in a new passage made in the spongy part of the urethra, for two inches beyond the stricture. We now passed a staff from the glans down the urethra, and another up from the last wound, to see at what distance the ends of the two instruments were, which would give us the length of the stricture. We found, by taking hold of the urethra between the finger and thumb on the outside, that the two ends were close together.   What was to be done next was our consideration; it immediately struck us that we might force our way through the stricture with safety.   The gentleman who assisted me in the operation passed a blowpipe one fifth of an inch in diameter (being not sufficiently furnished with instruments,) from the wound forwards to the stricture; and then I took a silver cannula, open at both ends, which had an iron piercer longer than itself, and passed it down to the stricture from the glans; and now the end of the cannula opposed the end of the blowpipe, and they were almost close upon one another. They were kept in this position, with the finger and thumb applied on the outside of the penis, like splints on a broken bone.   I then introduced the piercer and pushed it on, which went through the stricture into the hollow of the blowpipe.   Great care was taken not to push too forcibly, lest the two ends of the hollow tubes should slip by one another, which they would do if not held firmly, as actually happened twice in this case; but we succeeded the third time.   I then pushed on the cannula through the stricture, and with it pushed out the blowpipe. The next object was to pass a hollow bougie along the urethra to the bladder, to do which the small end of it was introduced into the cannula, which being pushed on forced out the cannula at the wound; we then passed a director into the other orifice of the urethra, leading on to the bladder, and put the end of the bougie into the groove of the director, and pushed it along the groove to the bladder; and before we withdrew the director we turned it round with its back to the bougie, that the end of the bougie might not stop against the end of the groove, and so be pulled out again.   After all this was done one stitch was made in the urethra, but the external wound in the skin was left for the passage of the urine, that it might not insinuate itself into the cellular membrane.   We dressed the wound superficially, and applied the T bandage, which was slit to go on each side of the scrotum, and just where it came to the scrotum we tied the two ends together, which supported the scrotum and kept it forwards on the penis; and the two ends that came from this knot on each side of the scrotum were tied to the circular part that came round the body.   The patient had some slight fever for a day or two, and the urine came partly through the bougie and partly by the side of it, through the wound.   A swelling of one testicle came on; likewise a swelling of the glands of the groin, pain in the belly, sickness, and at times vomiting, all which symptoms were owing to sympathy, and entirely went off in five or six days.   The water, in nearly the same time, came entirely by the natural passage. The bougie was changed from time to time till the cure was completed.

CHAPTER VI.

OF DISEASES IN CONSEQUENCE OF A PERMANENT STRICTURE IN THE URETHRA.

STRICTURES in the urethra produce almost constantly diseases in the parts beyond them; that is, in the part of the urethra between the stricture and the bladder. They bring on in most cases a gleet, as has been described, and often a considerable distension of the part of the canal beyond the stricture; also inflammation and ulceration, and in consequence of them diseases in the surrounding parts, as in Cowper's glands, the prostate, and the surrounding cellular membrane, forming abscesses there, and at last ulceration, for the purpose of making a new passage for the urine. The bladder is also often affected, and sometimes the ureters, with the pelvis of the kidneys, and in some cases the kidneys themselves. All these are effects of every permanent obstruction to the urine; some of them are methods which Nature takes to relieve the parts from the immediate complaints; such are the increase of the urethra beyond the stricture, and the enlargement of the ureters and pelvis of the kidneys, which are only to be considered as the parts accommodating themselves to the immediate consequence of the obstruction, which is the accumulation of urine. Of these complaints I shall take notice in their order.

§. 1. *Of the Enlargement of the Urethra.*

The urethra beyond the stricture I have observed is enlarged, because it is more passive than the bladder, and yields to the pressure of the urine. It is naturally passive while the bladder is acting, by which means it becomes distended in proportion to the force with which the bladder acts, and the resistance of the stricture. Its internal surface often becomes more irregular and fasciculated. It is also more irritable, the distension becoming often the immediate cause of spasms in that part, and these spasms are most probably excited with a view to counteract the effort produced by the action of the bladder.

§. 2. *Of the Formation of a New Passage for the Urine.*

When the methods recommended above for the removal of stricture have either not been attempted or have not succeeded, Nature endeavours to relieve herself by making a new passage for the urine, which, although it often prevents immediate death, yet, if not remedied, is productive of much inconvenience and misery to the patient through life. The mode by which Nature endeavours to procure relief is by ulceration on the inside of that part of the urethra which is enlarged and within the stricture. The ulceration commonly begins near or close to the stricture, although the stricture may be at a considerable distance from the bladder ; therefore we must suppose that there is some circumstance besides the distension of the urethra by the urine, which determines the ulceration to a particular part. This circumstance most probably arises immediately out of its vicinity to the stricture, and may be called contiguous sympathy. The stricture is often included in the ulceration, by which it is removed, the disease cured, and a stop sometimes put to the further ulceration ; but unluckily this is not always the case. We may observe that this ulceration is always on the side next to the external surface, as is common in abscesses.

As this ulceration does not arise from preceding inflammation, and as it cannot be said that the urine acts exactly as an extraneous body, because it is in its natural passage, we find that there is but very little inflammation of the adhesive kind attending these ulcerations. We must allow, however, that the urine produces the ulcerative disposition here, like matter on the inside of an abscess, although not so readily.

Whenever, therefore, the internal membrane and substance of the urethra are removed by absorption, the water readily gets into the loose cellular membrane of the scrotum and penis, and diffuses itself all over those parts, not having been previously united by the adhesive inflammation ; and as the urine has considerable irritating powers when applied to the common cellular membrane, the parts inflame and swell. The presence of the urine prevents the adhesive inflammation from taking place ; it becomes the cause of suppuration wherever it is diffused ; and the irritation is often so great, more especially in cases where the urine has been allowed to become very stale, that it produces mortification, first in all the cellular membrane, and afterwards in several parts of the skin, all of which, if the patient live, slough away, making a free communication between the urethra and external surface, and produce fistulæ in perinæo.

We may observe, however, that the want of the adhesive inflamma

tion in these ulcerations appears to be peculiar to that part of the urethra which lies between the membranous part and the glans penis; for
we find from experience that when this process takes place further back,
as in the prostate gland, a circumscribed abscess is generally formed.
This may arise from the difference in texture of the cellular membrane
of the parts, the first admitting of the diffusion of the urine very readily
from the looseness of its texture, the other producing adhesions before
the urine is allowed to pass, which adhesions afterwards exclude it.

It sometimes happens that the urine gets into the spongy substance
of the body of the urethra, and is immediately diffused through the
whole, even to the glans penis, producing mortification of all those
parts, as I have more than once seen.

When the urine has made its way into the cellular membrane, although
the ulceration of the urethra is in the perinæum, yet it generally passes
easily forwards into the scrotum, that part being composed of the loosest
cellular membrane in the body. When the seat of the ulceration is in
the membranous or bulbous part of the urethra, and the pus and urine
have found their way to the scrotum, there is always a hardness extended along the perinæum to the swelled scrotum, which is in the tract
of the pus.

Ulceration cannot be prevented but by destroying the stricture; but
when the water is in the cellular membrane, which is the state we have
been describing, the removal of the stricture will in general be too late
to prevent all the mischief although it will be necessary for the complete cure; therefore an attempt should be made to pass a bougie, for
perhaps the stricture may be included in the ulceration (as was mentioned before), and thereby allow a bougie to pass. When this is the
case, bougies must be almost constantly used to procure as free a passage
forwards in the right way as possible. Where the bougie will not pass,
I am afraid that the caustic, as described in the case of a stricture,
would in many cases be too slow in its operation, and in others it cannot be tried, as the situation of the stricture is often such as will not
admit of it.

While we are attempting the cure of the stricture every method is
to be used that removes inflammation, particularly bleeding. Great relief may be obtained by exposing the parts to the steam of hot water;
but this is merely a palliative cure. The warm bath, opium, and the
turpentines, given by the mouth, and also by the anus, will assist in
taking off any spasmodic affection; but all these are too often insufficient, and therefore immediate relief must be attempted, both to unload
the bladder, and prevent any further effusion of urine into the cellular
membrane. This must be done by an operation, which consists in

making an opening into the urethra somewhere beyond the stricture, and the nearer to the stricture the better.

The method of performing the operation is first to pass a director or some such instrument into the urethra, as far as the stricture; then to make the end of the instrument as prominent externally as possible, so as to be felt, which in such a case is often difficult, and sometimes impossible. If it can be felt, it must be cut upon, and the incision carried on a little further towards the bladder or anus, so as to open the urethra beyond the stricture; this will be sufficient to allow the urine to escape, and to destroy the stricture. If the instrument cannot be felt at first by the finger, we must cut down towards it, which will bring it within the feel of the finger, and afterwards proceed as above directed.

If the stricture in the urethra be opposite to the scrotum, it being impossible to make the opening there, it must be made in the perinæum, in which case there can be no direction given by an instrument, as one cannot be made to pass so far; therefore we must be guided by our knowledge of the parts. The opening being made, the stricture is to be searched for as described in the operation, in cases where a false passage has been made, by passing a probe from the wound forwards, towards the glans. The other steps of the operation will be nearly the same. In whichsoever way the operation is performed a bougie must be introduced, and the wound healed up over it. In my opinion a catheter answers this purpose better.

Great attention should be still paid to the inflammation, which arises in consequence of the urine having been diffused in the cellular membrane, as before described. Where the inflammation is attended with suppuration and mortification, it will be necessary, as well in this case as in that where no operation is required, to scarify the parts freely, to give an opening both to the urine and pus. Where mortification has taken place in the skin, the scarifications should be made in the mortified parts, if it can be done with equal advantage, and this with a view to prevent irritation.

In total suppressions of urine, from whatever cause, the urine should never be allowed to accumulate, and should either be drawn off frequently, or a catheter should be kept continually in the urethra and bladder, because we should on no account allow the bladder to be distended beyond an easy state; for if it be, it always brings on debilitating and alarming symptoms, as paralysis of that viscus. In many suppressions of urine, as in cases of strictures, it is impossible to draw off the water. In some cases where the urethra is ulcerated, and the urine gets into the cellular membrane of the penis and prepuce, so as to distend them much, producing a phimosis, it becomes impossible to find the orifice of the urethra. The following case illustrates most of the preceding doctrines.

A gentleman of a scrofulous habit had often had venereal gonorrhœas, which, being severe, commonly produced swellings, or knobs, along the urethra, upon which account he was advised to avoid this disease as much as possible. When in the country, in November 1782, he was attacked with a slight cold or fever, and a small discharge from the urethra, which he could not determine to be venereal. In this state he set out for London, but was seized on the road with a suppression of urine, which detained him two days at an inn. On his arrival in London I found him feverish. He spoke to me only of a discharge from the urethra; but as I did not conceive that the fever could arise from that cause, I desired him to be easy on that account. He was taken with a shivering fit, which made us suspect it might terminate in an intermittent, and we waited for the result. He still complained of the discharge, and mentioned a soreness in the perinæum, both when he made water and when he pressed it externally. On examining the perinæum, I found a fulness there, from which I suspected a stricture, and inquired particularly how he made water in common; he declared very well, which led me from the true cause. This swelling was regarded as the effect of an inflammation, either in consequence of the fever, the disposition of the part, or both, increased by sitting in a postchaise for several days. The part was fomented and poulticed, and leeches were applied several times. He had another shivering fit three days after the first, which, if his disease had been an intermittent, would have constituted a quartan; but he had another some hours after, which made us give up our suspicions of an intermittent. We now began to suspect that matter was forming in this part, although I could not feel anything like a fluctuation; nor was the pain of the throbbing kind, or so acute as we commonly find it in the suppurative inflammation. What in some degree surprised me was, that the swelling came forwards along the body of the penis towards the os pubis, while it seemed to be diminishing in the perinæum. He now began to find a difficulty in making water, with a frequent desire, which increased till there was a total suppression. I pressed on the lower part of the belly to determine whether or not the urine was secreted and accumulated in the bladder; but I could not find any fulness; nor did he then feel pain on such pressure: however, about twenty-four hours after he began to complain of a great desire to make water, and a pain in the lower part of his belly; and the hand being placed there, a fulness of the bladder was readily felt. It was now clear that the water ought to be drawn off; but as I still suspected mischief in the urethra as a cause in his complaint, I took

the necessary precautions. I provided myself with catheters and bougies of different sizes; and to be as much upon my guard as possible,
I introduced a bougie of a small size first, and found a full stop about
the bulbous part of the urethra; I then took a smaller, which passed, but
with difficulty. I afterwards passed a small catheter on to the stricture,
where it stopped; but as it was absolutely necessary that the water
should be drawn off, I used more force than I otherwise should have
done : it went on, but with difficulty, and I was not certain whether it
was in the natural passage or was making a new one.   When the bougie had gone so far as certainly (if in the right passage,) to have entered
the bladder, I found that no water came; I therefore pressed the lower
part of the belly, and the water immediately came out through the catheter, whence it appeared that the bladder had lost its power of contraction. The water was drawn off three times every day, that is, every
eight hours, to give as much ease to the bladder as possible; but still it
was necessary to press the belly, to assist the discharge of the urine;
and it was upwards of a fortnight before the bladder began to recover
its power of contracting. The swelling in the perinæum still continued,
advancing along the body of the penis, and spreading a little on the
pubes; it seemed to extend along the projecting part of the penis, and
at last filled the whole cellular membrane of the prepuce, but did not in
the least affect the scrotum. This swelling appeared to be owing to
the urine having found its way into the cellular membrane of the perinæum, and from thence proceeding along the side of the penis. When the
prepuce became much loaded with water, a very considerable phimosis
took place, which made the introduction of the catheter into the orifice
of the urethra very uncertain; so much did the swelled prepuce project
over the glans.   I was obliged to squeeze the water back into the body
of the penis, and introduce a finger, and feel for the glans, and on this
finger introduce the catheter; and in a few minutes I generally found the
orifice.

The nature of the case was now plain; for ulceration had taken place
beyond the stricture, and the swelling had arisen from the urine having
insinuated itself into the cellular membrane of the perinæum; and as
the urine escaped from the urethra, it was pushed forwards where the
cellular membrane was loosest, till it got to the very end of the prepuce
as before mentioned.

By this time he was become extremely low and irritable; his pulse
quick and small; his tongue brown, dry, and contracted; his appetite
gone, with great drought, bad sleep, and the first stages of a delirium
coming on. This discovery of the true state of the case gave a change
to the mode of treatment. Instead of evacuations to lessen inflamma-

tion, the bark and cordials were given, with as much food as his stomach would bear. Their effects on the constitution were almost immediate, and he began to recover, although but slowly. I made two
punctures in the phimosis at the extremity, with a view both to take off
the tension and to evacuate the urine from the cellular membrane, between the penis and the skin.

Blisters began to form on the skin of the penis, and at last mortification took place in several parts, especially on the prepuce, which I divided at the mortified parts, and thereby the glans became exposed, so
that the catheter could now be introduced easily.

Upon squeezing the swelling, from the perinæum forwards along the
penis, I could force out at the mortified parts, air, water, and some
matter. The cellular membrane under the skin was almost wholly mortified. When bounds were set to the mortification, the sloughing cellular membrane began to separate; and a good deal was cut away to
keep the parts clean, and to allow of a freer vent for the matter. Now
that separation was taking place, it was clear that no more water from
the bladder could insinuate itself any further into the surrounding cellular membrane; therefore it was not necessary to pass the catheter any
more, and the patient was allowed to make water whenever he had a
call, which when he did, the water came both ways, through the urethra and through the cellular membrane, at the openings where the skin
had sloughed off. As the sloughs separated they came forwards from
behind, at the side of the scrotum, so that I could draw them out; and
when most of the mortified cellular membrane was removed, I saw a
part, about the size of a sixpence, of the tendinous covering of the corpus cavernosum dead, which was also allowed to slough off. Most of
the water now came through the sore. The parts became more painful;
he was more restless, and one morning he had a shivering fit. I endeavoured to pass a bougie down the sore, between the skin and penis,
but could not: in the evening of the same day a gush of matter and
blood came out of the sore, which immediately relieved him, and he
began to mend again, and continued to do so, both in the parts and his
general health, the water coming both ways, but often varying in quantity between the two passages; more and more, however, came the right
way, till at last the new passage closed up entirely.

While the external parts were healing I passed a bougie occasionally,
to keep the passage clear and open. To find out the situation of the
internal opening, I ordered the patient to press on different parts of the
perinæum while he was making water, by which means he found that
by pressing upon a particular spot he could stop the water from flowing
through the new passage. He was directed, however, not to press too

hard, for fear of forcing together the sides of the natural passage. Upon erections, the penis was bent to the side that had suffered; but in time the parts gradually recovered their natural form.

§. 3. *Of Inflammation in the Parts surrounding the Urethra.*

Inflammation arising from distension and irritation of the urethra often extends considerably further than the surface of that canal, for the surrounding parts become the seat of inflammation, the situation of which will commonly be according to the situation of the stricture, pro-ducing the distension.   Thus we find the inflammation affecting the prostate gland, the membranous part of the urethra, the bulb, and pro-bably Cowper's glands, with other parts of the urethra between the bulb and the glans.   But inflammation in the surrounding parts of the ure-thra is not always a consequence of distension or stricture; it arises often from other irritations in this canal, such as violent gonorrhœas and very irritating injections.   When inflammation attacks these parts it is of the true adhesive kind, and therefore when suppuration takes place an abscess must be formed, unless the inflammation be resolved. The matter, according to a general principle in abscesses, points exter-nally; when the seat of the abscess is either in the prostate gland, membranous part, or in the bulb, the matter will point in the perinæum; or the abscess may be formed forwards in the scrotum, or before it, ac-cording to the situation of the stricture.

The seat of these abscesses is generally so near the inner surface of the urethra that the partition between them often gives way, and they open internally, as frequently happens in an abscess by the side of the rectum, so that the matter is at once discharged by the urethra, or car-ried back into the bladder to be discharged with the urine.   When the internal opening only takes place, I believe it is owing to the ulceration on the inner surface of the urethra, as has been already described; and in these cases also the stricture is sometimes involved in the abscess and ulceration, by which means the water will find a free passage for-wards; but the urine has also a free passage into the abscess, which we may suppose retards its healing, and often becomes the cause of its opening externally; but here, from the adhesive inflammation having taken place, the urine cannot insinuate itself into the surrounding cel-lular membrane, so as to produce the consequences mentioned in treat-ing of the way in which Nature endeavours to relieve herself.   In such cases we find that upon pressing the abscess externally the matter is squeezed into the urethra, and so out by the glans.   It sometimes hap-

pens that a catheter can be introduced into the opening of such an abscess, by which means it can be washed by injecting something through
the catheter, whereby probably it may be sooner healed. It more frequently happens that such abscesses open both internally and externally, discharging themselves both ways.

These ulcerations and suppurations, of both kinds, are to be considered as efforts of Nature, or, to speak more physiologically, as a natural
consequence arising from such irritation, by which, as the urine cannot
pass by the old passage, a new one is made to prevent further mischief.

Both these diseases, when they open externally, if not properly
treated, often lay the foundation for the complaint commonly called the
fistula in perinæo, which is owing to the bottom of the abscess having
a less disposition to heal than the external parts. It may be further
supposed, that the urine passing into the abscess by the inner orifice,
and making its escape into the external, keeps up a constant irritation
in the sore, which in some measure may prevent an union of the sides,
and rather dispose them to form themselves into a hard callous substance,
the inner surface of which loses the disposition to union, and assumes
the nature of an outlet.

But it is more than probable, that the cause which prevents these
abscesses from healing depends upon their first action often continuing
in full force; that is, a diseased state of the internal parts, as will be
further illustrated when we shall treat on the fistula in perinæo. They
often heal up at the orifice in the skin, especially if the water has a free
passage forwards; but if the internal opening is not perfectly consoli-
dated, some water will insinuate itself into the old sore, become the
cause of fresh inflammations and suppurations in the surrounding parts,
which frequently open externally in different places, not following the
old canal, although they sometimes communicate with it and form
branches, as it were, from the principal trunk. I have seen the scrotum, perinæum, and inside of the thigh, full of openings, which were
the mouths of so nany sinuses leading to the first-formed abscess.
When the abscess opens only externally, which is seldom the case, it is
to be considered as a common abscess.

When these inflammations arise from stricture, the difficulty in making water is increased in the time of the inflammation, which is generally
so great as to compress the sides of the urethra together for some way;
besides, the stricture itself will become tighter from being inflamed.
Inflammation in these parts, even when it does not arise from a stricture, brings on a suppression of urine; but in such cases a bougie or
catheter can be passed, the latter of which, in cases of obstruction arising from contiguous swellings, as tumours, inflammations, and swelled

prostate gland, is the proper instrument, as the sides of the urethra would be pressed together immediately upon withdrawing the bougie, by which the urine would be as much as ever prevented from following.

§. 4. *Of the Treatment of the Inflammation in the surrounding Parts.*

The inflammation of these parts is to be treated like other inflammations. Resolution is much to be wished for; but it is almost impossible it should take place where stricture is the cause. When the stricture is removed, either by ulceration or a bougie, we have only the inflammation to contend with; but this seldom happens, for the inflammation is but too often accompanied with suppuration.

When suppuration takes place, the sooner the abscess is opened externally the better, as that may in some cases be the means, though seldom, of preventing its opening internally; yet it may prevent the inner opening from becoming so large as it otherwise might be. The opening externally should be large; and if the stricture is not involved in the suppuration, then it must be destroyed, because there can be no cure while the water passes through the new opening. I have succeeded with the caustic even in strictures of long standing.

When the stricture will admit of the passage of a bougie through it, it is to be kept almost constantly in the urethra, and to be withdrawn only at the time of making water : this will allow the urine to pass more freely through the urethra, without escaping through the sore. The sore must be healed from the bottom*.

Hollow bougies are recommended in such cases, after the stricture is destroyed, to prevent the urine passing through the wound. This instrument admits of a constant dribbling of urine through it; but the bougie may be occasionally stopped up, and the urine permitted to pass when there is a desire to make water. It becomes under certain circumstances the worst instrument possible; for if its canal is not of a size sufficient to let the water pass as freely as the contraction of the bladder requires, the water will pass easily by the side of the bougie to the abscess, and, not getting forwards beyond the stricture, flow out at the abscess : to avoid this effect as much as possible, the hollow bougies

---

* Added: " In many such cases of abscess in perinæo, where the stricture has been destroyed, the passage at that part is so irregular that the catheter is the best instrument to use; and where the parts are much contracted, a flexible catheter may be readily introduced down to the stricture, and then a curved stilet passed into it which will admit of its being directed into the bladder. In this way I have sometimes succeeded when all other attempts have failed."—*Home.*

should be as large as the strictured part will allow, and its sides should be as thin as possible, that its passage may be the larger.   The elastic gum has these two properties in a higher degree than the spiral wire covered with waxed cloth.   But, as I doubt very much that the passage of the urine may be a hindrance to the healing of the sore, I am the less solicitous about such practice; for we find that after lithotomy the parts heal very readily; and even in this operation the external parts which are not diseased heal up very readily.   I suspect that the want of disposition to heal arises from the strictures not being sufficiently subdued, or the deeper parts not being in a healthy state.

When these suppurations are left to themselves, and no method tried to remove the stricture, and of course nothing introduced into the urethra, the stricture sometimes closes entirely, so that no water can pass forwards through the urethra; and therefore, before any attempt can be made to heal the fistulous orifices, a passage must be made through the united parts.   This cannot be done with a bougie; and if this union of the parts is before the bend of the urethra, which most commonly it is, nothing but the caustic can be applied with any prospect of success, as we shall mention more fully in treating of the fistula in perinæo.

§. 5. Of the Effects of Inflammation in the surrounding Parts upon the Constitution.

The effects which these attempts to form a new passage for the urine have upon the constitution are very considerable; much more so than what one would at first expect.   Those cases appear to be most formidable which begin by ulceration on the inner surface of the urethra, and where the water diffuses itself into the cellular membrane of the scrotum and penis.

Those where the inflammation is circumscribed are more of the true abscess, and therefore do much less mischief to the parts than when the urine is diffused in the cellular membrane.   In these last, if not soon relieved, the patient sinks, and a mortification comes on.   If, before the patient sinks, a separation of the slough takes place, this separation performs the operation of opening, and the patient may recover.   We should not, I believe, wait for such separation of the mortified part, but make an opening early, upon the first knowledge of a diffusion of water into the cellular membrane; and we should be guided as to situation by introducing a staff into the urethra on to the stricture.   But in some cases this cannot be done; for when the urine gets into the corpus spongiosum it produces mortification of all these parts, and renders the whole so indistinct that often no urethra can be found.

The effects that the circumscribed inflammation has upon the constitution is generally not so serious as the above; for mortification as seldom takes place in this as in abscesses in general. When the abscess is from the bulb backwards, there is generally a smart sympathetic fever, because the abscess will be of considerable size before it gets to the skin of the perinæum, and is generally attended with great pain; but this pain goes off by the formation of the matter, especially if opened early.

As there is a great disposition to violent action, attended with great weakness, in such cases, more especially in those of the first kind, it is advisable to give the bark early, and in considerable quantity; but I apprehend it is necessary to give along with it sudorifics, as some of the preparations of antimony, there being generally a good deal of fever. The bark gives strength, and also in some degree lessens irritability; but it should be assisted by other medicines.

§. 6. Of Fistulæ in Perinæo.

It often happens that the new passages for the urine do not heal, on account of the stricture not being removed; and even when the stricture is removed they frequently have no disposition to heal. In both cases they become fistulous, and produce fresh inflammations and suppurations, which do not always open into the old sore, but make new openings externally. These sometimes arise from the first external openings not being sufficiently large, so that they heal up long before the bottom, or long before the diseased urethra; and even when the external opening has been made as large as possible, it will often heal sooner than the bottom, and become fistulous at last.

It is very common for these diseases to affect the constitution so as to bring on complaints of an intermittent kind. I have seen several affected with regular agues, where the bark has produced no effect; but whenever the obstruction has been got the better of, or the fistulous orifice opened and in a state of healing, these complaints have entirely gone off.

To cure this disease it is necessary first to make the natural passage as free as possible, that no obstruction may arise from that quarter; and sometimes this alone is sufficient: for the urine, finding a free passage forwards, is not forced into the orifice, and the fistulæ heal up. The bougie may bring on an inflammation on the urethra at this part, and produce adhesions there ; but if this effect is not produced early, the bougie will rather do harm if applied too often, and too long at a time, as will be more fully explained.   But the dilatation of the stricture is not always sufficient; it is often necessary to perform an operation on the fistulæ, when they alone become the obstacle to the cure, which I shall now describe.

§. 7. Of the Operation for Fistulæ in Perinæo.

When the before-mentioned treatment is not sufficient for the cure of the new passages, a method should be followed similar to that used in the cure of fistulæ in other parts, by laying them freely open to the bottom, and even making the orifice in the urethra a fresh sore if possible.   This will be difficult in many situations of the internal orifice ; and the mode of opening, and other circumstances attending the operation, will vary according to the situation.

That as little of the sound part of the inner surface of the urethra may be opened as possible, and that the diseased part may be fully exposed, it is necessary to be well directed to the inner orifice, for which we have commonly two guides : one is a staff introduced into the urethra as far as is thought necessary, or as far as it will go (which will only be to the stricture, where the stricture still exists, or it may pass on to the bladder in cases where the stricture has been destroyed); the other guide is a probe passed into the fistulous orifice.   The probe should be first bent, that it may more readily follow the turns of the fistula, and be introduced as far as possible ; if it could be made to meet the staff so much the better, as then the operator could cut just what is necessary.   If the fistula is tolerably straight, so as to admit the passing a director, it is the best instrument for operating upon.   If neither the probe nor the director can be made to pass on to the staff, we must open as far as they go, and begin searching anew after the remainder of the passage with the same instrument, and pursue it till the whole fistulous canal is laid open.   If there are any sinuses, they are to be laid open if possible ; but it frequently happens that they cannot be followed by the knife, some running along the penis, where the scrotum is attached, others passing on towards the pubes, round the penis, while others are about the membranous part of the urethra.   In such cases some degree of violence may be used, and I have several times introduced my finger into these sinuses, and have torn the parts so as to produce a considerable inflammation, by which means they often suppurate, granulate, and unite.

If the situation of the internal orifice is opposite to the scrotum it will be difficult to get to it; but I imagine we may use great freedom with the external parts, whatever they are, for they are generally in a state of callosity.   However, this requires judgment.

In cases where the disease is before the membranous part and the stricture is not removed, a staff cannot be made to pass on to the inner orifice.   In such the fistulous opening must be followed by the introduction of a probe or director into it, and by dilatation upon the instrument till the urethra beyond the stricture is found; and then a probe must be passed on towards the glans, to meet the end of the staff at the stricture, similar to what is done in the operation where a false passage has been made by the mismanagement of the bougie.   The stricture must then be destroyed, and a bougie passed, as was recommended in that operation.

If either the ulceration or the abscess is formed in or near the prostate gland, then probably the stricture is near that part.   In that case a staff must be passed as far as possible, and a probe or director introduced into the external orifice, and the operation is to be directed accordingly.   The difference of the operation in this case from the former will be that we shall most probably be obliged to cut into the urethra on both sides of the stricture, therefore more of the canal must be exposed.

As this operation is the opening of all the fistulous canals, and also the destruction of the stricture, if there has been one, an instrument can afterwards, in every case, be passed into the bladder.   It will most probably always be proper to introduce an instrument into the bladder, and keep it there almost constantly, so as to preserve the passage of the urethra in a regular form, while the openings made are healing; and probably the catheter will be by much the best instrument, because it is not necessary to be withdrawn whenever the necessity to make water comes on, which a bougie must; and its introduction again is often not practicable, for its end will be apt to get into the wounds.

In such cases as require a hollow cannula to be left in the bladder for the purpose of drawing off the water, whether a catheter or hollow bougie, it is absolutely necessary it should be fixed there, or else it will in common come out by the actions of the part.   To effect this it is necessary to fix that end of the instrument out of the penis to some part of the body that is the least moveable.   What will answer extremely well is the common belt-part of the bag-truss, with only two thigh-straps fixed behind and made to tie or buckle before; and two or three very small rings or short tapes fixed to those straps where they pass between the thigh and scrotum; they should not be at a great distance from one another where they are fixed behind to the belt, for otherwise they are much altered in tightness by the motion of the thigh. If they have a flat spring in them so much the better*.

The common bag-truss for the scrotum answers extremely well, first by fixing two or three rings on each side of it along the side of the scrotum; and with a piece of small tape the ring of the cannula can be fastened to any one of those rings that is most convenient for its situation.

Whatever instrument is used for the purpose of keeping the passage clear and open while the sores are healing, whether the sores are in consequence of this operation, or in consequence of the causes of the fistulæ, which I have described, there is a limited time in many cases for its continuance; for if continued beyond a certain period, it frequently acts contrary to what was intended; at first it often assists the cure, but towards the last it may obstruct the healing of the sores by acting at the bottom of the wound as an extraneous body. Therefore, whenever the sores become stationary, I would advise the withdrawing of the instrument, and the introducing it only occasionally. The catheter will probably be still the best instrument for this purpose, as it will pass more readily, and draw off the water at the same time: however, I have often used a bougie, and by great care have passed it with success; and probably it will be proper to use it every now and then, even when all is healed, in order to determine whether or not the passage is free from disease.

The sore and the wound are to be at first dressed down to the bottom as much as possible, which will prevent the reunion of the parts just divided, and make the granulations shoot from the bottom so as to consolidate the whole by one bond of union.

When the urethra has suffered so much that abscesses have formed beyond the scrotum, the patient should ever after take great care to avoid a fresh gonorrhœa, for he seldom in that case escapes a return of the same complaints; and, indeed if he is not careful in many other respects, he is liable to returns of the same disease. If, notwithstanding this precaution, he should contract a gonorrhœa, everything heating is to be carefully avoided, particularly irritating injections.

The following case shows that keeping extraneous bodies in the urethra prevents wounds made into that canal from healing.

A man, aged twenty-six, came into St. George's Hospital March 2, 1783. He had laboured under a fistula in perinæo for near two years, arising from a stricture, attended with great pain and difficulty in making water. Four fistulous orifices were to be observed in the peri-

* Mr. Vanbutchell's springs would answer very well.

næum and scrotum. The smallest bougie could not be made to pass into the bladder after repeated trials. The caustic was then applied, but without success.

The operation for the fistula in perinæo was performed September 19. A catheter was first introduced as far as it would go, as a director, and all the sinuses were laid open to that catheter, which exposed near an inch in length of that instrument; then the catheter was in part withdrawn to expose that part of the urethra which was laid bare. The blood being sponged off, the orifice in the stricture was next searched for, and when found it was dilated. The catheter was now pushed on to the bladder, although with some difficulty, and the end of it was then fastened to a roller which went round the thighs; and the wound was distended with lint. He took an anodyne draught after the operation, and another at night. September 20, he had some pain in the head from the opiates; his pulse was natural, and he had slept tolerably well. On the 21st day the catheter slipped out, and the second introduction of it gave considerable pain. The anodyne was repeated. October 1. The catheter was still to be felt by introducing a probe into the wound. From this time to the 25th nothing material happened, excepting a piece of lint of the first dressing coming away through the urethra. November 20. The wound having for some time been stationary, and showing no disposition to heal, I conceived that the catheter was now acting as an extraneous body at the bottom of the wound, and therefore desired that it might be withdrawn, and passed occasionally; and no sooner was the wound free from it but it put on a healthy look, and by the 10th of December no urine came through the wound, but passed tolerably well through the urethra; and on the 12th the wound was quite healed, and his water came from him rather in a full stream and without pain, although we could never pass either catheter or bougie afterwards, probably from the new and old passages being irregular[a].

---

[a] [It is possible that some cases may occur where the operation which is described by the author may be required, but such cases are undoubtedly very rare. The complete removal of the stricture is in almost all instances followed by the spontaneous closure of the sinuses in the perinæum. Until the strictured portion is dilated to the same size with the rest of the urethra, there is little improvement. As soon as that is effected, the urine is no longer diverted into the sinus, but takes the more ready course of the natural passage; and the cause which maintained the fistula being thus removed, the opening gradually contracts, and in a short time heals, without any surgical treatment whatever.]

CHAPTER VII.

OF SOME OTHER AFFECTIONS OF THE URETHRA.

THE substance of the urethra is muscular, and it is therefore capable of contracting its canal, similar to an intestine, so as to shut it up entirely. This makes it subject to diseases peculiar to muscle in general; which is indeed the only proof we have of its being muscular.

§. 1. *Of the Spasmodic Affections of the Urethra.*

In a sound state of parts these muscles are never excited to violent actions, acting simply as sphincter muscles; but when irritated they are capable of acting violently, as is best seen in some cases upon the first use of injections, the urethra often refusing the injection entirely. This seems rather to be a salutary motion to hinder things from getting into the bladder; but there are often spasmodic contractions of these muscular fibres in different parts of the canal, shutting up the passage and obstructing the course of the urine, often not allowing a drop to pass. That this also is owing to spasm upon the muscular fibres is evident, because a large bougie will sometimes pass when it is at the worst. When the contraction is near the bladder it is called a strangury, and is often produced in a sound state of parts by irritating medicines, the power of which falls upon these parts, as cantharides; and when this part is in an irritable state, the spasm may be brought on by a vast number of things, such as most of the peppers, fermented liquors of all kinds, violent exercise, &c.

The urethra in cases of spasmodic stricture is more irritable than in the true stricture, which irritation indeed is in a great measure the cause of the spasm. Spasmodic strictures often bear so strong a resemblance to the cramp, that one would be apt to attribute them to the same cause as that which produces cramp. In such cases the spasm also goes off by tickling the part, similar to the removal of cramp.

In all cases of very irritable urethras, where spasms very readily take place, the patient should never long retain his urine when he has an inclination to void it; for I have seen cases where this alone has brought on the spasm: and indeed these parts, when in perfect health, will be

thrown into a spasmodic affection if the urine is too long confined in
the bladder; while at the same time a certain fulness of the bladder, or
a small degree of retention of the urine, will make the bladder contract
with more force, and the urethra will for the same reason relax more
freely; therefore in cases where there is a tendency to strangury there
is seldom any harm in waiting a little after the inclination comes on.

I may be allowed here to caution surgeons who have not had opportunities of seeing many of these cases, when they meet with permanent
strictures which are becoming troublesome, attended with frequency in
making water, and a difficulty in passing it often threatening strangury,
not to advise, or rather not to allow, their patients to take long journeys
either on horseback or in carriages, more especially in the winter. I
have known many patients labouring under such complaints taken ill in
the middle of a journey, and obliged to stop for days upon the road,
and who have continued in misery the remainder of the journey; and
after having arrived at the place of their destination, have been laid up
for months, and have suffered from most of the before-mentioned complaints.

§. 2. *Of the Cure of the Spasmodic Affection of the Urethra.*

It may not be improper to premise, that in diseases of the actions only
of the urethra and bladder, whether spasmodic and proceeding from too
great irritability, or paralytic (although two opposite diseases,) irritations on other parts have often wonderful effects, equally diminishing
the action in the one and increasing it in the other. The proof of this
will appear when we shall treat of the irritable and paralytic urethra
and bladder : for in either part, and in either case, we find blisters applied to the lower part of the small of the back or the perinæum, as also
many other applications to this part, often produce great effects*.

As spasm simply is not an alteration of structure, but is only a diseased or preternatural action arising from some irritation, it may be
made to cease instantaneously. In whatever part of the urethra the
spasm is, if time will allow, it is proper to try internal medicines, and
also external applications, to remove it. The internal medicines that

* That the parts concerned in the expulsion of the urine (as the bladder and urethra)
sympathize strongly with the skin of the perinæum I believe is commonly supposed,
from applications being often made to that part in cases of stoppages of urine.

A gentleman who had no complaint in these parts had a small fistula at the side of
the rectum, for which he often had occasion to sit over the steam of warm water and
vinegar; and this application to the perinæum never failed of making him void his
urine.

may be said to act immediately are opiates and turpentines*, given either by the mouth or the anus; but they are more immediate in their effects in the form of clyster, especially the opium. Bark is often had recourse to in spasmodic affections, in which it is thought to be of service; but in such affections of the urethra I think I have seen it frequently do harm.

The external applications are, the steam of warm water with spirits, the pediluvium, the warm bath, bladders of warm water applied to the perinæum, and similar applications. The crumb part of a new-baked loaf, warm from the oven, applied to the perinæum, has been found to give ease.

I have known a blister applied to the loins in a great measure remove the spasm from the urethra: it is equally effectual when applied to the perinæum. But in most cases these methods are too tedious; therefore when the case has been of some standing, before assistance has been called for, and requires immediate relief, recourse should be had to the catheter or bougie immediately

If the contraction is near the bladder, the catheter will answer best; but in most cases the bougie will be sufficient, and is a much safer instrument; for in many hands the catheter is a very dangerous one, requiring a dexterity only to be acquired by a thorough knowledge of the course of the canal, and a habit of passing it. The bougie has likewise this advantage, that in many cases, where the part spasmodically affected will not allow it to pass, it may be allowed to lie close to the stricture; for it is not always necessary for the bougie to pass through the constructured part: for a bougie which has only passed a very little way in the urethra has sometimes been effectual, if suffered to stay there till the desire of making water is perceived.

In such cases, even when the bougie passes into the bladder, it is necessary to let it stay in the passage till the inclination to make water comes on. If the water does not follow on the first attempt, it will be proper to make another; or if only part follows the bougie, it will be necessary to introduce it again. This circumstance, of the water following the bougie with more certainty if it is allowed to stay till the inclination comes on, is a proof that the disposition in the bladder to contracting removes in some degree the disposition to contraction in the urethra.

Some attention is necessary with respect to the passing of the bougie

* Dr. Home, in his experiments on this medicine, found that large doses brought on the strangury in women.

Strangury is the frequent effect of spirit of turpentine taken for some time.

in these cases: for the urethra being more irritable than common, it often resists the bougie before it reaches the true spasmodic part. When this is the case, force is not to be used; but we should rather wait a little with patience, and then make another attempt to push it on.   Dipping the end of the penis in very cold water often removes the spasm, and the water flows immediately and freely.

In most cases there is an uneasy sensation at the end of the penis, which leads the patient to rub those parts; and sometimes, though rarely, during the friction, the water will pass.   Gently irritating injections, thrown in only a little way, often give ease.   They may be supposed to act in a manner somewhat similar to a bougie that does not pass, and by irritating one part of the urethra to produce a relaxation in the other.   They act in some cases as a preventive.

§. 3. Of the Paralysis of the Urethra.

In opposition to the foregoing disease, there is the want of power of contraction of the urethra; but this is not so frequent a case as the former.   This disease is attended with symptoms contrary to those of the foregoing: the bladder is hardly allowed to be filled so as to give the stimulus of repletion, but the water dribbles away insensibly as fast as secreted by the kidneys; or if the bladder is filled so as to receive the stimulus for expulsion, then it immediately takes place, and the water flows, if the person does not act with the musculi acceleratores; but sometimes in such cases the power of contraction of these muscles is lost, and then the water will flow, whether the person will or not, there being little or no power of retention.   There is great difference in the degrees of violence of this disease.

§. 4. Cure of the Paralysis of the Urethra.

It is to be cured by stimulants, as a blister to the loins, or a blister to the perinæum.   It may be useful to immerse the feet in cold water. Tincture of cantharides, taken internally, fifteen or twenty drops once or twice a day, according to the effects, are of singular service in some cases.

A man came to St. George's Hospital with this complaint.   I ordered him the before-mentioned medicine, and it had such an effect as to bring on the contrary disease, or a spasmodic affection of the urethra, so that he could not make water when he had the inclination; but an injection of opium removed this complaint, and he was then well.   In this case a few drops less, probably, would have effected a cure without any inconvenience.

§. 5. *Of Caruncles or Excrescences in the Urethra.*

Strictures are not supposed to be the only causes of obstruction to the passage of urine in this canal; excrescences or caruncles are likewise mentioned by authors as happening frequently.   From the familiarity with which they talk of them, and the few instances in which they really occur, one would suspect that this cause of obstruction was originally founded in opinion, and not observation, and afterwards handed down as matter of fact.   If caruncles had been at first described from actual examination of cases, the language would have accorded with the appearances, and they would have been considered as seldom the causes of obstruction compared with strictures.   However, they do sometimes happen, although but rarely.   I have in all my examinations of dead bodies seen only two, and these were in very old strictures, where the urethra had suffered considerably.   They were bodies rising from the surface of the urethra like granulations, or what would be called polypi in other parts of the body.   It is possible they may be a species of internal wart; for I have seen warts extend some way into the beginning of the urethra, having very much the appearance of granulations.   Most probably it will not be possible in the living body to distinguish caruncles, excrescences, or risings in the urethra, from a stricture; for I cannot conceive that they can produce any new symptoms, or peculiar feel to the examiner.

§. 6. *Of the Cure of the Excrescence or Caruncle.*

I should very much suspect that this disease is not to be cured by the bougie; at least dilatation in such cases is not to be attempted, as there is no contraction.   If therefore the bougie is of any use, it must be in making the carnosity ulcerate from its pressure, which probably may be done by a large bougie pressing upon it with considerable force. But if this should not have the desired effect, I should certainly recommend or use the caustic, if the parts are so situated as to admit of the application; and from such practice I should not doubt of a cure.   But the difficulty lies in distinguishing the disease from the true stricture :

for although authors talk of caruncles as common, and give us the method of treatment, yet they have not told us how we are to distinguish
them from strictures.

I have never met with a caruncle in women.

CHAPTER VIII.

OF THE SWELLED PROSTATE GLAND.

ANOTHER disease of the parts surrounding the urethra, which is often
very formidable, is a swelling of the prostate gland. This is of more
serious consequence than any of the former causes of obstruction, because we have fewer methods of cure; for we cannot destroy it as we do
the stricture, nor can Nature relieve herself by forming new passages;
we have, however, often the means of temporary relief in our power,
which is not the case in the stricture; for most commonly we can draw
off the water by the catheter.

The swelling of the prostate gland is most common in the decline of
life. The use of this gland is not sufficiently known to enable us to
judge of the bad consequences that attend its diseased state, abstracted
from swelling. Its situation is such, that the bad effects of its being
swelled must be evident, as it may be said to make a part of the canal
of the urethra, and therefore when so diseased as to alter its shape and
size, it must obstruct the passage of the urine. When it swells it does
not lessen the surface of the urethra at the part like a stricture; on the
contrary, it rather increases it; but the sides of the canal are compressed
together, producing an obstruction to the passage of the urine, which
irritates the bladder and brings on all the symptoms in that viscus that
usually arise from a stricture or stone. From the situation of the gland,
which is principally on the two sides of the canal, and but little, if at
all, on the fore part, as also very little on the posterior side, it can only
swell laterally, whereby it presses the two sides of the canal together,
and at the same time stretches it from the anterior edge or side to the
posterior, so that the canal, instead of being round, is flattened into a
narrow groove. Sometimes the gland swells more on one side than the
other, which makes an obliquity in the canal passing through it.

Besides this effect of the lateral parts swelling, a small portion of it, which lies behind the very beginning of the urethra, swells forwards like a point, as it were, into the bladder, acting like a valve to the mouth of the urethra, which can be seen even when the swelling is not considerable, by looking upon the mouth of the urethra from the cavity of the bladder in a dead body.   It sometimes increases so much as to form a tumour*, projecting into the bladder some inches.   This projection turns or bends the urethra forwards, becoming an obstruction to the passage of a catheter, bougie, or any such instrument; and it often raises the sound over a small stone in the bladder, so as to prevent its being felt.   The catheter should for this part be more curved than is necessary for the other parts of the urethra.   In such cases I have frequently passed first a hollow elastic catheter till it has reached this point, and afterwards a stilet or brass wire properly curved, so as to go over the prostate gland.   The advantages of this method are, that if the hollow catheter passes, no more is necessary; and, if it does not, the curved wire will pass along the hollow bougie much easier, both to the surgeon and patient, than it would have done if it had been introduced at first with the hollow bougie over it; for it would endeavour to adapt the urethra to the curve; whereas, when introduced afterwards, the stilet acts only on the inside of the hollow bougie, which the patient hardly feels.

A gentleman had been often sounded for a stone, and yet no stone could be found; but it afterwards appeared that there was a stone, which, together with the swelling of the prostate gland, had been the cause of his death.

John Doby, a poor pensioner in the Charter-house, had been several years afflicted with the stone in the bladder, and was relieved from all the symptoms by an enlargement of this part of the prostate gland, preventing the stones from falling down upon the neck of the bladder and irritating those parts.   A twelvemonth after that the symptoms of the stone had gone off, he was attacked with a strangury, to relieve which many ineffectual attempts were made, both with the bougie and catheter; but it soon proved fatal.   Upon examination of the parts in the dead body, the prostate gland was found enlarged to a size six times greater than what it is in common, and the urethra, passing through it, was a slit about an inch and half in length, the two sides of which were close together, the upper end towards the pubes and the lower towards the rectum.   This slit was formed by the sides of the prostate gland only swelling, and the right side was the most enlarged, having its sur-

* Vide Plates XIII. and XV.

face next the urethra rounded or convex, and the left side was exactly fitted to it, having its surface hollowed in the same proportion. The small projecting point of the gland was so much enlarged as to come forwards into the cavity of the bladder, and fill up entirely the passage at the neck of it. The bladder itself was very much enlarged and thickened in its coats, and contained above twenty stones, most of them lying behind the projecting process of the prostate gland, and the rest lodged in small sacs, made by the internal membrane being pushed some little way between the fasciculi of muscular fibres.

The prostate gland, when swelled, generally becomes firmer in its consistence. The effects of these swellings are very considerable, for they squeeze the sides of the urethra close together, and the projecting point hinders in some degree the urine from entering the passage, and in many cases stops it entirely. Further, the increased firmness of the substance of the gland hinders it from yielding to the force of the urine, so that little or none can pass. It will be unnecessary to relate the particular symptoms which this disease occasions; they are such as arise from any stoppage of urine, producing an irritable bladder.

When a difficulty in making water takes place, a bougie is the instrument which the surgeon will naturally have recourse to, and if he finds the passage clear, which he often will, in such cases he may very probably suspect a stone. If search is made, and no stone felt, he should naturally suspect the prostate gland, especially if the sound or instrument used meets with a full stop, or passes with some difficulty just at the neck of the bladder. He should examine the gland. This can only be done by introducing the finger into the anus, first oiling it well, placing the fore part of the finger towards the pubes; and if the parts, as far as the end of the finger can reach, are hard, making an eminence backwards into the rectum, so that the finger is obliged to be removed from side to side, to feel the whole extent of such a swelling, and it also appears to go beyond the reach of the finger, we may be certain the gland is considerably swelled, and is the principal cause of those symptoms.

I have known cases where the common catheter has been pushed through the projecting part of the gland into the bladder, and the water then drawn off; but in one patient the blood from the wound passed into the bladder and increased the quantity of matter in it. The use of the catheter was attempted a second time, but not succeeding, I was sent for. I passed the catheter till it came to the stop, and then suspecting that this part of the prostate projected forwards, I introduced my finger into the anus and found that gland very much enlarged. By depressing the handle of the catheter, which of course raised the point, it passed over the projection; but unfortunately the blood had coagulated in the bladder, which filled up the holes in the catheter, so that I was obliged to withdraw it, and clear it repeatedly. This I practised several days; but suspecting that the coagulum must in the end kill, I proposed cutting him as if for the stone; but he died before it could be conveniently done, and the dissection, after death, explained the case to be what I have now described.

In some of those cases where this part of the gland swells into the bladder in form of a tumour, the catheter has been known not to bring off the water at times when it appeared to have passed; and upon the death of the patient, when the parts have been examined, it was imagined that the catheter, in the living body, had made its way into the tumour so as to have been buried in it at those times*.

From the knowledge of the above-mentioned facts, whenever I find the urine does not flow immediately upon introducing the catheter into the bladder, I have pushed it on and depressed the handle, so as to reach the fundus of the bladder with the end of the catheter, and have always succeeded. For the more ready introduction of the instrument, a catheter made flexible at the point only for about an inch is perhaps best, as it is more under the command of the hand than when wholly flexible.

If the bougie be used, it should be first warmed, and then very much bent at the point, and allowed to cool in this position, and passed quickly with the concave side upwards, before it loses the bend in its passage. But the bougie does not answer so well as the catheter, because, upon withdrawing the bougie the sides of the gland soon close again. I have known where the water has passed by the side of the bougie with more freedom than when it was pulled out, because the bougie gave a straightness to this part of the canal, which it had not when the bougie was withdrawn. The following case is a strong instance of the inconveniences arising from such a disease of the prostate gland.

A gentleman was attacked with a suppression of urine; a catheter could not be passed; but a bougie relieved him. He continued well for five years; but the same complaint returning, the bougie could not be passed, and the disease was supposed to be a stricture. A catheter however passed, although with a good deal of difficulty, and the bougie, though often tried, could not be passed, excepting once, just after using the catheter. I was sent for, and tried the bougie with as little success, and was obliged to have recourse to the catheter. I passed it with

* Vide Plate XV.

great ease, and the water was drawn off.   The late Mr. Tomkyns, who
had Daran's bougie, was called; but he was not more successful, and
was obliged to have recourse to the catheter; but such violence was
used as caused a good deal of blood to come from the urethra, and after
all it did not succeed.   I was again consulted, and passed the catheter,
but with much more difficulty than before, which made me believe that
the passage had been 'a good deal torn.   Upon taking out the catheter
I passed a large bougie into the bladder with great ease; this I allowed
to remain for three days, and the patient made water tolerably freely
by the side of it.   The moment I drew out the bougie I attempted to
pass another, but did not succeed, although I gave it the natural bend
of the passage.   Upon withdrawing those bougies that did not pass, I
observed that all of them had a bend at the point, contrary to the direction of the passage; this made me suspect that the place which stopped
the bougie was on the posterior surface, and that by being pushed on,
it bent forwards into the passage, and of course the point turned back.
I therefore took a thick bougie, and before I introduced it I bent the
point almost double, so that it could not catch at the posterior surface
of the urethra, where I supposed the stop to be: this point of the bougie rubbed all along the anterior and upper surface of the urethra, by
which means it avoided catching on the posterior surface, and it passed
with great ease into the bladder.   He made water by the side of the
bougie, as before.   He had been for some time troubled with fits of an
intermittent, which at first were very irregular, but became afterwards
more regular.   In one of the cold fits, the bougie, being in the urethra,
gave him great pain, and obliged him at last to pull it out, on which he
had immediate ease.   The sensation was as if it stretched the passage
too much, and it seemed to come out with difficulty.   This looks as if
there was a contraction of the urethra, as well as of the vessels of the
skin, in the cold fit; so that this disposition runs deep.   By giving the
bougie this bend he was able for the future to pass them with great
ease.   I may just observe, that by introducing the finger into the anus
I found the prostate gland much enlarged.

Many patients, while labouring under any of the before-mentioned
diseases of the urethra, and sometimes even after they have been cured
of them, find great pain in throwing forwards the semen, having a sensation as if it scalded.   This arises from the very irritable state which
the muscles of this part are in, giving great pain by their own action.

§. 1. *Of the Treatment of the Swelled Prostate Gland.*

The methods practised in the above cases afforded only temporary relief, yet such must be had recourse to in order to prevent the consequences of retaining the urine too long. As a temporary relief from pain, as also to remove spasm, opiate clysters should be thrown up once or twice a day. A certain cure, I am afraid, is not as yet discovered.

I have seen hemlock of service in several cases. It was given upon a supposition of a scrofulous habit. On the same principle I have recommended sea-bathing, and have seen considerable advantages from it, and, in two cases, a cure of some standing.

In one case in which I was consulted, the surgeon had found that burnt sponge had reduced the swelling of the gland very considerably.

This disease, like the stricture, produces complaints in the bladder; but in this the bladder is generally more irritable, perhaps from the cause being nearer to that viscus.

Diseases of the vesiculæ seminales are very familiarly talked of; but I never saw one. In cases of very considerable induration of the prostate gland and bladder, where the surrounding parts have become very much affected, I have seen these bags also involved in the general disease; but I never saw a case where it appeared that they were primarily affected.

In a case of a swelled prostate gland, with symptoms of an irritable bladder, in a young gentleman about twenty years of age, Mr. Earle tried a blister to the perinæum; but not finding the desired effect, and conceiving a greater irritation and discharge to be necessary, he passed a seton in the direction of the perinæum. The orifices were about two inches distant from each other. The symptoms of irritability in the bladder began to abate, and in time went entirely off. Upon examination of the prostate gland, from time to time, it was found to decrease gradually till it was nearly of the natural size. The seton was continued some months, and upon its being withdrawn the symptoms began to return. It was advised to introduce it again, which was accordingly done, but without the former good effects[a].

---

[a] [The enlargement of the prostate gland, as it occurs in old people, seldom, if ever, yields to surgical treatment: yet much may be done to prevent or alleviate the distressing effects which it produces on the neighbouring organs. In fact it is these effects only which give any importance to the malady. The disease of the prostate in most cases occasions no symptoms which are referrible to the gland itself. But it may impede the flow of the urine, or excite chronic inflammation of the bladder, and ultimately disease of the kidneys, or give rise to painful irritability of the rectum. The mode in which these consequences are produced, and the treatment by which they are to be obviated, are best detailed in the observations of Sir E. Home, on diseases of the prostate gland, to which work the reader is referred.]

CHAPTER IX.

OF THE DISEASES OF THE BLADDER, PARTICULARLY FROM THE BEFORE-MENTIONED OBSTRUCTIONS TO THE URINE.

ALL the diseases of the urethra, as also the diseases of the prostate gland, I have now treated of, and shall next consider the effects of them upon the bladder, as also the diseases of that viscus, independent of affections of the urethra.

The disease of the bladder arising from obstruction alone is increased irritability and its consequences, by which the bladder admits of little distention, becomes quick in its action, and thick and strong in its coats. But prior to the description of the effects of the diseases of the urethra on the bladder, it will be necessary, for the better understanding of the whole, to make some remarks upon those diseases of the two parts, in which we find that each affects the other; and these I shall consider without having any regard to the cause, but only to the general effects, when they are diseased. It may be observed, that every organ in an animal body is made up of different parts, the functions or actions of which are totally different from each other, although all tend to produce one ultimate effect. In most, if not in all, when perfect, there is a succession of motions, one naturally arising out of the other, which in the end produces the ultimate effect; and an irregularity alone in these actions will constitute disease, at least produce very disagreeable effects, and often totally frustrate the final intentions of the organs.

I may be allowed also to premise, that the natural width of the urethra gives such a resistance to the force or power of the bladder in expelling the urine, as is easily overcome by the natural action of the bladder; but when the canal is lessened, either by stricture, spasm, swelled prostate gland, or any other means, this proportion is lost, by which means the bladder finds greater difficulty than natural, and is of course thrown into an increased action to overcome the resistance, which becomes a cause of the irritability and increased strength of this viscus in such diseases.

It is to be understood, that in a sound state of these two parts, the bladder and urethra, the contraction of the one produces a relaxation of the other, and *vice versâ*; so that their natural actions are alternate, and they may be considered as antagonist muscles to one another.

Thus, when the stimulus of expulsion of the urine takes place in the bladder, which immediately produces contractions in it, the urethra relaxes, by which means the urine is expelled from the bladder, and allowed to pass through the urethra; and when the action ceases in the bladder, the urethra contracts again like a sphincter muscle*, for the purpose of retaining the urine which flows into the bladder from the kidneys till it gives the stimulus for expulsion again. But in many diseases of these two parts this necessary alternate action is not regularly kept up, the one not obeying the summons of the other. This irregularity arises perhaps oftener from disease in the urethra than in the bladder, for the action of the urethra depends upon the actions of the bladder; and if it is not disposed to obey the notices of the bladder, then there must be an irregularity as to time, which produces very troublesome symptoms.

We find in many diseases of the urethra, such as strictures and spasms, as also in diseases of certain parts belonging to this canal, such as the prostate and Cowper's glands, that there is a greater disposition in this canal for contraction than common, so that when the bladder has begun to act, the water is not allowed to flow, the urethra not immediately relaxing; and the moment such a symptom takes place, every other power takes the alarm, and is brought in to assist the bladder, such as straining violently with the abdominal muscles and muscles of respiration, from all which there is violent pain in the parts immediately concerned, especially in the glans penis†.

This disease has different degrees of violence. When slight, the distance in time between the contraction of the bladder and the relaxation of the urethra is but short, only giving a momentary pain and straining, before the urethra relaxes, and the water flows according to the dilatation of the urethra, which, in many of these cases, is but very small. In others the distance of time is very long, many straining for a considerable time before a drop will come; and what does come is often only in drops; and sometimes before the whole urine can be expelled in this way, the spasm of the urethra comes on again, and there is a full stop, which gives excruciating pain for a while; but at last the bladder is, as it were, tired, and ceases to act. But as the urine in such

---

* It may be remarked, that many sphincter muscles have two causes of action; one which may be called involuntary, depending on the natural uses and actions of the parts; the other is voluntary, where a greater degree of action can be produced by the command of the will: and when a diseased action takes place, it is probably of this voluntary action, for it is an increased action over the natural, which the voluntary is.

† Added: "A gentleman, whose bladder was in an irritable state, found, that by passing a bougie a little way into the urethra the irritation was taken off from the bladder, and he could retain the urine several hours."—*Home.*

cases is seldom all discharged, and often but a very little of it, the symptoms soon recur; and in this way, with a call to make water perhaps every hour out of the four-and-twenty, the patient drags on a miserable life.

The bladder, in all cases of obstruction, whether constant, as in the permanent stricture or swelled prostate gland, or only temporary, as in the spasmodic stricture, is generally kept distended, but much more so in the permanent stricture; and when the irritation of fulness comes on, which is very frequent, the contraction of that viscus becomes violent, in proportion to the resistance: the sympathetic contraction of the muscles of the abdomen takes place, and is also violent; yet the water at such times shall only dribble; and be discharged in small quantity; and in the spasmodic stricture often not a drop shall pass, so that the bladder is never entirely empty; and what does pass is no more than what is sufficient to take off the irritation of fulness, by which means these actions become more frequent, and consequently there is almost always a constant oozing of urine from the penis between the times of making water. This, however, is not always the case, for the bladder sometimes is so irritable as not to cease acting till it has evacuated the whole water; and even then it is not at ease, but still strains, though there is nothing to throw out, the action of the bladder becoming a cause of its own continuance.

In all such affections of the bladder there is a sensation of pain and itching combined in the glans penis*

If the symptoms are more urgent than what can be accounted for upon the supposition of a stricture or disease of the prostate gland, a stone is to be suspected.

§. 1. *Of the Treatment where the Actions of the Urethra and Bladder do not exactly alternate.*

The cure, where the disease arises from spasm alone, consists in removing the disposition to over-action in the urethra, and the irritable disposition of the bladder when the urethra does not obey it. Perhaps opiate clysters, as a temporary means of relief, are the very best medicines that can be administered. I have known a blister to the loins, or to the perinæum, remove the spasm, in a great measure, from the urethra.

---

* Added: "In diseases of the bladder the constitution is sooner affected by symptoms of dissolution than from the same apparent degree of disease in other parts; the patient becomes drowsy, insensible, and soon dies."—*Home.*

When the circumstance of the ultimate actions of these parts not being regular arises from stricture, swelled prostate gland, or any mechanical obstruction to the urine, then that cause must be removed, as has been fully described in the treatment of these diseases.

§. 2. *Of the Paralysis of the Bladder from Obstruction to the Passage of the Urine.*

We may observe that the bladder is a part easily deprived of its power of contraction; for we find in many debilitating diseases and long illnesses from any cause, as fever, gout, and considerable local diseases which debilitate, that the bladder often becomes paralytic, and the water must be drawn off. We may also observe, when the bladder has been distended considerably, from whatever cause, so as to have its contractile power destroyed, that there is a considerable extravasation of blood from the inner surface of the bladder, so that the water which is evacuated is often extremely bloody. I have seen in cases where the patient has died with this obstruction upon him, that the inner membrane of the bladder has been almost black, being loaded with extravasated blood; but this symptom of bloody urine goes off, as the bladder acquires again its power of contraction.

In the diseases of the urethra, before described, when not properly, or in time, attended to, and in cases of stricture, where Nature has not been able to relieve herself, the water must of course be retained in the bladder, which is perhaps always productive of another disease, that is, the loss of the power of contraction of that viscus. Although this one effect, the retention of urine, arises from very different causes, as before related, yet immediate relief must be given in all of them, which can only be effected by the evacuation of water. According to the nature of the obstruction, the mode of the evacuation will be different, and will be of two kinds, one by the natural passage by means of a hollow tube, the other by an artificial opening made into the bladder.

If the causes of suppression are either spasmodic affections of the urethra, a swelled prostate gland, inflammation in the surrounding parts of the urethra, or tumours pressing upon it, as happens in pregnant women, immediate relief may be procured by means of a catheter, because under such circumstances a catheter will most probably pass, the sides of the canal being merely forced together by spasm, or external pressure.

A bougie, although it will also pass under such circumstances, will not answer so well, because a bougie must be withdrawn before the water can flow, which will allow the cause of the obstruction to exert again its full force; and if the spasm should not now exist, yet the bougie will not answer, unless there be a power of action in the bladder; for it is with difficulty that the urine can be made to pass through the urethra, by pressing the abdomen only.

When the catheter is passed, it will be necessary to make the patient strain with his abdominal muscles, as also with his muscles of respiration, to squeeze out the water, the bladder having no power of contraction, and even this will not be sufficient, for it will be necessary to press on the region of the pubes, with the hand, to make the water flow.

In cases where there is a considerable degree of debility in the bladder, or in those cases where there is a considerable strangury and of long standing, and where a small quantity of urine in the bladder gives the stimulus of fulness to that viscus, which is always attended with considerable urgency to make water, and where only very small quantities are evacuated, the bladder not being emptied at each time of making it, and when a catheter, either rigid or flexible, can with readiness be passed, the question is, What is the best way upon the whole to evacuate the water? There are three ways in which it can be done, one, by allowing the parts to do their own business as much as they can, and this at first sight might be supposed to be the very best; but it is in some cases the very worst; for the frequency of the inclination to make water, arising from the water not being wholly evacuated each time, the evacuation not readily taking place, increases the effort, and for a few minutes produces excruciating pain, keeping up a considerable and almost constant irritation in all those parts, which few can bear. Another method is, to draw off the water each time with a catheter, but this in many cases is next to impracticable; for supposing the operation to be performed only twice or three times in the day, we shall find that this is oftener than what should be done. The third method is, to leave the catheter almost constantly in the bladder.

Which of these three methods is likely to give, on the whole, the least irritation must depend upon circumstances attending different cases. Where the frequency and the urgency is great, and the flowing of the water difficult, either the second or the third is to be pursued; and when the symptoms are such that a catheter must be passed very often, I believe it had better be left in, only taking it out occasionally. I think this is supported by observation and experience.

It sometimes happens in cases of swelled prostate gland, that the catheter cannot be passed without the utmost difficulty, and when this has been the case I have left it in the bladder, for fear of not being

able to pass it again, and continued it there till the bladder has sufficiently recovered its tone, which is known by its being able to throw the
urine through the catheter ; after which that instrument may be withdrawn.

If the spasm, in such cases as arise from that cause, should still continue after the bladder has recovered its tone, we must continue the
use of the catheter. But it often happens that the spasm leaves the
urethra before the bladder recovers its power of contraction, the disease
becoming then simply a paralysis of that viscus.

One of the first symptoms of the bladder beginning to regain its
power of contraction is, the sensation of fulness, or an inclination to
make water, and when that sensation comes on the patient should be
allowed to make water ; but not to force it, for that circumstance alone
will bring on the spasm if the urethra is not very ready to dilate. I
have seen however in some cases, that a slight sensation is not altogether
to be depended upon, for it required a little retention more effectually
to stimulate the bladder to action, and then the water has passed more
freely.

The spasmodic contraction of the urethra does not appear to give up
its action simply upon the stimulus or inclination to make water, and
not till the bladder begins to have the power of contraction ; for in cases
where the bladder is paralytic, and yet sensible of the stimulus arising
from being full, as it does not contract, the urethra does not relax, and
the water cannot be made to pass.

It would appear, that, as the bladder recovers of the paralysis, it is
not able to contain so much water as usual. Therefore the patients
are obliged to make water often, and of course in small quantities.

§ 3. Of the Cure of the paralysis of the Bladder, from Obstruction arising from Pressure or Spasm.

The removal of the causes of the paralysis of the bladder was fully
described when we were treating of the diseases which produce that
complaint, and the immediate relief, when the bladder is rendered inactive, has just now been considered; the paralysis itself is therefore
the only remaining thing to be attended to. In this disease there are
often contrary indications of cure, for a spasm is very different from a
paralysis ; and if the suppression is from spasm, and that still continues,
then what may be good for the paralysis, may be bad for the spasm.
As in such cases the water can be drawn off, the bladder should be first
attended to. Stimulants and strengtheners are useful ; blisters to the

loins to rouse the bladder to action, and blisters to the perinæum, to take off the spasm from the urethra, often succeed. Electricity is sometimes of singular service, when applied in such cases to the perinæum. Through the whole of the cure the urine must be drawn off frequently, because the bladder should not be allowed to be distended, which otherwise would be the consequence ; and the sensation arising from the distention of that viscus is a very oppressive one.

A gentleman was at times attacked with a difficulty in making water, which he paid no attention to, as it had always gone off; but at last he was obliged to have recourse to the catheter, which afforded only a temporary relief. The spasm continued, and I was sent for. When I passed the catheter, I was obliged to press the lower part of the abdomen to squeeze out the water, for the bladder appeared to give but little assistance. I ordered a blister to the loins, which gave some power of contraction to the bladder, and took off some of the spasm in the urethra, but still he was very little relieved. I then directed a blister to be applied to the perinæum, which immediately removed his complaint.

CHAPTER X.

OF A SUPPRESSION OF URINE—AND OPERATIONS FOR THE CURE OF IT.

In cases of total suppression of urine arising from strictures, or other causes where a catheter cannot be passed, and where every other method recommended is impracticable, an artificial opening must be made into the bladder for the evacuation of the water. There are three places where this opening may be made, and each has had its advocates, This operation has not been considered in all its circumstances in different patients, so as to direct the young surgeon in the variety of cases that may occur; for under some circumstances the operation is more advisable in one place than another; and indeed it may sometimes be next to impossible to perform it in a particular part.

The opening may be made first in the perinæum, where we now cut for a stone ; secondly, above the pubes, where cutting for the stone was

formerly practised; and thirdly, from within the rectum, where the
bladder lies in contact with the gut.

The first question, which naturally occurs, is, Which of those situations is the most proper for the safety of the patient, the evacuation of
the water, and the conveniency of operating, when no particular circumstance forbids either of the situations?

On the first view of the subject, one would be apt to prefer that
above the pubes, or from the rectum, as the bladder is nearer to either,
and the parts more adapted to an operation than from the perinæum,
where we must cut at random. These two situations, although the
most proper in this respect, under certain circumstances, yet may become the most improper, for they are subject to greater changes than
the perinæum.

The reasons that may render it very improper above the pubes are,
the persons being very fat, or the bladders not distending sufficiently
so as to rise above the pubes, which is common enough in diseases of
those parts.

In very fat people it will be found that the substance to be cut through
may be three or four inches, which will not only make the operation
very unpleasant, but often improper; for such thickness of parts will
make the swell of the bladder very obscure and uncertain; in many the
bladder is so diseased as to allow of but little distention, and in such
the symptoms of fulness come on very early, perhaps when there are
only a few ounces of water collected. But if the retention has been
for some considerable time, as twenty-four hours, then we may suppose
that the bladder has allowed of distention to a much greater degree,
which may in some cases be ascertained by introducing the finger into
the rectum.

But where the bladder distends, and the parts are so thin that it can
be plainly felt above the pubes, I see no material objection to this situation; and it has this advantage over the operation by the rectum,
that a catheter can more easily be introduced, and kept in, which will
be necessary to be done till the cause is removed.

It may be necessary here to mention some precautions respecting the
keeping the instrument in the bladder; as also the best kind to be used.
It must be a hollow tube, and should reach as far as the posterior surface of the bladder, for upon the contraction of that viscus its anterior
part recedes backwards and downwards from the abdomen towards its
fixed point, which may draw the bladder off from the tube. But as
the distance between the skin of the abdomen and posterior surface of
the bladder cannot be exactly ascertained, the cannula may be either
too long, or too short; if too long, its end may press upon the posterior

surface of the bladder and produce ulceration there, and in time work its way into the rectum. To avoid this mischief, as also the inconveniences arising from its being too short, and the bladder slipping off from its end, I would recommend the tube to be made with a curve, and to lie with its convex side on the posterior part of the bladder, which being a large surface, and following nearly the same curve as the cannula, less mischief is to be expected. The openings into the cannula may be made on the concave side.

It would probably be both safer and easier for the patient, to have the curved end of the catheter introduced into the urethra from the bladder. The passing of it into the urethra is very practicable; and we know that such a body lying in the urethra is not productive of any mischief. A common catheter passed in this way enters so far as to bring the handle almost flat to the belly; at most only a little bolster between the catheter and belly is necessary, and then with a piece of tape fixed to the handle of the catheter it might be fastened to the body; or a short catheter might be made with ears to fix the tape to *. In cases where the cannula has remained in the urethra some time, the artificial passage will become in some degree permanent, so that it may be taken out occasionally, and cleaned from any stony matter that may be attached to it. To avoid this part of the operation it has been recommended to have two cannulas, one within the other, that by drawing out the inner it may be cleaned, and again introduced; but in most cases it will also be necessary to withdraw the outer one, as its external surface will contract a crust.

The second method, or puncture by the anus, will more commonly admit of being performed than that above the pubes; for it does not require that distention of bladder which the other does, and is therefore not so often impracticable from that cause; and perhaps the only obstacle here is a swelled prostate gland. In many of these cases of diseases of the urethra, the prostate gland is very much swelled, which I can conceive may make the proper place for the puncture very uncertain; for the prostate gland, in such cases, will be pressed down towards the anus, before the bladder, and will be the first thing felt by the finger. Care must therefore be taken to distinguish the one from the other, which can only be done by getting the finger beyond the prostate gland,

---

* Where this operation is performed in consequence of a stricture, I have conceived that by passing a catheter into the urethra from the bladder till it comes to the stricture, and then passing another straight cannula from the glans down the urethra, that the two may nearly meet, only having the stricture between them; and a piercer may be passed down and forced into the end of the one from the bladder, and afterwards either a bougie or hollow catheter introduced.

which may not be practicable; and if practicable, it may not be an easy matter to distinguish the one from the other, as a thickened and distended bladder may seem to be a continuation of the same tumor. However, if the objections given to the performing it above the pubes exist, I should prefer operating by the rectum; for although the probability of succeeding here may not be apparently greater than above the pubes, yet the chances are in its favour.

I must however observe here, that the objections which I have started, are only raised in my own mind from my knowledge of the diseases of those parts, and not from cases of suppression of urine under all the before-mentioned circumstances having occurred to me in practice.

A case of a total suppression of urine arising from stricture, where no instrument could be passed by the natural passage, and where a puncture was made into the bladder, from the rectum, with success, is related in the Philosophical Transactions, by Dr. Hamilton of Kings-Lynn in Norfolk*.

What led Dr. Hamilton to do it here, was a difficulty which was found in passing the clyster-pipe into the rectum, which induced him to introduce his finger into the anus, and he found the bladder so prominent in the rectum as to give the hint of performing the operation there.

The man was put into the same position as in the operation for the stone, and a trochar was introduced upon the finger into the anus, and thrust into the lower and most prominent part of the tumor, in the direction of the axis of the bladder, and upon withdrawing the piercer the water flowed out through the cannula.

A straight catheter was then introduced through the cannula, lest the orifice in the bladder should be drawn off from the cannula.

Then the cannula was pulled out over the catheter, which was left in till the whole water was evacuated, and was then withdrawn.

The bladder, nothwithstanding this perforation, retained the water as usual, till the inclination to make it came on ; and when he performed the action of making water, the orifice in the bladder seemed to open, and it rushed out by the anus.   This continued about two days, when the water began to find its natural passage, and a bougie was introduced into the bladder, through the urethra, which gave a free passage for the water, and of course less came by the anus; so that on the sixth day after the operation the whole came by the natural passage. The man continued the use of the bougie till the stricture was dilated. Dr. Hamilton further remarks, that in those cases of suppression of urine,

* Philosophical Transactions for the year 1776, vol. lxvi. p. 578.

in general, he has found that calomel and opium, in large doses, answer better than anything he has tried.   He is convinced, from repeated trials, that the specific efficacy is in the calomel, as large doses of opium alone have proved ineffectual; but he does not say that calomel alone will answer.   He orders ten grains of calomel with two of opium, to be repeated in six hours if it has not answered in that time; and he says he has seldom been obliged to give a third dose.

This method of tapping the bladder was first suggested by Mons. Fleurant, surgeon to the Charité, at Lyons, in the year 1750.   The operation was performed at that time, and an account of it was afterwards published by Mons. Pouteau, in 1760, with the history of three cases, in all which the operation was performed by Mons. Fleurant. The propriety of performing the operation in this part occurred to him in a manner similar to that before related of Dr. Hamilton; for in introducing the finger into the rectum to examine the state of the bladder in a case where he was going to puncture in the perinæum, he found the bladder so prominent there, and so much within the reach of his instrument, that he immediately altered his intention, and performed it in this part.   He very readily drew off the water, and kept the cannula in, with a T bandage, till the urine came the right way, and then withdrew it, and all terminated well.   But there was a good deal of trouble on account of the cannula being left in on going to stool, as also from the constant dribbling of the water through it; all of which was prevented in Dr. Hamilton's case, by removing the cannula immediately upon the evacuation of the water.   This was productive of another good effect, which was the retention of the urine till the stimulus of fulness was given, and then it passed through the artificial as it would through a natural passage.   Should this be a constant effect in consequence of performing the operation here, I think it must be owned to be an unexpected circumstance which at first could not have been imagined*.

In another patient of Mons. Fleurant's, the cannula was kept in the anus and bladder thirty-nine days, without any inconveniency; so that the objection to this part of the operation cannot be material.   Pouteau mentions one case where he performed this operation, in the year 1752, and the man died†.   He says: "I was called to visit a poor man suffering under a retention of urine, so obstinate and violent that it had already the symptoms of what is called a reflux of urine into the blood; and the complaint had continued more than three days.   An empiric, to whose care he had been entrusted, after having very improperly given

* A history, with a description of this operation, was published by Mr. Reid, surgeon, of Chelsea, in 1778.

† Pouteau, Melanges de Chirurgie, printed at Lyons, 1760, p. 506—508.

him the most powerful diuretics, had likewise the rashness to search him. It appears probable that these attempts, which were made without success, must have increased the mischief. A catheter could not be passed into such parts by unskilful hands without increasing the inflammation. I only made three slight efforts to effect a passage into the bladder by the urethra, which appeared to be much diseased, as well by the effusion of blood as the extreme pain which these attempts produced. I determined at once to do as before, and plunged my trochar by the rectum into the bladder. The success was exactly the same; the bladder was entirely emptied, and I allowed the cannula to remain there a whole night and a day, during which time the urine flowed without intermission. Everything went on without any accident which could be supposed connected with the operation; and death, which happened next day, was entirely independent of it."

One must suppose, with Pouteau, that the death of the patient could not have arisen from this operation, but from the preceding diseases.

The bags called vesiculæ seminales, and the hæmorrhoidal vessels, have been mentioned as parts in danger of being wounded in the operation, and thereby proving troublesome; but if either of them are wounded, no inconvenience can arise. To avoid the vesiculæ seminales it is recommended to perforate high up, and directly in the middle of the bladder, between the two sides; and this situation is, at the same time, the one where the hæmorrhoidal vessels are the smallest, and therefore it is of less consequence if they are wounded.

It must appear from the following case, sent me by a gentleman, that a communication being kept up between the bladder and rectum is only inconvenient, and not so much so as might be expected.

" With respect to the sailor who passed his urine by the rectum, I have examined the few papers by me, but cannot find the particular remarks I made; however, as the case was singular, I recollect the man told me that, a few years before, (this was at Madras Hospital, in December 1779,) he had the venereal disease, very bad and long: that the urine came by the anus, but this passage healed up, and it came by the penis, and continued to do so till he caught the disease again, when the urine found its way a second time by the anus, and came that way for years. When he first came under my care, in the hospital at Bombay, February 1779, he felt no uneasiness or inconvenience from this manner of passing his urine: whenever he had an inclination to make water he sat down. I often made him lie upon his breast, with his legs drawn up, and the stream came through the anus with great force*."

* Added: "John Conway, a seaman belonging to the St. Antonia, was admitted into Haslar Hospital on the 24th November 1770, for the lues venerea. Besides the

In other cases, in consequence of abscesses forming between the bladder and rectum, where they have not healed up, there has been a reci-
procal passing of the contents of these cavities from the one to the other.

It only remains to speak of the puncture in the perinæum. An obstruction to the urine taking place in the natural passage prevents us
from introducing an instrument in most of those cases, and deprives us
of all the advantages we could receive from it as a guide in the operation; yet there may be cases of stricture where, by cutting into the
urethra beyond the stricture, the water will flow; but this must be done
without any guide or direction, and requires a nice and accurate knowledge of the parts. Or if the obstruction arises from the valvular projection of the prostate gland, a staff may be passed as far as this projection, and cut upon as for the stone, the surgeon only making a
similar incision, using a small gorget, or, in the room of that, a trochar
of a particular form might be run along it into the bladder; for although
the staff does not enter the bladder, yet the distance to pass through
without this guide is but small. If this cannot be done, a small and
deep incision may be made in the perinæum, with an imposthume lancet
towards the bladder; the point of the trochar is to be introduced by
this, the surgeon passing at the same time the forefinger of the other
hand into the anus, which will be a guide both for the direction of the
instrument, as also to avoid its point passing into the rectum. With
these precautions the error cannot be great.

I must own, however, that I have not seen cases enough to enable
me to give all the varieties that commonly happen, and of course to give
all the advantages and disadvantages of each method[a].

usual symptoms of that disease he had a communication between the bladder and rectum, which had continued four months. When he endeavoured to make water, the
water flowed both from the urethra and anus, coming from the anus in a small stream,
often to the quantity of a pint. It also flowed freely from the anus when he went to
stool, although none was voided by the urethra. In the beginning of the complaint
some portions of dead flesh, he said, had come away from the rectum, but when admitted into the hospital there was not any soreness remaining, or discharge of matter
from it, and the urine passed without pain: externally he never had any fistula pe-
entrating either into the bladder or rectum, and when disturbed with flatulence in the
bowels, did not perceive any wind to escape from the urethra."—*Home.*

*   [In cases of retention of urine from stricture, it is always more safe to open the
urethra than to puncture the bladder. The bladder is imbedded in loose cellular membrane, which envelopes it everywhere, and which must be wounded if the bladder is
punctured, whatever part be chosen for that operation. Now such a wound cannot be
made without great danger, because the urine is thus admitted into this loose cellular
texture, and frequently diffuses itself through it, producing extensive sloughing and
abscess. This is by no means a rare consequence of puncture of the bladder, and when
it occurs, is very generally fatal. The opening of the urethra is not attended with the

§. 1. *Of allowing a Catheter to remain in the Urethra and Bladder.*

In cases of debility of the bladder, and where a catheter passes with difficulty, or with great uncertainty, and in cases where it must be used frequently, and for a length of time, it will be necessary to keep an instrument in the urethra and bladder, so as to allow the water to pass through it freely. A common catheter, or one made of the elastic gum,

---

same risk, because the cellular membrane of the perinæum is generally loaded with fat, and the escape of the urine is in all cases direct and easy; and even if abscess should take place, it will be near the surface, and can be laid open with the greatest facility.

Under ordinary circumstances the urethra is collapsed, and is not easily found, unless some instrument is previously introduced as a guide: but in cases of retention of urine from stricture, it is always greatly dilated between the contracted part and the bladder, and there is not the same difficulty. As there is variety in the seat of stricture, there will be some variety also in the operation which is required.

When the obstruction is situated before the bulb, the distension of the urethra behind it may be distinctly felt in the perinæum, especially when the patient is straining to pass water. Under such circumstances nothing is easier than to open the dilated part of the passage with a common lancet.

But the stricture is much more frequently seated at the part where the membranous portion of the canal enters the bulb. In this case the difficulty is greater. Nevertheless, the dilated part of the urethra may generally be felt through the rectum, and more or less distinctly in the perinæum; and if a previous incision be made, as in lithotomy, through the superficial parts, it may be reached, and laid open. The operator may derive some assistance from the introduction of a sound into the urethra, as far as the stricture, which will point out the direction of the canal; but his principal guide must be the position of the pubes, since in this case the part which is to be punctured will lie immediately below the symphysis.

When the contraction is still further back, so as to be near the apex of the prostate gland, it may be impossible to feel any dilatation; and in this case the operation must be varied. A staff should be first introduced into the urethra, and passed down to the stricture. The groove of the staff should then be laid open for a small extent near its point, and this will enable the operator to introduce a probe, which may be passed on to the stricture, and without much trouble, made to penetrate it. When that has been effected, it will not be difficult to pass a catheter through the stricture into the bladder, and to draw off the water.

These operations are not applicable to cases where the obstruction arises from an enlarged prostate gland. In this case the mouth of the urethra is closed, and no urine is admitted into it: yet even here the operation of puncturing the bladder is more hazardous than the perforation of the enlarged prostate. A silver catheter may be forced forward through the prostate, and carried into the cavity of the bladder; and this has been done on several occasions, without being followed by serious consequences, or even by material inconvenience. The opening thus made has sometimes been permanent; at other times it has appeared to close, and the urine has been passed in the same manner as before the operation, and with equal facility.]

is perhaps the best instrument; but it must be fixed in the canal: this will be best done by its outer end being tied to some external body, as I shall now describe. When the catheter is fairly in the bladder, the outer end is rather inclined downwards, nearly in a line with the body. To keep it in this position we may take the common strap or belt-part of a bag-truss, with two thigh-straps either fixed to it or hooked to it, and coming round each thigh forwards by the side of the scrotum, to be fastened to the belt where the ears of the bag are usually fixed. A small ring or two may be fixed to each strap just where it passes the scrotum or root of the penis ; and, with a piece of small tape, the ends of the catheter may be fixed to those rings, which will keep it in the bladder. A bit of rag about four or five inches long, with a hole at the end of it, passed over the exterior end of the catheter, and the loose end allowed to hang in a bason, placed between the thighs, will catch the water which cannot disengage itself from the catheter, and keep the patient dry ; or if another curved pipe is introduced into the catheter it will answer the same purpose.

Under such treatment the bladder will never be allowed to be dis-tended; and when the patient wants to have the bladder in some degree emptied, he has only to strain with his abdominal muscles, by which means he will be able to throw out a great deal at each time.

As the bladder begins to recover its actions, the patient will find that an inclination to make water will come on, and at those times he will also find that the water will come from him without straining with the abdominal muscles ; when this takes place readily, the catheter may be taken out, and it will be found that he will be able in future to make water of himself. If it is necessary to keep in the catheter a consider-able time, it will be the cause of a great deal of slime and mucus being formed in the urethra and bladder; but I believe this is of no conse-quence. I have known a catheter kept in this way for five months without any inconveniency whatever.

In all cases where it is necessary to keep an extraneous body for a considerable time in the bladder, whether in an artificial passage or the natural one, it will be proper a few days after its first introduction to withdraw it, and examine whether it is incrusting, or filling up in its cavity with the calculous matter of the urine. If, after remaining in the bladder for some days, it has contracted none, we need be under no apprehension of its doing it; but if, as frequently happens, it should have collected a considerable quantity, then it will be necessary to have it occasionally withdrawn and cleaned. The best method probably of doing this is to put it in vinegar, which will soon dissolve the stony matter.

§. 2. *Of the increased Strength of the Bladder.*

The bladder, in such cases as have been described, having more to do than common, is almost in a constant state of irritation and action; by which, according to a property in all muscles, it becomes stronger and stronger in its muscular coats; and I suspect that this disposition to become stronger from repeated action, is greater in the involuntary muscles than the voluntary; and the reason why it should be so is, I think, very evident: for in the involuntary muscles the power should be in all cases capable of overcoming the resistance, as the power is always performing some natural and necessary action; for whenever a disease produces an uncommon resistance in the involuntary parts, if the power is not proportionally increased, the disease becomes very formidable; whereas in the voluntary muscles there is not that necessity, because the will can stop whenever the muscles cannot follow; and if the will is so diseased as not to stop, the power in voluntary muscles should not increase in proportion.

I have seen the muscular coats of the bladder near half an inch thick, and the fasciculi so strong as to form ridges on the inside of that cavity*; and I have also seen the fasciculi very thin, and even wanting in some parts of the bladder, so that a hernia of the internal coat had taken place between the fasciculi and formed pouches†. These pouches arise from the thin parts not being able to support the actions of the strong; as happens in ruptures at the navel or rings of the abdomen.

§. 3. *Of the Distention of the Ureters.*

It sometimes happens that the irritation from the distention of the bladder, and the difficulty in throwing out its contents, is so great that the urine is prevented from flowing freely into that viscus from the ureters, which become thereby preternaturally distended. The pelvis of the kidneys and infundibula are also enlarged; but how far this di-

---

* This appearance was long supposed to have arisen from a disease of that viscus; but upon examination I found that the muscular parts were sound and distinct, that they were only increased in bulk in proportion to the power they had to exert, and that it was not a consequence of inflammation, for in that case parts are blended into one indistinct mass.

† This is perhaps the cause of the stone being often found in a pouch formed in the bladder: for the bladder in cases of stone is often very strong, which arises from the violent contraction of that viscus, caused by the irritation of the stone on the sides of it; and also from the stone being often opposed to the mouth of the urethra in the time of making water.

latation of the ureters and pelvis is really owing to a mechanical cause
I am not so clear, or whether it is not a disposition for dilatation arising
out of the stimulus given by the bladder. In some cases of long standing, where the bladder was become very thick, and had been for a long
time acting with great violence, it had affected the mamillæ, so that the
surface of these processes produced a matter, and perhaps even the secreting organs of the kidneys, so that the urine secreted was accompanied with a pus, arising from the irritation being kept up in all these
parts.

The urine in the above cases is generally stale, even before it is
thrown out of the bladder, which when joined with the circumstance of
the linen being constantly kept wet, by the almost continual discharge
of urine, becomes very offensive, and it is hardly possible to keep the
patient sweet.

§. 4. *Of Irritability in the Bladder independent of Obstructions to the Passage of the Urine.*

Another disease of the bladder, connected with the present subject,
is, where that viscus becomes extremely irritable, and will not allow of
its usual distention. The symptoms of this disease are very similar to
those arising from obstructions to the passage of the urine in the urethra, but with this difference, that in the present disease the urine flows.
readily, because the urethra obeys the summons and relaxes; however,
there is often considerable straining, after the water is all voided, arising from the muscular coat of the bladder still continuing its contractions.

This irritability of the bladder often arises from local causes, as a
stone, cancer, or tumours forming on the inside, all which produce irritability of this viscus. In such cases the straining is violent, for the
cause still remains which continues to give the stimulus of something
to be expelled, and the bladder continues to contract till tired, as in the
cases of simple irritability, and then there is a respite for a time; but
this respite is of short duration, for the urine is soon accumulated.

This disease will in the end be fatal by producing hectic fever.

§. 5. *Of the Cure of simple Irritability of the Bladder.*

When the symptoms arise from irritability alone, and not from a
stone or any local affection, the nature of the complaint may not at first

be so obvious; temporary relief may, however, be procured by opium, which is most effectual in slight and recent cases; and if it be applied as near to the part as possible, its effects will be more evident; and therefore it may be given by clyster as well as by the mouth*.

I should, however, be rather inclined to rely on a blister applied to the perinæum, or to the lower part of the small of the back, or upper part of the sacrum if more convenient, than to any other method of cure.

In all cases, where there is an irritation of the bladder, the patient should never endeavour to retain his water beyond the inclination to make it. It hurts the bladder and increases its irritability; and indeed I am apt to think that this circumstance, even in sound parts, is often a predisposing cause of disease in this viscus and its appendage, the urethra: for I have known several cases where it has brought on the spasmodic stricture in the urethra in sound parts, and it is frequently an immediate cause of strangury in those who have either a stricture or a disposition to spasms in those parts.

A gentleman in perfect health, from retaining his urine beyond the inclination, in the playhouse, had all the symptoms of an irritable bladder brought on, which continued for several years, rendering him miserable.

§. 6. *Of a Paralysis of the Acceleratores Urinæ.*

In many irritations of the bladder, the urethra not only relaxes directly on the stimulus to make water being felt in that viscus, as has been described, but a paralysis sometimes takes place in the voluntary muscles of those parts, so that the will cannot command them to contract to hinder the inconveniences that may attend an immediate evacuation of that fluid. If we attempt to stop the water, which is an act of the will, it is in vain; the acceleratores will not obey, and the water flows.

A blister applied to the perinæum will have considerable effects in removing this complaint.

* Added: "I have known alum whey given, under which treatment the patient got well."—*Home.*

CHAPTER XI.

OF THE DISCHARGE OF THE NATURAL MUCUS OF THE GLANDS OF THE URETHRA.

THE small glands of the urethra and Cowper's glands secrete a slimy mucus, similar to the white of an egg not coagulated. This seldom appears externally, or flows from the urethra, but during the indulgence of lascivious thoughts, and is seldom or never attended to, excepting by those who are either under apprehensions of a gonorrhœa coming on, or imagine the last infection is not gone off entirely, and are therefore kept in constant terror by this natural discharge. They often find it in such quantity as to leave spots on the shirt, but without colour; and often after toying, the lips of the urethra are, as it were, glued together by it, from its drying there, which appearances alarm the mind of the patient without cause. Although this is only a natural discharge, and is secreted, at such times, under the same influence which naturally produces it, it must be owned that it is commonly much increased in those cases of debility arising from the mind, which is probably not easily to be accounted for. It would seem that the contest between the mind and the body increases this secretion, for it cannot be considered as a disease of the parts.

§. 1. *Of the Discharge of the Secretions of the Prostate Gland and Vesiculæ Seminales.*

This complaint is imagined to be the consequence of the venereal disease in the urethra; but how far this is really the case is not certain, though most probably it is not. It is a discharge of mucus by the urethra which generally comes away with the last drops of urine, especially if the bladder is irritable, and still more at the time of being at stool, particularly if the patient be costive, for under such circumstances the straining or actions of the muscles of those parts are more violent. It has generally been supposed that this discharge is semen, and the disease is called a seminal weakness; but it appears, from many experiments and observations, that the discharge is undoubtedly not semen. It is only the mucus secreted either by the prostate gland, by those bags improperly called vesiculæ seminales, or both; and it may not be improper to give here the distinguishing marks between these two fluids. First, we may observe the discharge in question is not of the same colour with the semen, and is exactly of the colour of the mucus of the prostate gland and of those bags. It has not the same smell, and indeed it hardly has any smell at all. The quantity, evacuated at one time is often much more considerable than the evacuation of semen ever is and it happens more frequently than it could possibly do were the discharge semen. It is a disease that often attacks old men, where one can hardly suppose much semen to be secreted; and we find that those who are affected with this disease are no more deficient in the secretion and evacuation of the semen, in the natural way, than before they had the disease. If the mind be at ease, this shall take place immediately after a discharge of semen as well as before, which could not be the case were it semen. Further, if those that labour under this complaint are not connected with women they are subject to nocturnal discharges from the imagination, as persons who are perfectly sound: and indeed most patients, when made acquainted with these circumstances, become very sensible that it is not the semen*.

It is not clear what the diseased state of the parts is upon which this discharge depends, whether there is a larger secretion of this mucus than natural, or whether it is entirely owing to a preternatural uncommon action of those parts; and if this last, why these parts should be put into action when the bladder, rectum, and abdominal muscles are thrown into action to expel their contents, is not easily explained. It is plain that the most violent actions of these parts are necessary to produce this evacuation; for it does not come with the first of the urine, nor in general with an easy stool.

As it was thought to be a seminal discharge, it was imagined to arise from a weakness in the organs of generation; and as frequent discharges of the semen in the natural way generally weaken, it was therefore imagined that this discharge must also weaken very considerably; and the imagination will operate so strongly as to make the patients believe they really are weakened. Whether the cause of such a discharge is capable of weakening, I will not pretend to say; but I believe that the discharge simply does not. Fear and anxiety of mind may really weaken the patient. In the cases I have seen of this kind the mind has been more affected than the body.

From my own practice, I can hardly recommend any one medicine,

---

* Added: "A gentleman has often a discharge of mucus from the urethra with the last drops of urine, and when he goes to stool, but after having connexion with women it does not take place."—*Home.*

or way of life, for removing this complaint. In one case I found considerable benefit from giving hemlock internally.

The idea that has been formed of the disease leads to the practice generally recommended, such as giving strengthening medicines of all kinds; but I never saw any good effects from any of them, and I should rather be inclined to take up the soothing plan to prevent all violent actions. Keeping the body gently open will in some degree moderate the discharge, and probably may effect a cure in the end.

CHAPTER XII.

OF IMPOTENCE.

THIS complaint is by many laid to the charge of Onanism at an early age; but how far this is just it will in many cases be difficult to determine; for, upon a strict review of this subject, it appears to me to be by far too rare to originate from a practice so general.

How far the attributing to this practice such a consequence is of public utility, I am doubtful, particularly as it is followed most commonly at an age when consequences are not sufficiently attended to, even in things less gratifying to the senses; but this I can say with certainty, that many of those who are affected with the complaints in question are miserable from this idea; and it is some consolation for them to know that it is possible it may arise from other causes. I am clear in my own mind that the books on this subject have done more harm than good.

In the cases of this kind that have come under my care, although the persons themselves have been very ready to suppose that the disease has arisen from the cause here alluded to, yet they did not appear to have given more into the practice than common; and in particular, the worst case I have ever seen was where but very little of this practice had ever been used, much less than in common among boys*.

Nothing hurts the mind of a man so much as the idea of inability to

---

* Added: "which is particularly pernicious from the frequency of the repetition, there being no want of opportunity."—*Home.*

perform well the duty of the sex.   If his scrotum hangs low it makes him miserable; he conceives immediately that he is to be rendered incapable of performing those acts in which he prides himself most.   It is certain that the relaxation or contraction of the scrotum is in some degree a kind of sign of the constitution; but it is of the constitution at large, not of those parts in particular.   Nurses are so sensible of the contraction of that part being a sign of health in the children under their care, that they take notice of it.   The relaxation of it in them cannot be supposed to arise from inability to perform those acts at one time more than another.   The face is one of the signs of the constitution, and has as much to do with those peculiar acts as the scrotum.   However, we must allow that this part is much more lax than what we should conceive was intended by Nature, even in young men who are well in health; but as this is very general, I rather suspect that it arises from the circumstances of the part being kept too warm, and always suspended, the muscles hardly ever being allowed to act, so that they have less force.   How far it is the same in those countries where the dress does not immediately suspend those parts, I have not been able to ascertain.   Warmth appears to be one cause, for we find that cold has generally an immediate effect; but this is perhaps owing to its not being accustomed to cold, which if it were, it might possibly become as regardless of it as it is of warmth.   What the difference is in this part, in a cold and warm climate, all other circumstances the same, I do not know.   But whatever may be the cause, if it is really in common more lax than intended by Nature, it is of no consequence as to the powers of generation.   The testicles will secrete, whether kept high or low[a].

§. 1. *Of Impotence depending on the Mind.*

As the parts of generation are not necessary for the existence or support of the individual, but have a reference to something else, in which the mind has a principal concern, a complete action in those parts cannot take place without a perfect harmony of body and of mind; that is, there must be both a power of body and disposition of mind; for the mind is subject to a thousand caprices, which affect the actions of these parts.

---

[a] [Sir E. Home has here added a note, in which he expresses a belief that Onanism is more hurtful than the author imagined, and that its being practised before the parts have arrived at maturity in weakly constitutions, may prevent their ever attaining their full power and development.   This opinion is not only in itself reasonable, but seems also to be confirmed by experience.]

Copulation is an act of the body, the spring of which is in the mind; but it is not volition; and according to the state of the mind so is the act performed. To perform this act well, the body should be in health, and the mind should be perfectly confident of the powers of the body; the mind should be in a state entirely disengaged from everything else; it should have no difficulties, no fears, no apprehensions; not even an anxiety to perform the act well; for even this anxiety is a state of mind different from what should prevail; there should not be even a fear that the mind itself may find a difficulty at the time the act should be performed. Perhaps no function of the machine depends so much upon the state of the mind as this.

The will and reasoning faculty have nothing to do with this power; they are only employed in the act, so far as voluntary parts are made use of; and if they ever interfere, which they sometimes do, it often produces another state of mind, which destroys that which is proper for the performance of the act; it produces a desire, a wish, a hope, which are all only diffidence and uncertainty, and create in the mind the idea of a possibility of the want of success, which destroys the proper state of mind, or necessary confidence.

There is perhaps no act in which a man feels himself more interested, or is more anxious to perform well, his pride being engaged in some degree, which, if within certain bounds, would produce a degree of perfection in an act depending upon the will, or an act in voluntary parts; but when it produces a state of mind contrary to that state, on which the perfection of the act depends, a failure must be the consequence.

The body is not only rendered incapable of performing this act, by the mind being under the above influence, but also by the mind being perfectly confident of its power, but conscious of an impropriety in performing it; this, in many cases, produces a state of mind which shall take away all power. The state of a man's mind, respecting his sister, takes away all power. A conscientious man has been known to lose his powers on finding the woman he was going to be connected with unexpectedly a virgin.

Shedding tears arises entirely from the state of the mind, although not so much a compound action as the act in question; for none are so weak in body that they cannot shed tears; it is not so much a compound action of the mind and strength of body, joined, as the other act is; yet if we are afraid of shedding tears, or are desirous of doing it, and that anxiety is kept up through the whole of an affecting scene, we certainly shall not shed tears, or at least not so freely as would have happened from our natural feelings.

From this account of the necessity of having the mind independent respecting the act, we must see that it may very often happen that the state of mind will be such as not to allow the animal to exert its natural powers; and every failure increases the evil. We must also see from this state of the case, that this act must be often interrupted; and the true cause of this interruption not being known, it will be laid to the charge of the body, or want of powers. As these cases do not arise from real inability, they are to be carefully distinguished from such as do; and perhaps the only way to distinguish them is to examine into the state of mind respecting this act. So trifling often is the circumstance which shall produce this inability depending on the mind, that the very desire to please shall have that effect, as in making the woman the sole object to be gratified.

Cases of this kind we see every day, one of which I shall relate, as an illustration of this subject, and also of the method of cure.

A gentleman told me that he had lost his virility. After above an hour's investigation of the case, I made out the following facts. That he had, at unnecessary times, strong erections, which showed that he had naturally this power; that the erections were accompanied with desire, which are all the natural powers wanted; but that there was still a defect somewhere, which I supposed to be from the mind. I inquired if all women were alike to him; his answer was, no; some women he could have connexion with as well as ever. This brought the defect, whatever it was, into a smaller compass; and it appeared there was but one woman that produced this inability, and that it arose from a desire to perform the act with this woman well, which desire produced in the mind a doubt, or fear of the want of success, which was the cause of the inability of performing the act. As this arose entirely from the state of the mind, produced by a particular circumstance, the mind was to be applied to for the cure; and I told him that he might be cured if he could perfectly rely on his own power of self-denial. When I explained what I meant, he told me that he could depend upon every act of his will, or resolution; I then told him, if he had a perfect confidence in himself in that respect, that he was to go to bed to this woman, but first promise to himself that he would not have any connexion with her for six nights, let his inclinations and powers be what they would, which he engaged to do, and also to let me know the result. About a fortnight after he told me that this resolution had produced such a total alteration in the state of his mind that the power soon took place; for instead of going to bed with the fear of inability, he went with fears that he should be possessed with too much desire, too much power, so as to become uneasy to him, which really happened; for he would have been

x 2

happy to have shortened the time; and when he had once broke the spell, the mind and powers went on together, and his mind never returned to its former state*.

§. 2. Of Impotence from a want of proper correspondence between the actions of the different organs.

I lately observed, when treating of the diseases of the urethra and bladder, that every organ in an animal body, without exception, was made up of different parts, whose functions, or actions, were totally different from each other, although all tending to produce one ultimate effect. In all such organs, when perfect, there is a succession of motions, one naturally arising out of the other, which in the end produces the ultimate effect; and an irregularity alone in these actions will constitute disease, at least will produce very disagreeable effects, and often totally frustrate the final intention of the organ. I come now to apply this principle to the actions of the testicle and the penis; for we find that an irregularity in the actions of these parts sometimes happens in men, producing impotence; and something similar, probably, may be one cause of barrenness in women.

In men the parts subservient to generation may be divided into two, the essential and the accessory. The testicles are the essential; the penis, &c., the accessory. As this division arises from their uses or actions in health, which exactly correspond with one another; a want of exactness in the correspondence, or susceptibility of those actions, may also be divided into two: where the actions are reversed, the accessory taking place without the first, or essential, as in erections of the penis, where neither the mind nor the testicles are stimulated to action; and the second is where the testicle performs the action of secretion too readily for the penis, which has not a corresponding erection. The first is called priapism, and the second is what ought to be called seminal weakness.

The mind has considerable effect on the correspondence of the actions of these two parts; but it would appear in many instances that erections of the penis depend more on the state of the mind than what the secretion of the semen does; for many have the secretion, but not the erection; but in such the want of erection appears to be owing to the mind only.

Priapism often arises spontaneously, and often from visible irritation

---

* Added: "Several similar instances have come under my care, but there is an evident objection to multiplying unnecessarily cases of this kind."—*Home.*

of the penis, such as the venereal gonorrhœa, especially when violent. The sensation of such erections is rather uneasy than pleasant; nor is the sensation of the glans at the time similar to that arising from the erections of desire, but more like to the sensation of the parts immediately after coition.   Such as arise spontaneously are of more serious consequence than those from inflammation, as they proceed, probably, from causes not curable in themselves, or by any known methods.

The priapism arising from inflammation of the parts, as in a gonorrhœa, is attended with nearly the same symptoms; but generally the sensation is that of pain, proceeding from the inflammation of the parts.   It may be observed, that what is said of priapism is only applicable to it when a disease of itself, and not as a symptom of other diseases, which is frequently the case*.

The common practice in the cure of this complaint is to order all the nervous and strengthening medicines, such as bark, valerian, musk, camphor, and also the cold bath.   I have seen good effects from the cold bath; but sometimes it does not agree with the constitution, in which cases I have found the warm bath of service.   Opium appears to be a specific in many cases, from which circumstance, I should be apt, upon the whole, to try a soothing plan.

Seminal weakness, or a secretion and emission of the semen without erections, is the reverse of a priapism, and is by much the worst disease of the two.   There is great variety in the degrees of this disease, there being all the gradations from the exact correspondence of the actions of all the parts to the testicles acting alone; in every case of the disease there is too quick a secretion and evacuation of the semen.   Like to the priapism, it does not arise from desires and abilities, although when mild it is attended with both, but not in a due proportion; a very slight desire often producing the full effect.   The secretion of the semen shall be so quick that simple thought, or even toying, shall make it flow.

Dreams have produced this evacuation repeatedly in the same night; and even when the dreams have been so slight, that there has been no consciousness of them when the sleep has been broken by the act of emission.   I have known cases where the testicles have been so ready to secrete that the least friction on the glans has produced an emission: I have known the simple action of walking, or riding, produce this effect, and that repeatedly in a very short space of time.

A young man, about four or five and twenty years of age, not so much

---

* Added: "A gentleman had a priapism for two years; it originated from an irritation in the bladder, which went off at the time the priapism came: it only takes place in the night, and mostly in his sleep, and immediately awakens him; having connexion makes it worse."—*Home.*

given to venery as most young men, had these last-mentioned complaints upon him. Three or four times in the night he would emit; and if he walked fast, or rode on horseback, the same thing would happen. He could scarcely have connexion with a woman before he emitted, and in the emission there was hardly any spasm. He tried every supposed strengthening medicine, as also the cold bath and sea-bathing, but with no effect. By taking twenty drops of laudanum, on going to bed, he prevented the night emissions; and by taking the same quantity in the morning, he could walk or ride without the before-mentioned inconvenience. I directed this practice to be continued for some time, although the disease did not return, that the parts might be accustomed to this healthy state of action; and I have reason to believe the gentleman is now well. It was found necessary, as the constitution became more habituated to the opiate, to increase the dose of it.

The spasms, upon the evacuation of the semen, in such cases are extremely slight, and a repetition of them soon takes place; the first emission not preventing a second; the constitution being all the time but little affected*. When the testicles act alone, without the accessory parts taking up the necessary and natural consequent action, it is still a more melancholy disease; for the secretion arises from no visible or sensible cause, and does not give any visible or sensible effect, but runs off similar to involuntary stools, or urine. It has been observed that the semen is more fluid than natural in some of these cases.

There is great variety in the diseased actions of these parts, of which the following case may be considered as an example.

A gentleman has had a stricture in the urethra for many years, for which he has frequently used a bougie, but of late has neglected it. He has had no connexion with women for a considerable time, being afraid of the consequences. He has often in his sleep involuntary emissions, which generally awake him at the paroxysm; but what surprises him most is, that often he has such without any semen passing through the penis, which makes him think that at those times it goes backwards into the bladder. This is not always the case, for at other times the semen passes forwards. At the time the semen seems to pass into the bladder he has the erection, the dream, and is awaked with the same mode of action, the same sensation, and the same pleasure, as when it passes through the urethra, whether dreaming or waking. My opinion is that the same irritation takes place in the bulb of the urethra

---

* It is to be considered that the constitution is commonly affected by the spasms only, and in proportion to their violence, independent of the secretion and evacuation of the semen. But in some cases even the erection going off without the spasms on the emission shall produce the same debility as if they had taken place.

without the semen, that takes place there when the semen enters, in consequence of all the natural preparatory steps, whereby the very same actions are excited as if it came into the passage; from which one would suppose that either semen is not secreted, or if it be, that a retrograde motion takes place in the actions of the acceleratores urinæ. But if the first be the case, then we may suppose that in the natural state the actions of those muscles do not arise simply from the stimulus of the semen in the part, but from their action being a termination of a preceding one making part of a series of actions. Thus they may depend upon the friction, or the imagination of a friction, on the penis, the testicles not doing their part, and the spasm in such cases arising from the friction, and not from the secretion.

In many of those cases of irregularity, when the erection is not strong, it shall go off without the emission; and at other times an emission shall happen almost without an erection: but these arise not from debility, but affections of the mind.

In many of the preceding cases, washing the penis, scrotum, and perinæum with cold water is often of service; and, to render it colder than we find it in some seasons of the year, common salt may be added to it, and the parts washed when the salt is almost dissolved.

CHAPTER XIII.

OF THE DECAY OF THE TESTICLE.

It would appear, from some circumstances, that the parts of generation are not to be considered as necessary parts of the animal machine, but only as parts superadded for particular purposes, and therefore only necessary when those particular purposes are to be answered; for we may observe that they are later of coming to maturity than any other parts, and are more liable to decay. Thus far in their natural properties they are different from most other parts of our body, the teeth only excepted, which are similar in some of those circumstances.

The testicles appear to be more subject to spontaneous disease than any other part of the body; but what is the most singular thing of all is the wasting of those bodies. One or both testicles shall wholly disappear, like to the thymus gland, or membrana pupillaris, &c. in the infant. This we do not find in any parts of the body which are essential to its œconomy, excepting the parts are of no further use and might become hurtful in the body, as in the instance of the membrana pupillaris. But the testicles do not undergo this change as if in consequence of an original property stamped upon them, as is the case of the thymus gland, whenever the age of the person is such as to render them useless, but are liable to it at any age ; and therefore the disposition is in the testicles themselves, independent of any connexion with the animal œconomy. An arm or leg may lose its action, and may waste in part, but never wholly.

Testicles have been known to waste in cases of rupture, probably from the constant pressure of the intestine. Mr. Pott has given us cases of this kind. I have seen in the hydrocele the testicle almost wasted to nothing, probably from the compression of the water ; but in all these the causes of wasting are obvious, and would probably produce similar effects in other parts of the body under the same circumstances ; but a testicle without any previous disease wastes wholly ; or at other times it inflames, either spontaneously, or from sympathy with the urethra, becomes large, and then begins to subside, as in the resolution of common inflammation of the body ; but does not stop at the former size, but continues to decay till it wholly disappears. The following cases are instances of this.

Case I.   A gentleman about nine years ago had a gonorrhœa, with a bubo, which suppurated. A swelling of one of the testicles came on, for which he used the common methods of producing resolution, and seemingly with success. All the other symptoms being removed, he thought himself quite well ; but some time after he found that the testicle, which had been swelled, was become rather smaller than the other, which made him now pay attention to it : this decrease continued till it wasted entirely. For some years past there has been no appearance of a testicle. He is not in the least different in inclination or powers from what he was before.

Case II : communicated by Mr. Nanfan.   " A gentleman, aged about eighteen, who never had any venereal complaint, has had two different attacks of the same nature, one in each testicle. February 3, 1776, after skating a few hours, without having to his knowledge received any injury from it, he was seized with a violent pain and inflammation of the left testicle, which in a few days increased much in size. A surgeon being sent for, followed the usual treatment in such cases of inflammation. In about six weeks the inflammation and swelling gradually subsided, some hardness only remaining. A mercurial plaster was now applied, which, after being worn for some time, was left off. The testicle ever since has continued gradually to decrease, and is no larger than a horsebean; indeed the body of the testicle is quite decayed, nothing remaining but what seems part of the epididymis. It appears to have no sense of pain, except when pressed, and is very hard and uneven on its surface. The spermatic chord is not in the least affected. October 20, 1777, he was seized in the same manner in the right testicle, without any apparent cause, whereupon I was applied to. He was immediately bled, took an opening mixture, after that a saline mixture, with tartar emetic; and a fomentation and embrocation of spiritus mindereri, and spiritus vini, was used. On the 27th a cataplasm was applied of linseed meal and aqua vegeto-mineralis. This treatment was persisted in till about the middle of November. The inflammation went off, and the testicle seemed much in the natural state. On December 19 I was applied to again; it seemed to be growing hard, and decreasing in size, much in the same manner as the other had done, which made him very unhappy. I ordered him some pills with calomel and tartar emetic, in hopes of increasing the secretion of the glands in general, and making some change in the testicle. At first this method seemed to be of service, but soon lost its effects, and the testicle began to decrease just as the other did." Mr. Adair and Mr. Pott were consulted with me, but nothing could be thought of that could give any hopes of success. I advised him to employ the parts in their natural uses, as much as inclination led him; but all was to no purpose, the testicle continued to decrease till not a vestige was left.

Case III: communicated by Dr. Cothom of Worcester. "A young man, aged sixteen, was suddenly seized with great coldness and shivering, attended with frequent rigors. During this paroxysm, which continued three hours, his pulse was small and contracted, and so exceedingly quick that the strokes of the artery were with difficulty counted. This period was succeeded by an intense heat, and a strong, hard, full, pulse, on which account he was copiously bled; a dose of cooling physic was immediately administered, and a clyster thrown up to promote its more speedy effects. In the evening the bleeding was repeated. All this day he complained of excruciating pain in his loins and the side of his belly, descending down into the scrotum. On examining the part affected, I saw an appearance of inflammation in the groin of the left side, and a great tension about the ring of the abdominal muscles, with an enlargement of the testicles. These parts were now ordered to be fomented with a discutient fotus, strongly impregnated with crude sal ammoniac, and to be bathed with spiritus mindereri and spiritus volat. aromat., before the application of each stupe; and he was directed to take six grains of the pulv. antimonialis, with fifteen grains of nitre every three hours; his food to be thin gruel, with fruit and lemon-juice, and his drink barley-water, with sugar and nitre.   Notwithstanding this antiphlogistic plan of frequent cooling physic, anodynes, three emetics, and thirteen blood-lettings, the fever continued, and the pain, inflammation, and tumour increased till the eighth day, including the first day of seizure, when seeing no hope of discussing the tumour, the testicle being nearly as large as a child's head, I attempted, by emollient fotuses and maturating cataplasms, to bring it to suppuration. On the 10th a fluctuation was perceptible, and on the 12th much more so, the scrotum having then put on a livid appearance.   I used every possible argument for permission to open it, but he being now quite easy, would not admit it.   On the 15th the patient was again attacked with rigors, coldness, and shivering, succeeded by a great feverish heat, which soon terminated in a profuse sweat; yet no pain attended this paroxysm.   In the evening, however, the tumour was so prominent that I was of opinion it would open spontaneously before morning, when I hoped to obtain his consent to enlarge the aperture; but this not happening, and all entreaties relating to the necessity of an incision proving ineffectual, I contented myself by giving the bark with elixir of vitriol.   From this time, after every paroxysm of fever, the testicle was observed to decrease.   Not being permitted to make an incision, and his strength and appetite continuing good, I began to entertain hopes of success without it, and advised him to persist in the use of the tonic and antiseptic plan, with the addition of stupes wet with the decoction of bark, to be constantly applied; by which means, at the end of thirty days from the first seizure, the pus was totally absorbed.   The testicle then appeared to be of the size of an hen's egg, and was as hard as a scirrhus.   I directed it to be rubbed, night and morning, with equal parts of the unguent. mercur. fort. and liniment. volat. camphorat., and ordered, internally, some mercurial alteratives, with a decoction of bark. By these aids his night sweats, and every other disagreeable symptom, gradually abated; he gathered strength, flesh, and spirits very fast, and the diseased testicle went on constantly decreasing, though very slowly, for near twelve months, at the expiration of which time there was no other appearance of it than a confusion of loose fibres, obvious to the feeling, in the upper part of the scrotum.   About a month ago the patient consented to my examining it.   Of the testicle there was not the least vestige; neither could I perceive the tunica vaginalis on that side in the groin; but upon the os pubis, and a little under it, I could embrace with my fingers and thumb the chord, and distinguish the vessels, which were without the least degree of hardness or scirrhosity; and if I pressed one in particular, I gave him exquisite pain for a moment.

He is in perfect health, of a strong robust constitution, and has fine healthy children; the only change which he has perceived in the constitution has been a propensity to grow fat, which neither temperance nor violent exercise on horseback, daily, with little rest, will prevent*.

* Added: "Case IV. A gentleman had a stricture, for which he passed a bougie; inflammation and swelling came upon one of the testicles; the inflammation was removed, and the swelling subsided; the testicle continued to diminish till it was extremely small.

"Case V. A gentleman had received a hurt upon one of his testicles in riding; it inflamed and swelled to a very great degree; the symptoms went off, and he considered himself well; it did not, however, remain of the natural size, but gradually diminished till it entirely disappeared.

"Case VI. A gentleman was lifted from the ground by the hands with a considerable jerk: he felt immediately a violent pain in the groin of the left side, and an inflammation and swelling came upon the right testicle; when this subsided, the testicle diminished to the size of a pea, and was very hard in its substance.

"Case VII. A gentleman, eighteen years of age, had a swelling brought upon one of his testicles by lying upon wet grass; it afterwards continued to diminish, till it was only one fourth of the natural size.

"Case VIII. A gentleman, twenty years of age, had been attacked at various times in the preceding eight years with violent pain and swelling in the right testicle and spermatic chord, which went entirely off, till two years ago there was a more violent seizure: for eight hours the pain was intolerable, and the swelling very great; it confined him six weeks. Since that time it has been diminishing in size and increasing in hardness: at present it is as small as a horsebean, and the spermatic chord is contracted. The left testicle has occasionally swelled, but always recovered its usual size. During the time he was affected with this pain, he has felt at intervals a pain about the neck of the bladder, especially when he made water, but not in any violent degree; he likewise frequently feels during these attacks a sensation like the circulation of some fluid within the testicles."—*Home.*

PART IV.

CHAPTER I.

OF CHANCRE.

I HAVE been hitherto speaking of the effects of this poison when applied to a secreting surface, and without a cuticle; of the intention of Nature in producing these effects; and of all the consequences, both real and supposed. I now mean to explain its effects when applied to a surface that is covered with a common cuticle, as the common skin of the body, which on such a surface will be found to be very different from those I have been describing. But I may be allowed here to remark, that the penis, the common seat of a chancre, is, like every part of the body, liable to diseases of the ulcerative kind, and from some circumstances, rather more so than other parts, for if attention is not paid to cleanliness, we have often excoriations, or superficial ulcers, from that cause; also, like almost every other part that has been injured, these parts, when once they have suffered from the venereal disease, are very liable to ulcerate anew. Since then this part is not exempted from the common diseases of the body, and as every disease in this part is suspected to be venereal, great attention is to be paid in forming our judgement of ulcers here.

Venereal ulcers commonly have one character, which however is not entirely peculiar to them, for many sores that have no disposition to heal (which is the case with a chancre,) have so far the same character. A chancre has commonly a thickened base, and although in some the common inflammation spreads much further, yet the specific is confined to this base. The future or consequent ulcers are commonly easily distinguished from the original, or venereal, which will be described hereafter.

It is an invariable effect, that when any part of an animal is irritated to a certain degree, it inflames and forms matter, the intention of which is to remove the irritating cause. This process is easily effected when it is on a surface whose nature is to secrete, but when on a surface whose nature is not to secrete, it then becomes more difficult, for another process must be set up, which is ulceration. This is not only the case in common irritations, but also in specific irritations from morbid poisons, as the venereal disease and smallpox. The variolous matter, as well as the venereal, produces ulcers on the skin; but when it affects secreting surfaces, a diseased secretion is the consequence; and this is different in different parts; on the tongue, inside of the mouth, uvula and tonsils, the coagulable lymph is thrown out in form of sloughs, somewhat similar to the putrid sore throat; but in the fauces, and all down the œsophagus, a thickish fluid, in appearance like matter, is secreted. When the irritation is applied to a surface whose cuticle is thin, and where there is a secretion naturally, as the glans penis or inside of the prepuce, there it sometimes only irritates, so as to produce a diseased secretion, as was described; but this is not always the effect of such irritation on such surfaces. They are often irritated to ulceration, and produce a chancre.

The poison has in general either no disposition, or not sufficient powers to blister or excoriate the common skin, for if it did, the symptoms most probably would be at first nearly the same, if not exactly so, with a gonorrhœa; that is, a discharge of matter from a surface, without a cuticle, newly inflamed; for it is reasonable to suppose that the poison would produce on that excoriated surface a secretion of matter, which would be at first a gonorrhœa, and which very probably would afterwards fall into the second mode of action or ulceration, and then become a chancre.

There are three ways in which chancres are produced; first, by the poison being inserted into a wound; secondly, by being applied to a nonsecreting surface; and thirdly, by being applied to a common sore. To whichever of these three different surfaces it is applied, the pus produces its specific inflammation and ulceration, attended with a secretion of pus. The matter produced in consequence of those different modes of application is of the same nature with the matter applied, because the irritations are the same in both.

The poison much more readily contaminates if it is applied to a fresh wound than to an ulcer, in this resembling the inoculation of the smallpox. Whether there are any parts of the skin, or any other part of the body, more susceptible of this irritation than others, in consequence of local application, is not yet ascertained.

This form of the disease, like the first, or gonorrhœa, is generally caught on the parts of generation, in consequence of a connexion between the sexes; but any part of the body may be affected by the application of venereal matter, especially if the cuticle is thin.

I have seen a chancre on the prolabium, as broad as a sixpence, caught the person did not know how*. The penis, and particularly the pre- puce, being the parts most commonly affected by this form of the dis- ease, are so constructed as to suffer much from it, especially when they are very susceptible of such irritation, for the construction alone pro- duces many inconveniences, besides considerable pain, while under the disease, and in general retards the cure.

The chancre is not so frequent an effect of the poison as the gonor- rhœa, and I think very good reasons may be assigned for it, although there are more modes than one of catching it, as I just now mentioned ; but the parts in two of them, to wit, the wound and the sore, are seldom in the way of being infected ; therefore when it is caught, it is commonly by the same mode of application with that of the gonorrhœa ; but as the cuticle cannot be affected by this poison, this covering acting as a guard to the cutis, it is often prevented from coming in contact with it ; and indeed it is almost surprising that the cutis should be affected by it where it has such a covering, excepting about the glans, the inside of the prepuce, or other parts of the body, where this covering is thin. The proportion which the cases of gonorrhœa bear to those of chancre is as four or five to one.

When it is caught in men it is generally upon the frænum, glans penis, prepuce, or upon the common skin of the body of the penis, and sometimes on the fore part of the scrotum ; but I think most frequently on the frænum, and in the angle between the penis and glans. Its af- fecting these parts arises from the manner in which it is caught, and not from any specific tendency in these parts to catch it more than others ; and its affecting the frænum, &c. more frequently than the other parts of the penis arises from the external form of this part, which is irregular, and allows the venereal matter to lie undisturbed in the chinks, by which means it has time to irritate and inflame the parts, and to produce the suppurative and ulcerative inflammation in them. But as this matter is easily rubbed off from prominent parts by every thing that touches them, it is a reason why such parts in general so often escape this disease.

The distance of time between its application and its effects upon the part is uncertain ; but, upon the whole, it is rather longer in appearing than the gonorrhœa ; however, this depends in some measure on the nature of the parts affected. If it be the frænum, or the termination of the prepuce into the glans, that is affected, the disease will in general

---

* That this sore was a chancre I made no doubt, for besides its diseased appearance, he had a bubo forming in one of the glands under the lower jaw, on the same side.
It is most probable that his own fingers were the conveyers.

appear earlier, these parts being more easily affected than either the glans, common skin of the penis, or scrotum; for in some cases, where both the glans and prepuce were contaminated from the same application of the poison, it has appeared earlier on the prepuce.

I have known cases where the chancres have appeared twenty-four hours after the application of the matter, and others where it has been seven weeks. A remarkable case of this kind was in a gentleman who had not touched a woman for seven weeks, when a chancre appeared. That this was a venereal chancre was proved, by his having had the lues venerea from it, and being under a necessity of taking mercury. An officer in the army had a chancre which appeared two months after he had had any connexion with a woman. After the last connexion he marched above an hundred miles, when the chancre broke out, and only gave way to mercury.

This, like most other inflammations which terminate in ulcers, begins first with an itching in the part; if it is the glans that is inflamed, generally a small pimple appears full of matter, without much hardness or seeming inflammation, and with very little tumefaction, the glans not being so readily tumefied from inflammation as many parts are, especially the prepuce; nor are the chancres attended with so much pain or inconvenience as those on the prepuce; but if upon the frænum, and more especially the prepuce, an inflammation more considerable than the former soon follows, or at least the effects of the inflammation are more extensive and visible. Those parts being composed of very loose cellular membrane, afford a ready passage for the extravasated juices; continued sympathy also more readily takes place in them. The itching is gradually changed to pain; the surface of the prepuce is in some cases excoriated, and afterwards ulcerates: in others a small pimple or abscess appears, as on the glans, which forms an ulcer. A thickening of the part comes on, which at first, and while of the true venereal kind, is very circumscribed, not diffusing itself gradually and imperceptibly into the surrounding parts, but terminating rather abruptly. Its base is hard, and the edges a little prominent. When it begins on the frænum, or near it, that part is very commonly wholly destroyed, or a hole is often ulcerated through it, which proves rather inconvenient in the cure, and in general it had better, in such cases, be divided at first*.

* Added: "The original excoriation or wound may heal, although contaminated, and afterwards become a chancre. A gentleman, in the act of copulation, tore the root of his prepuce all round, but in two days the whole healed; but one part broke out afterwards into a chancre, with a hard base, which readily yielded to mercury. This is similar to what takes place in inoculation for the smallpox."—*Home.*

If the venereal poison should be applied to the skin, where the cuticle is more dense than that of the glans penis, or frænum, such as that upon the body of the penis, or fore part of the scrotum (parts which are very much exposed to the application of this matter), then it generally appears first in a pimple, which is commonly allowed to scab, owing to its being exposed to evaporation. The scab is generally rubbed off or pushed off, and one larger than the first forms. I think there is less inflammation attending these last than those on the frænum and prepuce, but more than those upon the glans.

When the disease is allowed to go on, so as to partake of the inflammation peculiar to the habit, it becomes in many instances more diffused, and is often carried so far as to produce disagreeable symptoms, as phimosis, and sometimes paraphimosis, greatly retarding the cure; but still there is a hardness peculiar to this poison, surrounding the sores, especially those upon the prepuce.

When these ulcers are forming, and after they are formed, or in the state of inflammation, it is no uncommon thing for the urethra to sympathize with them, and give a tickling pain, especially in making water; but whether or not there is ever a discharge in the urethra from such a cause I will not determine; but if a discharge never takes place but when the disease really attacks the urethra, it would make us suppose that this sympathy is not really inflammatory; or if it is carried so far as to produce inflammation, yet that it is not of the specific kind. However, it is possible in those cases where there is a gonorrhœa preceded by a chancre, that this gonorrhœa may arise from sympathy, and is not a disease proceeding from the original contamination, nor from the matter of the chancre. That the sensation in the urethra, in those instances where there is no discharge, is from sympathy, and not from the urethra being attacked with the disease at the time that the matter laid the groundwork for the chancre, is evident from the following observation. I have seen it happen more than once, when the seat of the chancre had broke out a second time, and where no new or fresh infection had been caught, that the patient complained of the same tickling or slight pain in the urethra before any discharge had taken place in the beginning ulcerations. From the same connexion of parts I have seen a chancre coming upon the glans absolutely cure both a gleet and an irritation all along the passage of the urethra. So great was the previous irritation in this case, that I suspected a stricture; but, on passing a bougie, found none.

In consequence of the urethra sympathizing with the chancre, the testicles and scrotum will further sympathize with the urethra, and become affected. I have seen this sympathy extend over the whole pubes, and so strong, that touching the hairs gently on the pubes has given disagreeable sensations, and even pain.

In speaking of the local, or immediate effects of the venereal disease, I mentioned that they were seldom wholly specific, and that they partook both of the specific and the constitutional inflammation; and therefore it is always very necessary to pay some attention to the manner in which chancres first appear, and also to their progress, for they often explain the nature of the constitution at the time. If the inflammation spreads fast, and considerably, it shows a constitution more disposed to inflammation than natural. If the pain is great, it shows a strong disposition to irritation. It also sometimes happens that they begin very early to form sloughs; when this is the case, they have a strong tendency to mortification.

These additional symptoms mark the constitution and direct the future mode of treatment.

When there is a considerable loss of substance, either from sloughing or ulceration, a profuse bleeding is no uncommon circumstance, more especially if the ulcer is on the glans; for it would appear that the adhesive inflammation does not sufficiently take place there to unite the veins of the glans so as to prevent their cavity from being exposed, and the blood is allowed to escape from what is called the corpus spongiosum urethræ. The ulcers or sloughs often go as deep as the corpus cavernosum penis, where the same thing happens[a].

---

[a] [In this chapter the author has delineated with his usual sagacity and precision the true characters of a primary venereal sore. At least his description applies to a large majority of such cases. It is the more valuable as the points of distinction are not drawn merely from obvious appearances, which, though they strike the eye, are scarcely communicable by language, but from the laws which govern the effects of the venereal virus, and the operation of which may be traced even where the appearances are dissimilar.

Two consequences follow the application of the venereal virus, induration and ulceration. These two consequences seem to be distinct and independent; since, though they generally exist in conjunction, they are sometimes found separate, one or the other of them being in some cases wanting. The induration, though not always so obvious as the ulceration, is on the whole more constant, more characteristic, more peculiar and distinct in its appearance. The author has therefore rightly directed the attention more especially to the thickening as a distinction of a primary venereal sore.

The description given of this peculiar thickening by the author can scarcely be improved. It is " very circumscribed, not diffusing itself gradually and imperceptibly into the surrounding parts, but terminating rather abruptly." It retains these characters through all its stages, though they may be sometimes partially obscured by other concomitant circumstances.

The thickening in general precedes the ulceration. The first effect of venereal contamination is to produce this peculiar change in the texture of the part; the second effect is to produce ulceration of the indurated portion. The character of primary ve-

§. 1. *Of the Phimosis and Paraphimosis.*

These diseases arise from a thickening of the cellular membrane of the prepuce, in consequence of an irritation capable of producing con-

---

nereal infection is essentially induration passing afterwards into ulceration. In the earliest stage of the existence of a chancre this sequence is least discernible, there being frequently at that period superficial and incipient ulceration with very little apparent thickening. But in the progress of the disorder the two stages become in general very clearly distinguishable. If the sore be watched, it will be found that the thickening becomes daily more distinct and extensive, till the ulcer assumes the true venereal appearance of a sore situated on an indurated base. The induration everywhere encompasses the ulcer, being both beneath it and around it, forming as it were the bed of the sore, and at the same time encircling its margin, so as to connect it everywhere with the sound parts in the vicinity. In fact it marks the part most recently contaminated, which has not yet passed into ulceration. In the progress of the case, the induration spreads first, so that no parts are involved in the ulcer until they have previously passed through this change of texture. A primary venereal sore is scarcely ever stationary. The ulcer itself may be stationary; but careful observation will detect a gradual increase of the thickened base, which proves, no less certainly than the enlargement of the ulceration itself, that the virus is steadily extending.

These observations will explain certain occasional variations in the aspect of venereal sores, which, though sufficiently intelligible when closely examined, are exceedingly perplexing to those who form their diagnosis merely from the obvious appearances.

It is not very uncommon that a primary venereal sore should assume the following characters. A portion of the prepuce, of about the size of a silver penny, shall become slightly thickened so as to lose its natural flexibility; and perhaps the surface shall be slightly excoriated. In the course of a few days, if the part is kept very clean, the excoriation shall in many cases disappear, but the hardness shall progressively increase, assuming a more defined character, and at last forming a large flat mass of the size of half-a-crown, so inflexible and rigid that the prepuce cannot be everted without difficulty. There shall be no tenderness, no inflammation, sometimes no ulceration at all, at other times only a slight dark-coloured excoriation of the surface. Yet the case shall be venereal. If the usual anti-venereal remedies are not employed, all doubts on this subject shall be removed at the end of eight or ten weeks by the appearance of distinct secondary symptoms.

In this case the aspect of the part bears no obvious resemblance to that of a common chancre; yet the difference is more apparent than real. The venereal virus produces the usual induration; but, from the slowness of its progress and the absence of inflammation, the indurated portion does not pass into ulceration. With this single exception, the course of the disease is the same as that of an ordinary chancre. The increase of the hardness is progressive, until mercury is employed. As soon as the constitution is affected by the remedy, the thickened mass begins to diminish in size, and it gradually disappears from the circumference to the centre, exactly like the induration left by a chancre. As a still further proof of the identity of the diseases, it may be stated, that, notwithstanding the absence of ulceration, the contiguous surface is often similarly affected. A similar induration will be produced in the part of the glans with which the original tumour is in contact, or on the opposite nympha when this affection is situated on the nympha in the female.

Again, the deviation from the usual course may be of an opposite kind. The ulcera-

siderable and diffused inflammation, which, when it does happen, is generally in consequence of a chancre in this part. This irritation,

---

tion may be so rapid as to overtake the induration, and to destroy it as quickly as it is formed. Sores are frequently seen, especially on the external prepuce, which spread rapidly, sometimes by sloughing and sometimes by ulceration, with profuse discharge and some surrounding inflammation, but with little or no characteristic hardness. But the absence of this distinctive character of venereal sores is only accidental, and is occasioned by the rapid progress of the ulcer : for if the extension of the sore be checked by local means, which may often be effected, the surrounding induration shall appear, and shall become daily more palpable ; until its further progress is stopped by such remedies as act directly on the virus, and thus remove the cause from which it arises.

It is evident that these occasional variations do not affect the truth of the general position, that the natural result of venereal infection is induration passing into ulceration. But in the practical application of this principle as a criterion of the real nature or a sore, some circumstances must be taken into the account, which often modify the appearances and perplex the diagnosis.

The true venereal induration is "circumscribed, and terminates abruptly." But when much inflammation is present these characters will not be discernible. The specific thickening will be confounded in the general thickening from inflammation, and will not be distinguishable from that which may attend an ordinary sore. Its existence cannot be distinctly and indubitably ascertained till the general inflammation is removed or palliated ; and then, when the surrounding lymph is absorbed, there will still remain at the seat of the sore a hardened base and a hardened circumference, having a well-defined abrupt margin.

Sores that are ill-conditioned may produce surrounding thickening, although free from all specific virus. If the surface is sloughy, the base may be indurated. In such cases it is sometimes impossible to say at once with certainty whether the thickening is to be ascribed to the presence of the venereal virus, or is the mere consequence of the ill-conditioned state of the sore. The opinion should generally be suspended, and local means should be used for the removal of the slough. When this is effected, in common sores, the hardness which was produced by its irritation will disappear also : in venereal sores, notwithstanding a similar change of the surface has been produced, the induration will nevertheless remain, and continue to spread, and ultimately the sore will again become foul and perhaps sloughy.

It is evident therefore that the distinction is to be drawn less from the appearance of the sore at any one moment than from its course and progress. Many circumstances may at any one time confuse the appearances, and may deceive the surgeon ; but it is scarcely possible that he can err, if he watches the progress of the case, and uses means to obviate the causes of error. If the sore be venereal, he will be able to detect the changes which mark the contamination, viz. first, induration ; and secondly, ulceration.

It is not meant that the other characters of venereal sores are to be disregarded in forming the diagnosis. The bright red areola which encircles them ; the mode of extension which is equally in all directions ; the disposition of the discharge from them to produce similar sores on the surfaces with which it is allowed to come in contact ; these all form important distinctions, and should by no means be overlooked. But it often happens that these tests cannot be applied. The red areola is often obscured by surrounding inflammation, and altogether undistinguishable. Sores which are not venereal often spread regularly and evenly from a centre. Where attention is paid to cleanliness and the discharge is not allowed to collect, no other sores will be produced, and the

however, and inflammation sometimes attacks the prepuce, even when
the disease is in the form of what I suspect to be a gonorrhœa of the
glans and prepuce*, sometimes even in the common gonorrhœa, but
most frequently of all from a chancre in the prepuce.   When this disease or tumefaction takes place in consequence of a chancre, I suspect
that there is an irritable disposition in the habit; for it is plain there
is more than the specific action, the inflammation extending beyond
the specific distance[a].

It may be observed here, that the prepuce is no more than a doubling
of the skin of the penis when not erected, for then it becomes too large
for the penis, by which provision the glans is covered and preserved
when not necessary to be used, whereby its feelings are probably more
acute.   When the penis becomes erect it in general fills the whole skin,
by which the doubling forming the prepuce in the non-erect state is
unfolded, and is employed in covering the body of the penis.

The diseases called phimosis and paraphimosis, being a thickening
of the cellular membrane of this part, they will commonly be in proportion to the inflammation and distensibility of the cellular membrane
of the part.   The inflammation often runs high, and is frequently of the
erysipelatous kind; besides, in such parts where the cellular membrane
is so very loose, the tumefaction is considerable, and the end of the prepuce being a depending part the serum is accumulated in it, which in
many inflammations is allowed to pass from the inflamed to some more

* See page 169, where this gonorrhœa is mentioned.

---

original chancre will remain single.   The character and course of the induration form
on the whole that criterion which is most certain and most generally observable.

But it must not be forgotten that there is a class of venereal sores to which the above
description does not apply.   In the sores usually called phagedenic, the progress of the
ulcer is not preceded by the venereal induration, nor is such induration left after it is
cicatrized.   The other points of discrimination fail also.   The extension is irregular,
one edge generally spreading while another is healing: and the discharge does not infect the parts on which it is suffered to rest.   Yet undoubtedly these sores are the consequences of impure connexion, and are followed by secondary symptoms; and it is
therefore difficult to deny their venereal origin, though the laws which they observe are
very different from those which regulate the course of a common chancre.   They are
comparatively rare.   The description of the author is applicable to forty-nine cases out
of fifty; and its practical value is scarcely diminished by the occasional occurrence of
phagedenic sores, which may be readily known by the characters which peculiarly belong to them, and of which a more particular description will be given hereafter.]

[a] [Any ulcer on the internal prepuce may produce phimosis, because it may be attended by so much thickening as to destroy the natural flexibility of the prepuce.   A
chancre is more likely to produce it than any other sore, because it is necessarily accompanied by induration, and that of a kind which is much more obstinate than the
thickening of a common inflammation.]

depending part, as in an inflammation of the leg or thigh, where the foot commonly swells or becomes œdematous in consequence of the descent of the serum extravasated above.

A natural contraction of the aperture of the prepuce is very common, and so strong in some that those under such construction of parts have a natural and constant phimosis. Such a state of parts is often attended with chancres, producing very great inconveniences in the time of the cure; and in those cases of considerable diffused inflammation, a diseased phimosis, similar to the other, unavoidably follows; and, whether diseased or natural, it may produce the paraphimosis simply by the prepuce being brought back upon the penis; for this tight part acting as a ligature round the body of the penis, behind the glans, retards the circulation beyond the ligature, producing an œdematous inflammation on the inverted part of the prepuce. When the paraphimosis takes place in consequence of a natural tightness only, although attended with chancres, yet it has nothing to do with the constitution, this being only accidental; however, in either case a paraphimosis is to be considered as in some degree a local violence.

This natural phimosis is so considerable in some children as not to allow the urine to pass with ease; but in general becomes larger and larger as boys grow up, by frequent endeavours to bring it over the glans, by which the bad consequences that would otherwise ensue in it when affected with disease are often prevented.

This part of the prepuce, although in most men it is loose enough to produce no inconvenience in a natural state, yet it sometimes contracts without any visible cause whatever, and becomes so narrow as to hinder the water from getting out, even after it has got free from the urethra, so that the whole cavity of the prepuce shall be filled with the urine, and give great pain. The cases that I have seen of this kind have been principally in old men.

When the prepuce is in its natural position it then covers entirely the glans, and is commonly a little loose before it; but when it begins to swell and thicken, more and more of the skin of the penis is drawn forwards over the glans, and the glans at the same time is pushed backwards by the swelling against its end. I have seen the prepuce projecting from such a cause more than three inches beyond the glans, and its aperture much diminished.

The prepuce often becomes in some degree inverted by the inner skin yielding more than the outer, having a kind of neck where the outer skin naturally terminates. From the tightness and distension of the parts in a state of tumefaction it becomes impossible to bring it back over the penis, so as to invert it and expose the sores on the inside.

Such a state of the prepuce is very often productive of bad consequences, especially when the chancres are behind the glans; for the
glans being between the orifice of the prepuce and the sores, it there
fills up the whole cavity of the prepuce, between the chancres and
opening, and often so tightly, that the matter from the sores behind
cannot get a passage forwards between the glans and prepuce, by which
means there is an accumulation of matter behind the corona glandis,
forming an abscess which produces ulceration upon the inside of the
prepuce. This abscess opens externally, and the glans often protruding
through the opening, throws the whole prepuce to the opposite side,
the penis appearing to have two terminations.

On the other hand, if the prepuce is loose, wide, and is either accustomed to be kept back in its sound state or is pulled back to dress the
chancres, and is allowed to remain in this situation till the above tumefaction takes place, then it is called a paraphimosis; or if the prepuce
is pulled forcibly back after it is swelled, it is then brought from the
state of a phimosis, as before described, to that of a paraphimosis.

This last-described situation of the prepuce is often much more
troublesome, and often attended with worse symptoms, than the former,
especially if it should have been changed from a phimosis to a paraphimosis. The reason of which is, that the aperture of the prepuce is naturally less elastic than either the internal inverted part or the external
skin; therefore when the prepuce is pulled back upon the body of the
penis, that part grasps it tighter than any other part of the skin of the
penis, and more so in proportion to the inflammation: the consequence
of which is, the swelling of the prepuce is divided into two, one swelling close to the glans, the other behind the stricture or neck. This
stricture is often so great as to interrupt the free circulation of the
blood beyond it, which also assists in increasing the swelling, adds to
the stricture, and often produces a mortification of the prepuce itself,
by which means the whole diseased part, together with the stricture, is
sometimes removed, forming what may be called a natural cure*.

In many cases the inflammation not only affects the skin of the penis,
in which is included the prepuce, but it attacks the body of the penis
itself, often producing adhesions and even mortification in the cells of
the corpora cavernosa, either of which will destroy the distensibility of

---

* A young man came into St. George's Hospital with a paraphimosis in consequence
of chancres on the inside of the prepuce. All the parts before the stricture, formed by
the prepuce, mortified and dropped off. I ordered nothing but common dressings, and
it healed very readily, and he left the hospital cured of the local complaint. Whether
or not absorption had taken place previous to the mortification I do not know, as I
never heard more of him.

those parts ever after, giving the penis a curve to one side in its erections. This sometimes takes place through the whole cellular substance of the penis, producing a short and almost inflexible stump.

The adhesions of those cells do not proceed from venereal inflammation only; they are often the consequences of other diseases, and sometimes they take place without any visible cause whatever.

A gentleman, sixty years of age, who has been lame with the gout these twenty years past, has for these eighteen months had the penis contracted on the left and upper side, so as to bend that way very considerably in erections, which erections are more frequent than common.

Quere: Is the gout the cause of this, by producing adhesions of the cells of one corpus cavernosum, so as not to yield to or allow of the influx of blood on that side? And is the irritation of the gout the cause of the frequency of the erections?

CHAPTER II.

OF CHANCRES IN WOMEN.

WOMEN are subject to chancres; but, from the simplicity of the parts, the complaint is often less complicated than in men. For in this sex we have only the disease and constitutional affection, and no inconvenience arising from the formation of the parts.

When the matter is introduced into the vagina or urethra it there irritates a secreting surface, as I described when treating of the disease in general and of women in particular; but when it is lodged in the inside of the skin of the labia or nymphæ those parts are often only affected with gonorrhœa; but, like the glans penis in men, they are also capable of ulceration. Ulcerations are generally more numerous in women, because the surface upon which they can form is much larger: we find them on the edge of the labia, sometimes on the outside, and even on the perinæum.

Ulcers that are formed on the inside of the labia or nymphæ are never allowed to dry or scab; but on the outside they are subject to have the matter dry upon them, which forms a scab similar to those on the body of the penis or scrotum.

The venereal matter frqm such sores is very apt to run down the
perinæum to the anus, as in a gonorrhœa, and excoriate the parts, especially about the anus where the skin is thin, and often produces chancres
in those parts.

Chancres have been observed in the vagina ; which I suspect not to
have been original ones, but to have arisen from the spreading of the
ulcers on the inside of the labia[a].

This form of the disease, like the gonorrhœa, both in women and in
men, is entirely local, the constitution having no connexion with it but
sympathetically, and I believe much more seldom in this than in the
former.

CHAPTER III.

GENERAL OBSERVATIONS ON THE TREATMENT
OF CHANCRES.

THE inflammation from the venereal poison, when it produces ulceration, generally if not always continues till cured by art, which I observed
was not the case with the gonorrhœa. It will perhaps not be an easy
task to account for this material difference in the two kinds of disease ;
but I am inclined to think that as the inflammation in the chancre spreads
it is always attacking new ground, which is a succession of irritations,
and is the cause that it does not cure itself.

Chancres, as well as the gonorrhœa, are perhaps seldom or never
wholly venereal, but are varied by certain peculiarities of the constitution at the time. The treatment therefore of them, both local and constitutional, will admit of great variety; and it is upon the knowledge
of this variety that the skill of the surgeon principally depends.   On
this account the concomitant symptoms are what require particular
attention. Mercury is the cure of the venereal symptoms abstractedly

---

[a] [Original chancres do occasionally occur within the vagina, being situated either
on the membrane lining the vagina or on the os uteri itself. These chancres can only
be detected by the use of a speculum. However, sores on these internal parts are extremely rare, notwithstanding the degree in which they are exposed to the contact of
the venereal virus during coition.]

considered; but there is no one specific for the others, the treatment of which must vary according to the constitution. From hence we must see that no one kind of medicine joined with mercury will be likely to succeed in all cases, although the different pretended secrets are of this kind, some cases not requiring anything excepting mercury, others requiring a something besides, according to their nature, which in many cases it will not be an easy matter to find out from the appearances of the chancre itself, but which must be discovered by repeated trials.

Probably from the before-mentioned circumstances it is, that a chancre is in common longer in healing than most of the local effects from the constitutional disease, or lues venerea, at least longer than those in the first order of parts; and this is found to be the case notwithstanding that the cure of a chancre may be attempted both constitutionally and locally, while the lues venerea can in common only be cured constitutionally. It is commonly some time before a chancre appears to be affected by the medicine. The circulation shall be loaded with mercury for three, four, or more weeks before a chancre shall begin to separate its discharge from its surface, so as to look red and show the living surface, but when once it does change, its progress towards healing is more rapid. A lues venerea shall in many cases be perfectly cured before chancres have made the least change.

Upon the same principle some attention should be paid to internal medicines, and it should be considered whether weakening, strengthening, or quieting medicines should be given; for sometimes one kind, sometimes another, will be proper.

Chancres admit of two modes of treatment: the object of one is to destroy or remove them by means of escharotics or by extirpation, that of the other is to overcome the venereal irritation by means of the specific remedy for that poison.

I have endeavoured to show that chancres are local complaints: this opinion is further confirmed by their being destroyed or cured by merely a local treatment. But in chancre, as well as in a gonorrhœa, it has been disputed whether mercury should ever be applied locally to them or not; some have objected to it, while others have practised it, and probably the dispute is not yet generally settled.

Upon the general idea which I have endeavoured to give of the venereal disease it can be no difficult task to determine this question.

It is to be observed that in the cure of the chancres we have two points in view: the cure of the chancre itself and the prevention of a contamination of the habit.

The first, or the cure of the chancre, is to be effected by mercury applied either in external dressings, or internally through the circula-

tion, or in both ways. The second object, or preservation of the constitution from contamination, is to be obtained, first, by shortening the
duration of the chancre, which shortens the time of absorption, and also
by internal medicine, which must be in proportion to the time that the
absorption may have been going on.

If the power of a chancre to contaminate the constitution, or, which
is the same thing, if the quantity absorbed is as the size of the chancre
and the time of absorption, which most probably it is, then whatever
shortens the time must diminish that power or quantity absorbed; and
if the quantity of mercury necessary to preserve the constitution is as
the quantity of poison absorbed, then whatever lessens the quantity absorbed must proportionally preserve the constitution. For instance, if
the power of a chancre to contaminate the constitution in four weeks is
equal to four, and the quantity of mercury necessary to be given internally, both for the cure of the chancre and the preservation of the constitution, is also equal to four, then whatever shortens the duration of
the chancre must lessen in the same proportion the quantity of the mercury; therefore, if local applications along with the internal use of
mercury will cure the chancre in three weeks, then only three fourths
of the mercury is necessarily wanted internally. Local applications
therefore, so far as they tend to shorten the duration of a chancre,
shorten the duration of absorption, which also shortens the necessity of
the continuance of an internal course of mercury, all in the same proportion. For example: if four ounces of mercurial ointment will cure
a chancre and preserve the constitution in four weeks, three ounces will
be sufficient to preserve the constitution if the cure of the chancre can
be by any other means forwarded so as to be effected in three weeks.
This is not speculation, but the result of experience, and the destruction of chancres confirms it[a].

§. 1. *Of the Destruction of a Chancre.*

The simplest method of treating a chancre is by destroying or extir-
pating it, whereby it is reduced to the state of a common sore or wound,
and heals up as such. This only can be done on the first appearance of

---

[a] [The author's experience on this point seems to be at variance with that of others.
It does not appear that in practice it is safe to make the period of the healing of the
sore a measure of the length of the mercurial course. General experience would seem
to show that a mercurial course for primary symptoms, even though it be commenced
before the chancre has existed a week, cannot be continued for a less period than a
month, without exposing the patient to imminent danger of a subsequent relapse.]

the chancre, when the surrounding parts are not as yet contaminated, because it is absolutely necessary that the whole diseased part should be removed, which is done with difficulty when it has spread considerably. It may be done either by incision or by caustic. If the chancre appears upon the glans, touching it with the lunar caustic is preferable to incision, because the hæmorrhage by such a mode would be considerable from the cells of the glans.

The common sensation of the glans is not very acute, therefore the caustic will give but little pain. The caustic to be used should be pointed at the end like a pencil, that it may only touch those parts that are really diseased. This treatment should be continued till the surface of the sore looks red and healthy, after having thrown off the last sloughs; after it has arrived at this state, it will be found to heal like any other sore produced by a caustic.

If the sore is upon the prepuce, or upon the common skin of the penis, and in its incipient state, the same practice may be followed with success; but if it has spread considerably, it is then out of the power of the caustic, when only applied in this slow manner, to go so deep as to keep pace with the increasing sore, but it is very probable that the lapis septicus may answer very well in such cases. When this cannot be conveniently used, incision will answer the purpose effectually.

I have taken out a chancre by dissection, and the sore has healed up with common dressings. However, as our knowledge of the extent of the disease is not always certain, and as this uncertainty increases as the size of the chancre, it becomes necessary in some degree to assist the cure by proper dressings, and therefore it may be prudent to dress the sore with mercurial ointment. From such treatment there is but little danger of the constitution being infected, especially if the chancre has been destroyed almost immediately upon its appearance, as we may then reasonably suppose there has not been time for absorption. But, as it must be in most cases uncertain whether there has been absorption or not, this practice is not always to be trusted to, and from that circumstance perhaps never should; and therefore, even in those cases where the chancre has been removed almost immediately, it would be prudent to give some medicine internally, the quantity of which should be proportioned to the time and progress of the sore; but if it has spread to a considerable size before extirpation, then mercury is absolutely necessary, and perhaps not a great deal is gained by the extirpation*.

* [The treatment of chancres by caustic or extirpation is more beautiful in theory than commendable in practice. It is impossible to know with certainty to what distance the virus has extended, and the whole of the contaminated parts may not there-

§. 2. *Of the Cure of Chancres.—Local Applications.*

The cure of a chancre is a different thing from its destruction, and consists in destroying its venereal disposition, which being effected, the parts heal of course as far as they are venereal.

Chancres may be cured in two different ways, either by external applications, or internal through the circulation. The same medicine is necessary for both these purposes, that is mercury.

I have shown that a gonorrhœa and a chancre have so far the same disposition as to form the same kind of matter, yet I have also observed that mercury has no more power in curing the gonorrhœa than any other medicine, and therefore it might be supposed that mercury would have no effect in the present complaint; but we find that in a chancre it is a specific, and will cure every one that is truly venereal: but as other dispositions take place so other assistance is often necessary, as will be taken notice of in the history of the cure. The action of this medicine must be the same in whatever way it is given, for its action must be upon the vessels of the part, in one way acting only externally, in the other internally*.

For external local applications mercurial ointments are the common

---

* This is well illustrated by the application of some medicines locally to parts whose actions are immediate and visible; and by throwing the same medicine into the constitution the same immediate and visible effect is produced: for instance, if ten grains of ipecacuanha is thrown into the stomach of a dog, it will in a short time make him vomit, from its local applications to that viscus; and if a solution of five grains is thrown into a vein it will produce vomiting before we can conceive it to have got to the vessels of the stomach. The same effects are produced from an infusion of jalap thrown into the veins that are commonly produced when taken into the stomach and bowels.

---

fore be destroyed by the caustic. This defect is not always evident at the time. The sore may cicatrize under the caustic, yet the virus may not be extirpated, and the general system may be subsequently affected. Again, caustic seems to increase the disposition to absorption, so that if the object is not attained by the first application it will not in general be achieved by its repetition. Hence it happens, in very many instances, that the use of caustic is followed immediately by a bubo, and at a more remote period by secondary symptoms; and the patient, who might have been cured in the first instance by a moderate course of mercury, is subsequently exposed to the necessity of passing through a protracted course, which is not only attended with much trouble and annoyance, but which cannot be employed without considerable risk to the general health. The treatment by caustic should therefore be reserved for those cases where, from peculiar circumstances, an immediate course of treatment must be avoided at all risks.

When caustic is supposed to be successful the sores are for the most part not chancres, but simple pustules or herpetic vesicles.]

dressings ; but if the mercury were joined with watery substances instead of oily, by mixing with the matter the application would be continued longer to the sore, and would prove more effectual. This is an
advantage that poultices have over common dressings. I have often
used mercury rubbed down with some conserve in the room of an ointment, and it has answered extremely well. Calomel, used in the same
way, and also the other preparations of mercury mixed with mucilage
or with honey, answer the same purpose. Such dressings will effect
a cure in cases that are truly venereal ; but perhaps we seldom have a
constitution quite free from some morbid tendency.

Some will have an indolent disposition, to counteract which it will
be right to join with the mercury some warm balsam in a small proportion, or as much red precipitate as will only stimulate, without acting as an escharotic ; and sometimes both may be necessary.

Calomel mixed with some salve, or any other substance which will
suspend it, is more active than common mercurial ointment, and in such
cases as require stimulating applications it will answer better.

Many other applications are recommended, such as solutions of
blue vitriol, verdigris, calomel, with the spiritus nitri dulcis, and many
others.

But as all of these are only of service in remedying any peculiar disposition of the parts, having no specific power on the venereal poison,
and as such dispositions are innumerable, it becomes almost impossible
to say what will be effectual in every disposition : some will answer in
one state of the sores, some in another. It may be found oftentimes
that the parts affected are extremely irritable : in such cases it will be
necessary to mix the mercury with opium, or perhaps preparations of
lead, as white or red lead, to diminish the action of the parts.

The oftener the dressings are shifted the better, as the matter from
the sore separates the application from the diseased parts, by which
means the effects are lost or diminished. Three times every day in
many cases is not oftener than necessary, especially if the dressings are
of the unctuous kind ; for they do not mix, like watery dressings, with
the matter, so as to impart some of their virtues to it, which would in
a proportional degree affect the sore.

Chancres, after having their venereal taint corrected, often become
stationary, and having acquired new dispositions, increase the quantity
of disease in the part, as will be taken notice of hereafter. When they
become stationary only they may often be cured by touching them
slightly with the lunar caustic. They seem to require that the surface
which has been contaminated, or the new flesh which grows upon that
surface, should be either destroyed or altered before it can cicatrise ;

and it is suprising often how quickly they will heal after being touched, and probably once or twice may be sufficient.

§. 3. *Of the Treatment of Phimosis in consequence of or attended with Chancre.*

From the history which I have given of the disease we must see that a phimosis may be of two kinds : one natural, with the disease super-added, the other brought on by disease. The first may be increased by the disease; but if otherwise, it is not so troublesome as the other. Such as arise from the disease, I have observed, depend upon the peculiarity of the constitution. In either case it is often not practicable to apply dressings to the chancres on the inside of the prepuce.

A phimosis should be prevented, if possible ; therefore, upon the least signs of a thickening of the prepuce, which is known by its being retracted with difficulty and pain, the patient should be kept quiet; if in bed so much the better, as in a horizontal position the end of the penis will not be so depending, but may be kept up. If confinement in bed cannot be complied with, then the end of the penis should be kept up to the belly, if possible; but this can hardly be done when the person is obliged to walk about, for the extravasated fluids, descending and remaining in the prepuce, contribute often more to render the prepuce incapable of being drawn back than the inflammation itself.

When the diseased phimosis completely takes place the same precautions may be followed; but as the sores cannot be dressed in the common way, we must have recourse either to dressings in forms of injections, or the operation for the phimosis. If we use injections only, they should be often repeated, as they are only temporary applications.

The dressings, in form of injections, should be mercurial, either crude mercury rubbed down with a thick solution of gum arabic, which will assist in retaining some of the injection between the glans and prepuce ; or calomel with the same, and a proportion of opium. In the proportion of these no nicety is required; but if a solution of corrosive sublimate is made use of as an injection some attention is to be paid to its strength. About one grain of this to an ounce of water will be as much as the sensation of the part will allow the patient to bear, and if this gives too much pain it may be lowered by adding more water.

After the parts are as well cleaned as possible with this injection, it will be necessary to introduce other mercurial applications of some kind, to remain there till the parts want cleaning again, which will be very soon. Such as are mentioned before will answer this purpose very well;

but I have my doubts about the propriety of using any irritating medicines or injections in such cases.

As often as he voids his urine the patient may wash the parts, by pressing the orifice of the prepuce together, so as to oblige the water to run back between the prepuce and glans; immediately after this the patient should use the mercurial applications, otherwise this operation of washing may do harm, as it will wash away the former application of mercury; but in many cases the parts are so sore as not to allow of this practice.

A poultice of linseed meal alone, or of equal parts of this and bread, should be applied. This poultice is to be made with water, to which one eighth of laudanum has been added. But previous to this, and immediately after the cleaning, it would be very proper to let the penis hang over the steam of hot water, with a little vinegar and spirits of wine in it, which is the neatest way of applying fomentations.

The oftener this is practised the better, for thus a mercurial application is kept in contact with the diseased parts a greater number of the hours out of the twenty-four, than otherwise could be were the matter allowed to lie on the parts.

When to the above-mentioned symptoms a bleeding of the chancre is added, I do not know a more troublesome complaint, because here the cells or veins have no great disposition for contraction*. Oil of turpentine gives the best stimulus for the contraction of vessels of all kinds; but where bleeding arises from an irritable action of the vessels, which is sometimes the case, then sedatives are the best applications. Whatever is used in such a state of the prepuce must be injected into the part.

When in consequence of the treatment the inflammation begins to go off, and the chancres to heal, it will be necessary to move the prepuce upon the glans as much as they will allow of, to prevent adhesions which sometimes happen when there have been chancres on both surfaces opposite to each other. Indeed the practice here recommended is such as will in general prevent such consequences.

If this has not been properly attended to, and the parts have grown together, the consequences may not be bad; but it must be very disagreeable to the patient, and a reflection upon the surgeon.

I have seen the opening into the prepuce so much contracted from all these internal ulcers healing and uniting, that there was hardly any

* I suspect that where chancres bleed profusely, the blood comes either from the glans, when there are chancres there, or from the spongy substance of the urethra, where the chancre has begun about the fraenum, for we seldom see profuse bleedings from the prepuce when its inside is the seat of the chancre, and can be exposed; but indeed in such cases the inflammation is not violent.

passage for the water.   If the passage in the prepuce so contracted be
in a direct line with the orifice of the urethra, then a bougie may be
readily passed; but this is not always the case : it often happens that
they are not in a direct line, therefore an operation becomes necessary.
The operation consists in either slitting up part of the prepuce, or removing part of it ; but as these parts have become very indistinct from
the adhesions, either the slitting it up, or removing part of it, becomes
a difficult operation.   Whenever the urethra is discovered, or can be
found out by a bougie, that is to be introduced, and its application repeated till the passage becomes free, and has got into the habit of keeping so.

I observed formerly that this tumefaction sometimes produced a confinement of the matter formed by the chancre, and that while this effect
lasted no subsiding of the inflammation or tumefaction could take place ;
that therefore those diseases continued to exist, and that the part thus
circumstanced came under our definition of an abscess ; that is, the formation of matter in a state of confinement.   Although it never has been
considered in this light, yet the necessary treatment shows it to be
such.   This consists in laying it open from the external orifice to the
bottom where the matter lies, as in a sinus, so as to discharge it.   However, the intention annexed to this practice was not to allow of the discharge of the matter of the sore, but to admit of the applications of
dressings to it, for it has been recommended and practised where there
was no particular confinement of matter, which I have not found to be
necessary merely for that purpose, as we are in possession of an internal remedy ; and if the opening produces no other good but the allowing of the application of dressings, it is not so material, because the
sores may be washed with an injection through a syringe.

§. 4. Of the common Operation for the Phimosis produced by Chancres.

The common operation for the phimosis is slitting the prepuce nearly
its whole length, in the direction of the penis; but even this is sometimes thought not sufficient, and it is directed to cut the prepuce in two
different places, nearly opposite to one another.   When it was thought
proper to be done in this way, it was imagined that it was seldom necessary to cut the whole length of the prepuce.   It will in some degree
depend on circumstances which practice is to be followed.   If it is a
natural phimosis without tumefaction, and the chancre is near the orifice of the prepuce, which in such cases it most probably will be, as the

glans is not denuded in coition so as to have chancres deeper seated, then it may be necessary only to go as far as the chancres extend.

From the common situation of the chancre, this disease of the phimosis arises more commonly from the tumefaction of the parts; and from the idea I have endeavoured to give of the inconveniences arising from this phimosis, where the chancres are placed behind the corona, producing a confinement of the matter behind the glans, slitting open the prepuce a little way cannot be sufficient, for in such cases it must be exposed to the bottom, or no good can arise from the operation.

Although this operation will not take off the tumefaction of the prepuce, so as to allow it to be brought back, yet it will allow of a free discharge of the matter, and also in some cases it will allow of dressings being applied to the sores, but not in all, for the tumefaction will not now allow more of an inversion of the prepuce than before, and in such the sores cannot have dressings applied to them.

In many cases it will be found that so violent an operation is improper, for it often happens that, while the inflammation is so very considerable, there is danger of increasing it by this additional violence, of which mortification may be the consequence; while on the other hand there are cases where a freedom given to the parts would prevent mortification, so that the surgeon must be guided by the appearances and other circumstances. Besides these reasons for and against the operation arising from the disease itself, it will not always be consented to by the patients themselves, for some have such a dread of operations that they will not submit to cutting instruments; however, in those cases where the matter is confined it will be absolutely necessary to have an opening somewhere for the discharge of it. This is often produced by the ulcerative process going on on the inside, which makes an opening directly through the skin, laterally, which affords a direction for the surgeon: therefore the opening may be made directly into the cavity of the prepuce, through the skin, on the side of the penis, by a lancet; or a small caustic may be applied there, for which the lapis septicus is the most convenient.

The opening will allow of the discharge of the matter, and also admit any proper wash to be thrown in. But this opening should not be a large one, as in many cases the consequence of this lateral opening proves very troublesome; for from the tumefaction of the prepuce the glans is squeezed on all sides, and rather more backwards upon the body of the penis than in any other direction, by which means it is often forced through this opening, whereby the glans is directed to one side, and the prepuce to the opposite, having a forked appearance. Besides, this state of the parts tightens the skin of the penis round the root of the glans, acting there somewhat like a paraphimosis, and sometimes makes the whole prepuce mortify and drop off, which is often a lucky circumstance; but if this is not the consequence, then amputation of the prepuce becomes necessary: however, this should not be done till all inflammation is gone off, and the chancres are cured, when probably the tumefaction of the prepuce will have considerably subsided.

A mortification of the prepuce is sometimes a consequence of chancres when attended with violent inflammation, even without any previous operation; and I have seen cases where the glans and part of the penis have mortified, while the prepuce has kept its ground. But I should suspect in all such cases that there is some fault in the constitution, and that the inflammation is of the erysipelatous, not of the true suppurative kind.

I have seen the mortification go so far as to remove the whole of the diseased prepuce, and the parts have put on so favourable an appearance that I have treated it as a common sore, and no bad consequences have happened. In this case the disease performed what is often recommended in other diseases of this part, that is, circumcision; but this is not always to be trusted to, for if absorption of the venereal matter has taken place previous to the mortification, a lues venerea will be the consequence, although the parts heal very readily.

§. 5. *Of the Constitutional Treatment of Phimosis.*

In those cases where violent inflammation has attacked the seat of a chancre, producing phimosis, as before described, and often so as to threaten mortification, a question naturally occurs, what is to be done? Is mercury to be given freely to get rid of the first cause? or does that medicine increase the effect while it destroys the cause? Nothing but experience can determine this.

I should incline to believe that it is necessary that mercury should be given, for I am afraid our powers to correct such a constitution, while the first cause subsists, are weak. However, on the other hand, I believe the mercury should be given sparingly, for if it assists in disposing the constitution to such symptoms we are gaining nothing, but may lose by its use. I therefore do suppose that such medicines as may be thought necessary for the constitution should be given liberally, as well as the specific. Bark is the medicine that probably will be of most general use; opium in most cases of this kind will also be of singular service. The bark should be given in large quantities, and along with it mercury, while the virus is still supposed to exist. Or if the in-

flammation has arisen early in the disease, they may be then given together, so as to counteract both diseases, and not allow the inflammation to come to so great a height as it would otherwise do if mercury
was given at first alone. This inflammation may be so great in many
cases, or be so predominant, that mercury may increase the disposition,
and therefore become hurtful. Where this may be supposed to be the
case, bark must be given alone[a].

§. 6. *Of the Treatment of the Paraphimosis from Chancres.*

A prepuce in the state of inflammation and tumefaction, and which
has been either kept back upon the body of the penis while inflaming,
or pulled back when inflamed, seldom can be again brought forwards
while in this state, therefore becomes also the subject of an operation,
which consists in dividing the same part, as in the phimosis, only in a
different way, arising from its difference of situation, the intention of
which operation is to bring the prepuce, when brought forwards, to the
state of a phimosis that has been operated upon. This operation becomes
more necessary in many cases under this disease than under the phimosis, because its consequences are generally worse; since, besides the
real disease, viz. inflammation, tumefaction, ulceration, &c., there is a
mechanical cause producing its effects, by grasping the penis, which

---

[a] [In many cases of phimosis mercury is not necessary, because in many cases the
affection arises not from a venereal chancre, but from a common sore: as, for instance,
from that sort of ulceration which the author has denominated gonorrhœa of the glans
and prepuce. When the sore is a chancre mercury must be used, and the sore will
seldom be overcome without it, because washes and other topical applications, as well
as diaphoretics and purgatives internally, though they exercise a certain degree of power
over the inflammation, do not reduce the genuine venereal thickening. If the surgeon
is in doubt as to the real nature of the sore within, he may suspend the use of mercury
till the inflammation has been partly subdued by other means, and he has acquired evidence of its true character, from the obstinacy of the contraction, or the distinct per-
ception of the chancrous induration. But the presence of active inflammation forms
no objection to the employment of mercury. On the contrary, under such circumstances, mercury will in all cases be beneficial. Even when the prepuce is sloughing,
it is not in general contraindicated, provided the bright arterial colour of the part, and
the state of the pulse and of the skin, show that the arterial action is above the natural
standard. The sloughing in such cases arises either from the confinement of matter
within the prepuce, or from the excessive violence of the inflammation. In the first
case it will be stopped by making an opening with a lancet at the part where the abscess
is pointing; in the second case it will be most effectually limited by quickly subduing
the inflammation; and this may be best accomplished by absolute rest, by the internal
use of antimony and mercury, and by the frequent injection of saturnine washes under
the prepuce.]

can of itself produce inflammation where the prepuce is naturally tight, as has been observed. From whatever cause it arises, it often produces mortification in the parts between the stricture and the glans if it is not removed. This removal sometimes happens naturally by the ulceration of the strictured part, but an operation is generally necessary, and it is more troublesome than in the former case, because the swelling on each side of the stricture covers or closes in upon the tight part, and makes it difficult to be got at.

The best way appears to be to separate the two swellings as much as possible where you mean to cut, so as to expose the neck; then take a crooked bistory which is pointed, and passing it under the skin at the neck, divide it; no part of the two swellings on the sides need be divided, for it is the looseness of the skin in these parts which admits of their swelling. When this is done the prepuce may be brought forwards over the glans; but as this disease arose from chancres which may require being dressed, and as the state of a phimosis is a very bad one for such treatment, it may be better, now that the stricture is removed, to let it remain in the same situation till the whole is well.

If the paraphimosis has arisen from a natural tightness of the prepuce, and its being forced back from accident, then no particular treatment after the operation is necessary but to go on with the cure as recommended in chancres. It is indeed probable that in consequence of the violence produced by the position of the prepuce, as also by the operation, a considerable inflammation may ensue; but as this will be an inflammation in consequence of violence only, local treatment for the inflammation will be sufficient.

But if it is a paraphimosis in consequence of a diseased phimosis, then the same mode of treatment becomes equally necessary as was recommended in the phimosis attended with considerable inflammation; and probably rather more attention is necessary here, as violence has been added to the former disease.

§. 7. Of the Cure of Chancres by Mercury given internally.

While chancres are under local treatment, as before described, it is necessary to give mercurials internally, both for the cure of a chancre and the prevention of a lues venerea; and we may reasonably venture to affirm, that the venereal disposition of chancre will hardly ever withstand both local and internal mercurials.

In cases of chancres where local applications cannot easily be made, as in cases of phimosis, internal mercurials become absolutely necessary, and more so than if they could be conveniently and freely applied externally. However, even in such cases, internal mercurials will in the end effect a cure, so that we need seldom if ever be under any apprehension of not curing such a disease.

In every case of a chancre, let it be ever so slight, mercury should be given internally, even in those cases where they were destroyed on their first appearance. It should in all cases be given the whole time of the cure, and continued for some time after the chancres are healed; for as there are perhaps few chancres without absorption of the matter, it becomes absolutely necessary to give mercury to act internally, in order to hinder the venereal disposition from forming*.

How much mercury should be thrown into the constitution in the cure of a chancre, for the prevention of that constitutional affection, is not easily ascertained; as there is in such cases no disease actually formed so as to be a guide, it must be uncertain what quantity should be given internally. It must in general be according to the size, number, and duration of the chancres. If large, we may suppose that the absorption will be proportioned to the surface, and if long continued, the absorption will be according to the time; and if they have been many, large, and continued long, then the greatest quantity is necessary.

The circumstances therefore attending the chancre must be the guide for the safety of the constitution, especially in those cases where some stress in the cure is laid upon the external remedy.

The mercury given to act internally must be thrown in either by the skin or stomach, according to circumstances.

The quantity in either way should be such as may in common affect the mouth slightly, which method of giving mercury will be considered hereafter.

When the sore has put on a healthy look, when the hard basis has become soft, and it has skinned over kindly, it may be looked upon as cured.

But in very large chancres it may not always be necessary to continue the application of mercury either for external or internal action till the sore is healed; for the venereal action is just as soon destroyed in a large chancre as it is in a small one, for every part of the chancre being equally affected by the mercury, is equally easily cured. But the skinning is different; for a large sore is longer in skinning than a small

---

* Added: " When chancres are attended with a great degree of inflammation and swelling of the neighbouring lymphatic glands, there are peculiarities in the constitution which are unfavourable to the use of mercury; it should therefore in such cases be used with caution, and joined with such remedies as will make it less irritating to the constitution."—*Home.*

one. A large chancre therefore may be deprived of its venereal action long before it is skinned over; but a small one may probably skin over before the venereal poison is entirely subdued. In the latter case, both on account of the chancre and constitution, it will be erring on the safe side to continue the medicine a little longer, which will most certainly in the end effect a cure; for we may reasonably suppose that the quantity of mercury capable of curing a local effect, although assisted by local applications, or of producing in the constitution a mercurial irritation sufficient to hinder the venereal irritation from forming, will be nearly as much as will cure a slight lues venerea.

I have formerly laid it down as a principle, that no new action will take place in another part of the body, however contaminated, whilst the body is under the beneficial operation of mercury; but there are now and then appearances which occur under the cure that will at first embarrass the practitioner. I have suspected that the mercury flying to the mouth and throat has sometimes produced sloughs in the tonsils, and these have been taken for venereal. The following cases in some degree explain this.

A young gentleman had a chancre on the prepuce, with a slight pain in a gland of one groin, for which I ordered mercurial ointment to be rubbed into the legs and thighs, especially on the side where the gland was swelled, and the chancre to be dressed with mercurial ointment. While he was pursuing this course the chancre became cleaner, the hardness at the base went off, and the pain in the groin was entirely removed. About three weeks after the first appearance of the disease he was attacked with a sore throat, and on looking into the mouth I found the right tonsil with a white slough, which appeared to be in its substance, with only one point yet exposed. From my mind being warped by the opinion that these complaints proceeded from the chancre, I immediately suspected that it was venereal; and the only way that I could account for this seeming contradiction, in one part healing while another was breaking out, was, that the healing sore was treated locally as well as constitutionally, while the tonsil, or the constitution at large, was only treated constitutionally, which was insufficient.

Soon after this another gentleman was under my care for venereal scurfs, or eruptions on his skin, for which he used mercurial friction till his mouth became sore; and in this state he continued for three weeks, in which time the eruptions were all gone, discolourations being left only where the eruptions had been, yet at the end of three weeks a slough formed in one of the tonsils, exactly as in the former case. This made me doubtful how far such cases were venereal. I ordered the friction to be left off, to see what course the ulcers would take: the slough came out and left a foul sore. I waited still longer, and in a day or two it became clean and healed up.

The first-mentioned case I did not see to an end; but I learned that the patient continued the mercury and got well, and the ulcer in the throat was supposed to be venereal; but, from the circumstances of the other case, I now very much doubt of that.

It is more than probable that these effects of mercury only take place in constitutions that have a tendency to such complaints in the throat. I know this to be the case with the last-mentioned gentleman; and it is also probable that there may be an increased disposition at the time, either in consequence of the mercury or some accidental cause. I have reason to suppose that mercury in some degree increases this disposition, which I shall further take notice of when treating of the cure of the lues venerea.

In the cure of chancres I have sometimes seen, when the original chancre has been doing well and probably nearly cured, that new ones have broken out upon the prepuce, near to the first, and have put on all the appearance of a chancre; but such I have always treated as not venereal. They may be similar to some consequences of chancres, which will be taken notice of hereafter.

As swellings of the absorbent glands take place in consequence of other absorptions besides that of poisons, we should be careful in all cases to ascertain the cause, as has been already described; and here it may not be improper still to observe further, that in the cure of chancres, swellings of the glands shall arise, even when the constitution is loaded with mercury sufficient for the cure of the sores; but then the mercury has been thrown into the constitution by the lower extremity, and therefore there is great room for suspicion that such swellings are not venereal, but arise from the mercury; for a real bubo, from absorption of venereal matter, if not come to suppuration, will give way to mercury rubbed into the leg and thigh. In such cases I have always desisted from giving the mercury in this way when I could give it by the mouth.

CHAPTER IV.

OF THE CURE OF CHANCRES IN WOMEN.

THE parts generally affected with chancres in this sex are more simple than in men, by which means the treatment in general is also more simple; but in most cases they require nearly the same, both in the local application of mercury, and in throwing it into the constitution. It may be supposed, however, that it will be necessary in many cases to throw into the constitution more mercury than in men, because in general there are more chancres, and the surface of absorption of course larger.

As it is difficult to keep dressings on the female parts, it is proper they should be washed often with solutions of mercury; perhaps corrosive sublimate is one of the best, as it will act as a specific, and also as a stimulant when that is wanted; but in chancres that are very irritable, the same mode of treatment as was recommended in men is to be put in practice. Afterwards the parts may be besmeared with a mercurial application, either oily or watery, to be frequently repeated, according to the circumstances of the case.

If the ulcers should have spread, or run up the vagina, great attention should be paid to the healing of them; for it sometimes happens that the granulations contract considerably, so as to draw the vagina into a small canal; at other times the granulations will unite into one another, and close the vagina up altogether; therefore in such cases it will be necessary to keep some substance in the vagina till the sores are skinned, for which purpose probably lint may be sufficient.

CHAPTER V.

OF SOME OF THE CONSEQUENCES OF CHANCRES, AND THE TREATMENT OF THEM.

AFTER the chancres have been cured, and all venereal taint removed, it sometimes happens that the prepuce still retains a considerable degree of tumefaction, which keeps up the elongation and tightness which it acquired from the disease, so that it cannot be brought back upon the penis to expose the glans.

For this perhaps there is, in many cases, no cure; however, it is necessary to try every possible means. The steam of warm water, fomentations with hemlock, and also fumigations with cinnabar, are often of singular service in this case.

But if the parts still retain their size and form, it may be very proper to remove part of the overgrown prepuce; how much, must be left to the discretion of the surgeon. I should suppose that all that part which projects beyond the glans penis may be cut away.

The best way of removing it is by the knife; but great care should be taken to distinguish first the projecting prepuce from the glans. When this is perfectly ascertained, the penis being held horizontally, an incision may be made on the upper surface, and followed down with caution; because if the incision should be too near the glans there may be danger of cutting it.

The parts may be allowed to heal with any common dressings, as it is to be considered as a fresh wound; however it will not heal so readily as a fresh wound made in an entirely sound part, because the operation consists in taking away only a superfluous part of a diseased whole; and what is left is diseased, but not so as to produce any future mischief.

Some care may be necessary in the healing of the parts, for it is very possible that the cicatrix may contract, and still form a phimosis. This will be best prevented by the patient himself if he brings the prepuce often back upon the penis; but it should not be attempted till the part is nearly healed; and it is to be performed with great care, and slowly.

§. 1. *Of Dispositions to new Diseases during the cure of Chancres.*

Chancres, both in men and women, often acquire new dispositions in the time of the cure, which are of various kinds, some of which retard the cure, as described, and, when the parts are cured, leave them tumefied and indolent, as in the enlarged prepuce. In others a new disposition takes place, which prevents the cure or healing of the parts, and often produces a much worse disease than that from which it arose. They also become the cause of the formation of tumours on these parts, which will be taken notice of hereafter.

Such new dispositions take place oftener in men than in women, probably from the nature of the parts themselves. They seldom or

never happen but when the inflammation has been violent, which violence arises more from the nature of the parts than the disease, and therefore belongs more to the nature of the parts or constitution than to the
disease.   However, I can conceive it may also take place where the inflammation has not been violent.

In general they are supposed to be cancerous, but I believe they seldom are, although it is not impossible that some may be so.

Of this kind may be reckoned those continued and often increased
inflammations, suppurations, and ulcerations, becoming diffused through
the whole prepuce, as also all along the common skin of the penis,
which becomes of a purple hue; the cellular membrane everywhere on
the penis being very much thickened, so as to increase the size of the
whole considerably.

The ulceration on the inside of the prepuce will sometimes increase
and run between the skin and the body of the penis, and eat holes
through in different places till the whole is reduced to a number of
ragged sores.   The glans often shares the same fate, till more or less of
it is gone; frequently the urethra at this part is wholly destroyed by
ulceration, and the urine is discharged some way further back.   If a
stop is not put to the progress of the disease, the ulceration will continue till the parts are entirely destroyed.   I suspect that some of these
cases are scrofulous.

As this is an acute case, immediate relief should be given, if possible;
but as it may arise from various peculiarities in the constitution, and as
these peculiarities are not at first known, no rational method can be here
determined.   The decoction of sarsaparilla is often of service in such
cases, but requires to be given in large quantities.

The German diet-drink* has been of singular service; I knew a case
of this kind cured by it, after every known remedy had been tried.   The
extract of hemlock is sometimes of service.   I have known sea-bathing
cure these complaints entirely.   A gentleman came from Ireland with
a complaint of this kind, and after having tried every common and
known method without effect, as sarsaparilla, hemlock, German diet-

---

* The following formulæ have been much recommended as diet-drinks.   Take of
crude antimony, pulverized, tied up in a bit of rag; pumice-stone, pulverized, tied up
in the same, of each one ounce; China-root, sliced; sarsaparilla-root, sliced and bruised,
of each half an ounce; ten walnuts, with their rinds, bruised; spring water four pints,
boil to half that quantity; filter it, and let it be drunk daily in divided doses.

Take sarsaparilla, Saunders-wood, white and red, of each three ounces; liquorice
and mezereon, of each half an ounce; lignum rhodium, guaiacum, sassafras, of each
one ounce; crude antimony, two ounces; mix them and infuse them in boiling water,
ten pints, for twenty-four hours, and afterwards boil them to five pints, of which let
the dose be from a pint and a half to four pints a day.

drink, and after having used a great variety of dressings (which were all at last laid aside, and opium only retained to quiet the pain), he bathed in the sea and got well. It may be sometimes necessary to pass a bougie, to hinder the orifice of the urethra from closing or becoming too small in the time of healing in such cases[a].

---

[a] [The description of the author is so vague that it is difficult to know with certainty what species of sore he here intends to designate. But it is probable that he chiefly refers to those sores which are called *phagedenic*, and which are of sufficient importance to require a particular description.

The name phagedenic has been given to them because they have been supposed to be the same with the ulcers described by Celsus under the name of phagedæna. Though the correctness of this supposition may be questioned, yet there is a convenience in retaining a name which not unaptly characterizes the ulcer, whether we regard the occasional rapidity of its progress, or the most remarkable features which distinguish its aspect.

It can scarcely be doubted that phagedenic ulcers arise from the application of a virus, since there is no satisfactory evidence that they ever occur where the party has not been exposed to infection, and since they are as constantly followed by secondary symptoms, as the genuine forms of chancre which have been previously described. Nor, though much attention has been paid to the subject, has it been possible to trace such a constant distinction as would establish that the virus which produces them is different from that which gives origin to the common Hunterian chancre. The characters of the phagedenic sore are very different from those of a common chancre; and if there is a diversity of virus, this diversity should be constant, and should be capable of being traced equally in the giver and the recipient; in the party from which the infection is derived, as well as in that to which it is communicated. But it has not been found possible to ascertain that this is the case. On the contrary, the phagedenic sore has in several instances appeared to have been derived from individuals who have suffered from the common forms of chancre.

The phagedenic sore begins with slight tumefaction of the part, and slight excoriation of the surface. This excoriated surface soon becomes foul, being covered with a yellow slough, and discharging a watery sanies of a brownish tinge. As the sore destroys the part on which it is situated the surface becomes uneven, and the outline of the sore irregular in shape, and, as it were, scolloped. These appearances are produced by the mode of progress, which is not regular and uniform in every direction, but proceeds in some parts more rapidly than in others. The central part, and perhaps one of the edges, then ceases to spread, and becomes clean, while on other sides the foul character remains, and the sore continues to extend. The part which is spreading is always somewhat tumefied, but the tumefaction is that of common inflammation, and is not distinctly defined, like that of an ordinary chancre. It does not terminate abruptly, but passes imperceptibly into the surrounding structure. In fact it is merely caused by the irritation of the spreading sore: the clean edge is altogether free from it. As soon as a part cleans, the tumefaction subsides, though the ulceration may remain long afterwards unhealed. The tumefaction cannot be said to precede the ulceration; it rather attends the sloughing, if that can be called sloughing which is in general only foul ulceration.

The phagedenic sore may destroy any part on which it is placed, but its ravages involve the cellular membrane more readily than either the prepuce or the body of the penis. The consequence is, that in most cases it burrows between the body and the

§. 2. *Of Ulceration resembling Chancres.*

It often happens that after chancres are healed, and all the virus gone, the cicatrices ulcerate again, and break out in the form of chancres.

---

skin of the penis, dissecting in its course the corpora cavernosa from the integuments, and creeping upwards between these parts, often as far as the os pubis. Under these circumstances, the bottom of the sore cannot be fully exposed; the part which is within view is generally clean, and sometimes slowly healing, while the portion which is concealed is foul and yellow, and secretes large quantities of a thin brownish discharge. This spreading edge is attended by the usual tumefaction, which may be felt externally as a hard ring encircling the body of the penis, marking the distance to which the sore has extended, and in the progress of the complaint approaching nearer and nearer to the root of the penis. As long as this thickened edge is to be felt, so long the sore is spreading. If the bottom of the sore cleans and tends to heal, the improvement may be known by the subsidence of this thickening, as immediately and as certainly as if the whole of the surface were exposed to view.

Under common circumstances the phagedenic sore spreads by foul ulceration, and eats its way very slowly, and almost imperceptibly. But it is subject to occasional accesses of sloughing, in which large portions of the prepuce, the glans, or the corpus spongiosum, mortify and separate. There are few cases of long standing in which such sloughing has not occurred; and in most instances a portion of the urethra has been destroyed by it, and an opening has been formed, at which the urine escapes, about an inch above the natural meatus. The suddenness of these attacks, and the irremediable destruction which they occasion, render it necessary that the treatment should always be conducted with a view to their occurrence.

The discharge from the phagedenic sore is profuse and unhealthy; but it does not seem, like the discharge of the common chancre, to affect the surfaces with which it comes into contact. It is common that the prepuce and the glans should be almost constantly bathed in it; yet it is very rarely or never that other sores arise on these parts in consequence. Again, the contiguous surfaces are not affected. The sore may be situated on the body of the penis, while the prepuce in contact with it shall remain free from ulceration. It is not uncommon that the phagedenic sore should be situated on one side of the meatus urinæ, and should destroy a considerable portion of the glans before it is arrested; yet the affection will not extend to the other side of the meatus, although the ulcerated surface is allowed to remain perpetually in contact with it.

The phagedenic sore is attended with some, but not with acute inflammation. The pain, except during an attack of sloughing, is not very severe. The prepuce is usually red, sometimes purple, almost always loaded with serum, and tumid; but it is not generally indurated, or firm to the touch; nor is the colour of that bright scarlet which attends acute phimosis from common chancre. Yet there is more constitutional disturbance: the pulse is usually quick and excitable, the skin hot, the appetite indifferent, and the sleep restless and disturbed.

It is rare that a suppurating bubo should arise from a phagedenic sore. A gland in the groin sometimes enlarges, but it is seldom very painful, and generally subsides spontaneously in less than a week.

The secondary symptoms which follow the phagedenic sore are peculiarly severe and intractable. They commonly consist of rupia, sloughing of the throat, ulceration of the nose, severe and obstinate muscular pains, and afterwards inflammation of the peri-

Although this is most common in the seat of the former chancres, yet it is not always confined to them, for sores often break out on other parts of the prepuce; but still they appear to be a consequence of a venereal complaint having been there, as they seldom attack those who never had gonorrhœa or chancres. They often have so much the appearance of chancres, that I am persuaded many are treated as venereal that are really not such: they differ from a chancre in general by not

---

osteum and bones. Similar complaints will follow the ordinary chancre; but when they follow a phagedenic sore they are very difficult to be cured; and it is not uncommon that the constitution of the patient should at length give way under them, and that the case should terminate fatally.

If the description of these sores is compared with that of a common chancre, which has been given in a former chapter, the distinction is sufficiently evident. The common chancre is preceded and followed by induration of a peculiar character, which holds its course in some measure independently of the ulceration itself. No such induration is found in the phagedenic sore: the thickening which does occur does not differ from that which is met with in other sores, and is merely an attendant on the unhealthy state of the ulcer. The common chancre spreads equally in all directions. The phagedenic sore spreads irregularly, and frequently heals at one edge while it is spreading at another. The common chancre tends to multiply and to produce similar ulcers on the surfaces which are in contact with it. The phagedenic sore remains single, and the contiguous surfaces are unaffected. There is also a difference, though less clearly defined, in the secondary symptoms which follow these two species of sore, and a different treatment must be adopted in the cure.

If the phagedenic sore is treated with a full course of mercury, it is most frequently found that the improvement in the first instance is more immediate and more decided than in the case of a common chancre. In a very few days the inflammation subsides, the surface cleans, and the sore begins to heal. But this amendment is usually only temporary: it generally happens that in a few days more, if the mercury is continued, and especially if the effect on the system is at all excessive, the aspect changes, the colour of the surrounding parts becomes dark and purple, sudden sloughing comes on, and the whole surface of the sore, and often much of the prepuce and of the penis, is involved in it. On the other hand, if mercury is entirely avoided, and such treatment only is adopted as would be employed in a common sore, the ulcer obstinately retains its unhealthy character, and makes constant, though less rapid, progress by foul ulceration.

Mercury is of great service in the treatment of the phagedenic sore, but if its depressing defects are allowed to come on, the consequence is, almost always, sloughing. It must therefore be so employed as to avoid these effects: it must be administered in those doses, and in those forms which least depress the circulation; and it must be combined with such medicines as are calculated at the same time to support the system. The oxymuriate of mercury, given in the dose of an eighth of a grain twice in the day, and in unison with decoction of sarsaparilla, is the safest and most efficient preparation. But even in this form the effect must be watched; and if the integuments in the neighbourhood of the sore should become pale or livid, or if much general languor is induced, the remedy must be intermitted, and resumed only after these symptoms of impending sloughing have disappeared.

It must not be omitted, that the internal use of the hydriodate of potass has often great effect on this form of disease.]

spreading so fast, nor so far; they are not so painful, nor so much inflamed, and have not those hard bases that the venereal sores have, nor do they produce buboes. Yet a malignant kind of them, when they attack a bad constitution, may be taken for a mild kind of chancre, or a chancre in a good constitution*.

Some stress is to be laid upon the account that the patient gives of himself; but when there is any doubt, a little time will clear it up. I have seen the same appearances after a gonorrhœa, but that more rarely happens. It would appear that the venereal poison could leave a disposition for ulceration of a different kind from what is peculiar to itself. I knew one case where they broke out regularly every two months, exactly to a day.

As they are not venereal, their treatment becomes difficult; for the cure consists more in preventing a return than in the healing up of the present sores.

They require particular attention; for although they are not dangerous, they are often troublesome, keeping the mind in suspense for months.

I have tried a great variety of means, but with little success; yet they have in general got well in the end. In the following case, the lixivium saponarium produced a speedy cure.

A gentleman had three sores broke out on the prepuce, which had very much the appearance of mild chancres. As I was doubtful of their nature, I waited some time, and only ordered them to be kept clean. As they did not get well, several things were tried. Mercurial dressings were applied, but they always produced considerable irritation, and it was necessary to leave them off. The mercurius calcinatus was given by way of trial, and to secure the constitution, but the sores continued the same. They were eat down with the lunar caustic, which appeared to have a better effect than any other thing tried; but still they were not healed at the end of five months. I ordered forty drops of the lixivium saponarium to be taken every evening and morning in a bason of broth. After using it three days he observed a considerable alteration in the sores, and in six they were perfectly skinned over. He had formerly had such sores often, which had always been treated as venereal; but he began to doubt whether they really were so, from their getting so soon well in the present instance by the lixivium.

I knew a gentleman who had these sores breaking out and healing again for years. By bathing in the sea for a month or two, they healed up, and never afterwards appeared.

* Added: " I have seen several that have puzzled me extremely."—*Home.*

§. 3. *Of a Thickening and Hardening of the parts.*

In some cases the parts do not ulcerate, but appear to thicken and become hard or firm; both the glans and prepuce seem to swell, forming a tumour or excrescence from the end of the penis, in form a good deal like a cauliflower, and, when cut into, showing radii running from its base or origin towards the external surface, becoming extremely indolent in all its operations. This gives more the idea of a cancer than the first, being principally a new-formed substance. However, it is not always a consequence of the venereal disease, for I have known it to arise spontaneously.

This disease appears to be a tumour of so indolent a kind that I do not know any medicine that stands the least chance of performing a cure. I have amputated them, and have also seen the same thing done by others, from the idea of their being cancerous, and the remaining part of the penis has healed kindly.

In most of these cases a considerable part of the penis must be removed. Immediately after the amputation, a suitable catheter should be introduced into the urethra; for if no such precaution is made use of, the consequences must be troublesome; for the first dressings become cemented to the orifice by the extravasated blood, and prevent the patient's making water, which must be attended with obvious inconveniences. This was the case with a patient whose penis I amputated.

§. 4. *Of Warts.*

Another disposition which these parts acquire from the venereal poison is the disposition to form excrescences or cutaneous tumours, called warts. This disposition is strongest where the chancres were, and indeed chancres often heal into warts; but perhaps the parts acquire this disposition from the venereal matter having been long in contact with their surfaces, for it often happens after gonorrhœas, where there had been no chancres; and probably it is only in those cases where the venereal matter had produced the venereal stimulus upon the glans and prepuce, forming there what may be called an insensible gonorrhœa.

A wart appears to be an excrescence from the cutis, or a tumour forming upon it, by which means it becomes covered with a cuticle, which, like all other cuticles, is either strong and hard or thin and soft, just as the cuticle is which covers the parts from whence they arise. They are radiated from their basis to the circumference, the radii appearing at the surface pointed or granulated, much like granulations that are healthy, except that they are harder and rise above the surface. It would appear that the surface on which each is formed has only the disposition to form one, because the surrounding and connecting surface does not go into the like substance: thus a wart once begun does not increase in its basis, but rises higher and higher. They have an increasing power within themselves: for, after rising above the surface of the skin, on which they are not allowed to increase in breadth at the basis, they swell out into a round thick substance, which becomes rougher and rougher.

This structure often makes them liable to be hurt by bodies rubbing against them; and often from such a cause they bleed very profusely, and are very painful.

These excrescences are considered by many not as simply a consequence of the venereal poison, but as possessed of its specific disposition, and therefore they have recourse to mercury for the cure of them; and it is asserted that such treatment often removes them. Such an effect of mercury I have never seen, although given in such a quantity as to cure in the same person recent chancres and sometimes a pox.

As these substances are excrescences from the body, they are not to be considered as truly a part of the animal, not being endowed with the common or natural animal powers, by which means the cure becomes easier. They are so little of the true animal, and so much of a disease, that many trifling circumstances make them decay; an inflammation in the natural and sound parts round the wart will give it a disposition to decay; many stimuli applied to the surface will often make them die. Electricity will produce action in them which they are not able to support; an inflammation is excited round them, and they drop off.

From this view of them, the knife and escharotics must appear not always necessary, although these modes will act more quickly than any other in many cases, especially if the neck is small. In such-formed warts perhaps a pair of scissors is the best instrument; but where cutting instruments of any kind are horrible to the patient, a silk thread tied round their neck will do very well; but, in whichsoever way it is separated, it will be in general necessary to touch the base with caustic.

Escharotics act upon warts in two different ways, namely, by deadening a part and stimulating the remainder; so that by the application of escharotic after escharotic the whole decays tolerably fast, and it is seldom necessary to eat them down to the very root, as the basis or root often separates and is thrown off. This however is not always the case, for we find that the root does not always separate, and that it will grow again; therefore in such cases it is necessary to eat down lower than the general surface to remove the root.

Any of the caustics, such as the lapis septicus, as also the metallic salts, such as the lunar caustic, blue vitriol, &c., have this power. The rust of copper and savine-leaves mixed are one of the best stimulants.

After they have been to appearance sufficiently destroyed, they often rise anew, not from any part being left, but from the surface of the cutis having the same disposition as before. This requires a repetition of the same practice, so as to take off that surface of the cutis.

§. 5. *Of Excoriations of the Glans and Prepuce.*

It very often happens that the surface of the glans and inside of the prepuce excoriate, becoming extremely tender, and then a matter oozes out. The prepuce in such cases often becomes a little thickened, and sometimes contracts in its orifice, both which circumstances render the inversion of it difficult and painful. Whether this complaint ever arises from a venereal cause is not certain, as it often takes place where there never has been any venereal taint.

This disease is in the cutis; and under such a disposition it has no power of forming a good cuticle. It is very similar to a gonorrhœa in this part, but is not venereal.

Drawing the prepuce back, and steeping the parts in a solution of lead, often takes off the irritation, and a sound cuticle is formed. Spirits diluted often produce the same effect; the unguentum citrinum of the Edinburgh Dispensatory, lowered by mixing with it equal parts of hog's-lard, is often of singular service in such cases. But there are cases which bid defiance to all our applications, in which I have succeeded by desiring the person to leave the glans uncovered, which produced the stimulus of necessity for the formation of a natural cuticle.

PART V.

———◆———

CHAPTER I.

OF BUBO.

A KNOWLEDGE of the absorbing system, as it is now established, gives us considerable information respecting many of the effects of poisons, and illustrates several symptoms of the venereal disease, in particular the formation of buboes. Prior to this knowledge we find writers at a loss how to give a true and consistent explanation of many of the symptoms of this disease. The discovery of the lymphatics being a system of absorbents has thrown more light on many diseases than the discovery of the circulation of the blood: it leads in many cases directly to the cause of the disease.

The immediate consequence of the local diseases, gonorrhœa and chancre, which is called bubo, as also the remote, or lues venerea, arise from the absorption of recent venereal matter from some surface where it has either been applied or formed. Although this must have been allowed in general ever since the knowledge of the disease and of absorption, yet a true solution of the formation of bubo could not be given till we had acquired the knowledge of the lymphatics being the only absorbents. Upon the old opinion, of absorption being performed by the veins, the lues venerea could easily have been accounted for, because it could as readily be produced by the absorbing power of the veins, if they had such, as by the lymphatics; but the difficulty was to say how the bubo was formed. There they seemed to be at a loss to account for this disease, yet they sometimes expressed themselves as if they had some idea of it, although at the same time they could have no clear notions of what they advanced: nor could they demonstrate what they said from the knowledge of the parts and their uses.

Buboes are by some imputed to the stopping of a gonorrhœa, or, as they express it, driving it to the glands of the groin, conformably to the idea they had of the cause of the swelling of the testicle. But this is not just, for we know of no such power as repulsion; and if it was driven there it could not be by stopping the formation of matter, but by increasing the absorption, of which they had no idea.

When we examine the opinion of authors concerning the formation of bubo, prior to the knowledge of the power of absorption in the lymphatics, we shall find them making use of terms which they could not possibly understand. For instance, Heister says, "They are of two kinds, one venereal, and the other not; but he does not say that the venereal arises only from impure coition.

Astruc says, p. 326, that some buboes arise immediately from impure coition, and these he calls essential; others from suppressed gonorrhœa, or a small discharge, or from chancres of the penis, and these he calls symptomatic; lastly, that they arise spontaneously without any immediate previous coition, and are a pathognomonic sign of a hidden pox.

In p. 327 he shows the impossibility of this last happening from what we now call or understand by a lues venerea; but in p. 328 he explains what he calls a latent lues venerea, which is local affection produced as he supposes from a lues venerea, but which most probably never yet happened; and if ever they had arisen from such a cause, even the absorption of their matter could not produce a venereal bubo, as will be explained. In short, as he understood not the true absorbing system, his ideas are become now unintelligible*.

We find Cowper, Drake, and Boerhaave, as well as Astruc, speaking of the vitiated lymph not passing the glands, therefore inflaming them; also of the inspissated lymph passing, either by the circulation of the blood, that is, from the constitution to these glands, (an opinion held by some to this day,) or by a shorter course, viz. the lymphatic vessels which go to the inguinal glands. They also speak of the swelling of the inguinal glands,˙ or venereal buboes, from the contagion being communicated by the resorbent lymphatics. Drake even speaks more pointedly; and, if we consider him no further, he would almost make us believe that he knew that the lymphatics were the absorbents; but as he has no such ideas when treating of those vessels expressly, we are not to give him credit for it. His words are: "The venereal bubo may very likely take its rise from some parts of the contagious matter of claps sucked up by the lymphatics of the penis, and thence imported to the inguinal glands, where they deposit their liquor; and thence it well behoves the surgeon to be as early as may be in the opening of such tumours, before by the exporting vessels of that class the poison is carried further into the blood, which very probably may be the case where such tumour ariseth immediately upon the stopping of a gonor-

* The above extracts are from the English edition, published in the year 1754.

2 A 2

rhœa, as does the hernia humoralis. But when the same appears some months after that was removed, we are to suppose, as in cases of other poisons laying hold of the blood, by the strength of Nature it is thrown forth, either by means of the lymphatics of the blood-vessels themselves, if not spewed out of the nervous tubes, as Wharton surmised, and deposited in these emunctories."

Here he compares it to the formation of a hernia humoralis, which plainly shows that he understood neither of them.

Even so late as the year 1748, we do not find any new ideas on this subject: Freke says, "By sealing up the mouths of the glands of the urethra, the poison is thence, by the ducts leading to the inguinal glands, conveyed to them."

In the year 1754, eight years after Dr. Hunter had publicly taught his opinion of the lymphatics being a system of absorbents, we find a treatise on this disease by Mr. Gataker, where as little new is advanced on this subject as in any of the former.

When we come so low down as the year 1770, in an abridgement of Astruc, by Dr. Chapman, (2nd edit.) in which he introduces his own knowledge and ideas, we find the absorbing power of the lymphatics brought in as a cause of the formation of buboes; but by this time the knowledge of the lymphatics being the system of absorbents was in this country generally diffused.

The doctrine of absorption being now perfectly understood, we have only to explain the different modes in which it may take place.

The venereal matter is taken up by the absorbents of the part in which it is placed; and although the absorption of the matter and the effects after absorption are the same, whether from the matter of the gonorrhœa or chancre, yet I shall divide the absorption into three kinds, according to the three different surfaces from which the matter may be absorbed, beginning with the least frequent.

The first and most simple is where the matter either of a gonorrhœa or chancre has only been applied to some sound surface, without having produced any local effect on the part, but has been absorbed immediately upon its application. Instances of this I have seen in men, and such are perhaps the only instances that can be depended upon; for it is uncertain in many cases whether a woman has a gonorrhœa or not. I think however I may venture to affirm that I have seen it in women, or at least there was every reason to believe that they had neither chancre nor gonorrhœa preceding, as there was no local appearance of it, nor did they communicate it to others who had connexion with them.

It must be allowed that this mode of absorption is very rare; and if we were to examine the parts very carefully, or inquire of the patients very strictly, probably a small chancre might be discovered to have been the cause, which I have more than once seen. For, when we consider how rarely it happens from a gonorrhœa, in which the mode of absorption is similar, we can hardly suppose it probable that it should here arise from simple contact, the time of the application of the venereal matter being commonly so very short. We might indeed suppose the frequency to make up for the length of time, which we can hardly allow, for the same frequency should give the chance of producing it locally. Therefore very particular attention should be paid to all the circumstances attending such cases.

There is however no great reason why it should not happen, and the possibility of it lessens the faith that is to be put in the supposition that the disease may be years in the constitution before it appears; for whenever it does appear in a lues venerea its date is always carried back to the last local affection, whether gonorrhœa or chancre, and the latter connexions are never regarded.

The second mode of absorption of this matter is more frequent than the former, and it is when the matter applied has produced a gonorrhœa; and it may happen while the complaint is going on, either under a cure or not. Some of the matter secreted by the inflamed surfaces having been absorbed and carried into the circulation, produces the same complaints as in the former case, by which means the person gives himself the lues venerea.

The third mode is the absorption of the matter from an ulcer, which may be either a chancre, or a bubo. This mode is by much the more frequent, which, with many other proofs, would show that a sore or ulcer is the surface most favourable for absorption. Whether ulcers in every part of the body have an equal power of absorption I have not been able to determine; but I suspect that an ulcer on the glans is not so good a surface for absorption as one on the prepuce, although I have seen both buboes and the lues venerea arise from the former, but not so often as from the latter.

To these three methods may be added a fourth, absorption from a wound, which, I have already remarked, is perhaps not so frequent as any of the former.

As the venereal poison has the power of contaminating whatever part of the body it comes in contact with, it contaminates the absorbent system, producing in it local venereal complaints. It is hardly necessary to observe, that what is now commonly understood by a bubo, is a swelling taking place in the absorbing system, especially in the glands, arising from the absorption of some poison, or other irritating matter; and when such swellings take place in the groin they are called buboes, whether from absorption or not, but are most commonly supposed to be venereal, even although there has been no visible preceding cause. This has been so much the case, that all swellings in this part have been suspected to be of this nature; femoral ruptures and aneurisms of the femoral artery have been mistaken for venereal buboes.

I shall call every abscess in the absorbing system, whether in the vessels or the glands, arising in consequence of the absorption of venereal matter, a bubo.

This matter, when absorbed from either of the four different surfaces, which are common surfaces, wounds, inflamed surfaces, and ulcers, is carried along the absorbent vessels to the common circulation, and in its passage often produces the specific inflammation in these vessels, the consequence of which is the formation of buboes, which are venereal abscesses, exactly similar in their nature and effects to a chancre, the only difference being in size. As the absorbents with the glands are immediately irritated by the same specific matter which has undergone no change in its passage, the consequent inflammation must therefore have the same specific quality, and the matter secreted in them be venereal*.

As this system of vessels may be divided into two classes, the vessels themselves and their ramifications and convolutions, called the lymphatic glands, I shall follow the same division in treating of their inflammations.

Inflammation of the vessels is not nearly so frequent as that of the glands. In men such inflammations, in consequence of chancres upon the glans or prepuce, generally appear like a chord leading along the back of the penis from the chancres. Sometimes they arise from the thickening of the prepuce in gonorrhœas, that part in such cases being generally in a state of excoriation, as was described when I treated of that form of the disease. These chords often terminate insensibly on the penis, near its root, or near the pubes; at other times they extend further, passing to a lymphatic gland in the groin: this chord can be easily pinched up between the finger and thumb, and it often gives a thickness to the prepuce, making it so stiff at this part as to make the inversion of it difficult, if not impossible, producing a kind of phimosis.

I think I have observed this appearance to arise as frequently from the gonorrhœa, when attended with the before-mentioned inflammation and tumefaction of the prepuce, as from chancres; which, if my obser-

---

* I do not know how far this reasoning will hold good in all cases of poisons, for I very much suspect that the bubo, that is sometimes formed in consequence of inoculation of the smallpox, does not produce variolous matter. The natural poisons, in producing buboes, certainly do not form a poison similar to themselves.

vation is just, is not easily accounted for. I have observed that absorption is more common to ulcers than inflamed surfaces, or at least the formation of a bubo in the gland, and its effects in the constitution, are more common from an ulcer; but it may be remarked, that the inside of the prepuce, from whence this chord appears to arise, is in an excoriated state. It is possible that this effect may arise from the lymphatics sympathizing with the inflammation of the urethra, but I believe the affection is truly venereal; or it is possible that even the absorption of the coagulable lymph, which was produced from the venereal inflammation, and which is the cause of the tumefaction, may have the power of contamination, as appears to be the case in the cancer.

The thickening, or the formation of this hard chord, probably arises from the thickening of the coats of the absorbents, joined with the extravasation of coagulable lymph, thrown in upon its inner surface, as in inflamed veins.

This chord often inflames so much as to suppurate, and sometimes in more places than one, forming one, two or three buboes, or small abscesses in the body of the penis. When this is going on we find in some parts of this chord a circumscribed hardness; then suppuration takes place in the centre, the skin begins to inflame, the matter comes nearer to it, and the abscess opens like any other abscess.

I have seen a chain of these buboes, or little abscesses, along the upper part of the penis, through its whole length.

This may be supposed to be exactly similar to the inflammation and suppuration of a vein after being wounded and exposed.

Inflammation of the glands is much more frequent than the former, and arises from the venereal matter being carried on to the lymphatic glands, the structure of which appears to be no more than the ramifications and reunion of the absorbent vessels, by which means they form these bodies.

From this structure we may reasonably suppose that the fluid absorbed is in some measure detained in these bodies, and thereby has a greater opportunity of communicating the disease to them than to the distinct vessels, where its course is perhaps more rapid, which may account for the glands being more frequently contaminated.

Swellings of these glands are common to other diseases, and should be carefully distinguished from those that arise from the venereal poison. The first inquiry should be into the cause, to see if there is any venereal complaint at some greater distance from the heart, as chancres on the penis, or any preceding disease on the penis; to learn if mercurial ointment has been at all applied to the legs and thighs of that side, for mercury applied to those parts, for the cure of a chancre, will sometimes tumefy the glands, which has been supposed to be venereal. We should further observe, if there be no preceding disease in the constitution, such as a cold, fever, &c., the progress of the swelling with regard to quickness is also to be attended to, as also to distinguish it from a rupture, lumbar abscess, or aneurism of the crural artery.

Perhaps these bodies are more irritable, or more susceptible of stimuli than the vessels. They are certainly more susceptible of sympathy; however, we are not yet sufficiently acquainted with the use of these glands to be able to account satisfactorily for this difference.

It would appear in some cases that it is some time after the absorption of the venereal matter before it produces its effects upon the glands; in some it has been six days at least. This could only be known by the chancres being healed six days before the bubo began to appear; and in such cases it is more than probable that the matter had been absorbed a much longer time before, for the last matter of a chancre most probably is not venereal; and indeed it is natural to suppose that the poison may be as long before it produces an action on the parts, when applied in this way, as it is either in the urethra or in forming a chancre, which I have shown to be sometimes six or seven weeks.

The glands nearest to the seat of absorption are in general the only ones that are attacked, as those in the groin, when the matter has been taken up from the penis in men: in the groin, between the labia and thigh, and the round ligaments, when absorbed from the vulva, in women. I think there is commonly but one gland at a time that is affected by the absorption of venereal matter, which, if so, becomes in some sort a distinguishing mark between venereal buboes and other diseases of these bodies. We never find the lymphatic vessels or glands, that are second in order, affected, as those along the iliac vessels or back; and I have also seen when the disease has been contracted by a sore, or cut upon the finger, the bubo come on a little above the bend of the arm, upon the inside of the biceps muscle; and in such where the bubo has come in that part, none has formed in the armpit, which is the most common place for the glands to be affected by absorption.

But this is not universal, although common, for I was informed by a gentleman who contracted the disease in the before-mentioned way, that he had buboes both on the inside of the biceps muscle and in the armpit. Another case of this kind I have heard of since; why it is not more common is perhaps not easily explained.

It might be supposed that the matter was weakened, or much diluted by the absorptions from other parts by the time it gets through these nearest ramifications, and therefore has not power to contaminate those which are beyond them; but it is most probable that there are other reasons for this. I once suspected that the nature of the poison was altered in these glands as it passed through them, which was the reason why it did not contaminate the second or third series of glands; and also why it did not affect the constitution in the same way as it did the parts to which it was first applied; but this explanation will not account for the next order of glands to suppurating buboes not being affected by the absorption of venereal matter. It appears to me that the internal situation of the other glands prevents the venereal irritation from taking place in them; and this opinion is strengthened by observing when one of these external glands suppurates and forms à bubo, which is to be considered as a large venereal sore or chancre, that the absorption from it, which must be great, does not contaminate the lymphatics or glands next in order, by the venereal matter going directly through them.

If this be true, then the skin would seem to be the cause of the susceptibility of the absorbents to receive the irritation. Whether the skin has the power inherent in itself, or acquires it from some other circumstance, as air, cold, or sense of touch, is not easily ascertained; but whichever it be, it shows that the venereal matter of itself is not capable of irritating, and that it requires a second principle to complete its full effect, that is, a combination of the nature of the poison and the influence of the skin, and that influence must be by sympathy, and therefore weaker than if acting in the same part, that is, the skin itself, which perhaps is the reason why the venereal matter does not always affect those vessels and glands, while it always does the skin, if inserted into it.

The situation of buboes arising from the venereal disease in the penis is, in men, in the absorbent glands of the groin; if a gonorrhœa is the cause of a bubo, one groin is not exempted more than the other; both may be affected: but if a bubo arises in consequence of a chancre, then the groin may be generally determined by the seat of the chancre, for if the chancre is on one side of the penis, then the bubo will commonly be on that side: however, this is not universally the case; for I have known instances, although but few, where a chancre on one side of the prepuce or penis has been the cause of a bubo on the opposite side, which, if arising from that chancre, is a proof that the absorbents either anastomose, or decussate each other. If the chancre be on the frænum, or on the middle of the penis, between the two sides, then it is uncertain which side will be affected.

The situation of the glands of the groin is not always the same, and therefore the course of the absorbent vessels will vary accordingly I have seen a venereal bubo, which arose from a chancre on the penis, a considerable way down the thigh; on the contrary, I have seen it often as high as the lower part of the belly, before Poupart's ligament, and sometimes near the pubes, all of which three situations may lead to some variations in the method of cure; therefore it may be proper to attend to them.

As the disease most commonly arises from copulation, the situation of buboes is generally in the groin; but as no part of the body, under certain circumstances, is exempt from this disease, we find the nearest external glands between the part of absorption and the heart, everywhere in the body share the same fate with those of the groin, especially if external.

CHAPTER II.

OF BUBOES IN WOMEN.

The same diseases in the absorbents, in consequence of the absorption of the venereal matter, take place in this sex as well as in men. I never saw but one case where the absorbent vessels were diseased; but this is nearly in the same proportion as in men, when I consider the proportion the number of the one sex bears to that of the other who apply to me for a cure of the venereal disease in any form. The case was a gonorrhœa, with violent itching and soreness when the patient sat or walked; but she had very little pain in making water. When I examined the parts, I could see no difference between them and sound parts, excepting that the left labium was swelled, or fuller than the other, and a hard chord passed from the centre of that labium upwards to the os pubis, and passed on to the groin of the same side, and was lost in a gland as high as Poupart's ligament. It was not to be felt but by pressing the parts with some force, and it gave considerable pain upon pressure.

The swelling of the labium appeared to be somewhat similar to the swelling of the prepuce in similar cases in men, so that they would appear to arise from the same cause.

One would naturally suppose that what has been said of this complaint in the lymphatic glands in men, would be wholly applicable to women, and also that nothing peculiar to women could take place; but the seat of absorption is more extensive in this sex, and the course of some of the absorbents is also different, from whence there are three situations of buboes in women, two of which are totally different from those in men, and these I suspect to be in the absorbents.

The third situation of buboes in this sex is similar to that in men, and therefore they may be divided into three, as in men.

When buboes arise in women where there is no chancre, it is more difficult to know whether they are venereal or not than in men; for when they arise in men without any local complaint it is known that no such complaint exists, and therefore the bubo cannot be venereal, excepting by immediate absorption; but in women it is often difficult to know whether there be any infection present or not; and therefore in order to ascertain the nature of the bubo attention must be paid to its manner of coming on, progress, and other circumstances.

When chancres are situated forwards, near to the meatus urinarius, nymphæ, clitoris, labia, or mons Veneris, then we find that the matter absorbed is carried along one or both of the round ligaments, and the buboes are formed in those ligaments just before they enter the abdomen, without, I believe, ever going further. These buboes I suspect not to be glandular, but inflamed absorbents; and if so, it strengthens the idea that it is only an external part that can be affected in this way.

When the chancres are situated far back, near the perinæum, or in it, the matter absorbed is carried forwards along the angle between the labium and the thigh to the glands in the groin; and often in this course there are formed small buboes in the absorbents, similar to those on the penis in men; and when the effects of the poison do not rest here, it often produces a bubo in the groin, as in men.

CHAPTER III.

OF THE INFLAMMATION OF BUBOES, AND THE MARKS THAT DISTINGUISH THEM FROM OTHER SWELLINGS OF THE GLANDS.

THE bubo commonly begins with a sense of pain, which leads the patient to examine the part, where a small hard tumour is to be felt*.

* It must be remarked here, that whenever a person has either a gonorrhœa or a

This increases like every other inflammation that has a tendency to suppuration; and, if not prevented, goes on to suppuration and ulceration,
the matter coming fast to the skin.

But we find cases, where they are slow in their progress, which I
suspect either arises from the inflammatory process being kept back by
mercury or other means, or being retarded by a scrofulous tendency,
such a disposition in the parts not so readily admitting the true venereal action.

At first the inflammation is confined to the gland, which is moveable
in the cellular membrane; but as it increases in size, or as the inflammation, and more especially the suppuration, advances, which in all
cases produce rather a common than a specific effect, the specific distance
is exceeded; the surrounding cellular membrane becomes more inflamed,
and the tumor is more diffused. Some buboes become erysipelatous, by
which means they are rendered more diffused and œdematous, and do
not readily suppurate, a circumstance often attending the erysipelatous
inflammation.

To ascertain what a disease is, is the first step in the cure; and when
two or more causes produce similar effects, great attention is necessary
to distinguish one effect from another, so as to come at the true cause
of each.

The glands of the groin, from their situation, are liable to suspicion,
for besides being subject to the common diseases, they become exposed
to others, by allowing whatever is absorbed to pass through them; and
as the route of the venereal poison to the constitution is principally
through them, and being oftener ill from this cause than any other, they
often are suspected of this disease without foundation.

To distinguish with certainty the true venereal bubo from swellings
of those glands arising from other causes, may be very difficult. We
must, however, examine all circumstances, to ascertain in what the bubo
differs from the common diseases of those glands, whether in the groin
or elsewhere, in which examination the apparent causes are not to be
neglected. I have already given the character of the venereal bubo in
general terms; but I shall now be more particular, as the two are to be
contrasted.

The true venereal bubo, in consequence of a chancre, is most commonly confined to one gland. It keeps nearly its specific distance till

chancre, he becomes apprehensive of a bubo; and as there are in the gonorrhœa, and
sometimes in the chancre, sympathetic sensations in or near the groin, they are suspected by the patient to be beginning buboes, and the hand is immediately applied to
the part; and if he feels one of the glands, although not in the least increased, the suspicions are confirmed, from a belief that he has no such parts naturally.

suppuration has taken place, and then becomes more diffused*. It is rapid in its progress from inflammation to suppuration and ulceration. The suppuration is commonly large for the size of the gland, and but one abscess. The pain is very acute. The colour of the skin which the inflammation attacks is of a florid red.

It may be observed, that the buboes in consequence of the first mode of absorption, viz. where no local disease has been produced, will always be attended with a greater uncertainty of the nature of the disease than those attended or preceded by a disease in the penis, because a simple inflammation and suppuration of these glands are not sufficient to mark it to be venereal; but as we always have this disease in view when the glands of the groin are the seat of the disease, the patient runs but little risk of not being cured, if it should be venereal; but I am afraid that patients have often undergone a mercurial course when there has been no occasion for it.

It will perhaps be difficult to find out the specific difference in the diseases themselves; but I think that such buboes as arise without any visible cause are of two kinds; one similar to those arising from chancres or gonorrhœa; that is, inflaming and suppurating briskly. These I have always suspected to be venereal; for although there is no proof of their being so, yet from these circumstances there is a strong presumption that they are.

The second are generally preceded and attended with slight fever, or the common symptoms of a cold, and they are generally indolent and slow in their progress. If they are more quick than ordinary, they become more diffused than the venereal, and may not be confined to one gland. When very slow they give but little sensation, but when more quick, the sensation is more acute, though not so sharp as in those that are venereal; and most commonly they do not suppurate, but often become stationary. When they do suppurate it is slowly, and often in more glands than one, the inflammation being more diffused, and commonly small in proportion to the swelling. The matter comes slowly to the skin, not attended with much pain, and the colour is different from that of the other, being more of the purple. Sometimes the suppurations are very considerable, but not painful.

Now let us see what other causes there are for the swelling of these glands besides venereal infection, to which I have ascribed one of the modes of swelling; for there must be other causes to account for the other modes of it.

---

* It may be observed here, that the glands and surrounding parts being dissimilar, inflammation does not so readily become diffused as when it takes place in a common part.

The first thing to be attended to is, whether or not there are any venereal complaints; and if not, this becomes a strong presumptive proof
that they may not be venereal, but proceed from some unknown cause.
If the swelling is only in one gland, very slow in its progress, and gives
but little or no pain, it is probably merely scrofulous; but if the swelling is considerable, diffused and attended with some inflammation and
pain, then it is most probable that there is a constitutional action con-
sisting in slight fever, the symptoms of which are lassitude, loss of appetite, want of sleep, small quick pulse, and an appearance of approaching
hectic. Such swellings are slow in their cure, and do not seem to be
affected by mercury, even when very early applied.

A gentleman had all the symptoms of a slight fever; the pulse a little
quick and hard, loss of appetite, and of course loss of flesh; a listless-
ness, and a sallow look. While he was in this state a swelling took
place in the glands of one of the groins. He immediately sent for me,
because he imagined it to be venereal. From the history of the case, I
gave it as my firm opinion it was not; in this he had not much faith.
The swellings were not very painful, and, after having acquired a considerable size, they became stationary. To please him, I gave him a
box of mercurial ointment, to be rubbed on the leg and thigh only of
the side affected, that it might have a sufficient local effect, and as little
go into the constitution as possible; but it did not appear to be of any
service to the swellings in the groin, they remaining stationary, and almost without pain. His friends became uneasy, and sent their surgeons
to him, who, without knowing he was my patient, and of course without
knowing my opinion, imagined that the disease was venereal, and talked
of giving mercury. With respect to the cure, I thought he should go
to the sea and bathe.

Allowing the chance of the disease being venereal or not venereal to
be equal, I reasoned upon that ground. His present want of health
could not be supposed to arise from any venereal cause, as it was prior
to the swelling in the groin; and therefore though the swelling might
be venereal, he was not at present in a condition to take mercury, as a
sufficient quantity of that medicine, for the cure, might kill him: and if
it should not be venereal, that still a greater quantity of mercury must
be given than what was necessary if it were venereal; because its not
giving way readily would naturally make the surgeon push the mercury
further; and, besides this disagreeable circumstance, the disease in the
groin might be rendered more difficult of cure. But by going to the sea
his constitution would be restored; and if the disease in the groin proved
to be venereal, he would be in a proper condition to go through a mercurial course, and by that means get rid of both diseases by the two

methods. But if I should be right in my opinion, that there was no-thing venereal in the case, then he would probably get well by the sea-bathing alone.

These arguments had the desired effect: he went directly to the sea, and began to recover almost immediately. About a fortnight after, a small suppuration took place in one of the glands. I directed that a poultice should be made with sea-water, and applied; and, in case of the breaking of the abscess, that it should not be further opened, but poul-ticed till healed. In six weeks he came back perfectly recovered in every respect.

The above-mentioned appearance, with the constitutional affections, I have seen take place when there were chancres, and I have been puz-zled to determine whether it was sympathetic, from a derangement of the constitution, or from the absorption of matter.

I have long suspected a mixed case, and I am now certain that such exists. I have seen cases where the venereal matter, like a cold or fever, has only irritated the glands to disease, producing in them scro-fula, to which they were predisposed.

In such cases the swellings commonly arise slowly, give but little pain, and seem to be rather hastened in their progress if mercury is given to destroy the venereal disposition. Some come to suppuration while under this resolving course, and others, which probably had a venereal taint at first, become so indolent that mercury has no effect upon them, and in the end get well either of themselves or by other means, which, I imagine, may have induced some to think that buboes are never venereal. Such cases require great attention, that we may be able to determine them properly; and I believe this requires in many cases so nice a judgement that we shall be often liable to mistakes.

Buboes are undoubtedly local complaints, as has been explained.

How far the lymphatic glands are to be considered as guards against the further progress of this or any other disease caught by absorption, is not easily determined. We must, however, allow that they cannot prevent the poison from entering the constitution in cases where it pro-duces buboes, for whenever it affects these glands in its course, it pro-duces the same disease in them which is capable of furnishing the con-stitution with an increased quantity of the same kind of poison.

CHAPTER IV.

GENERAL REFLECTIONS ON THE CURE OF BUBOES.

FROM what has been offered on the history of buboes, it will be needless here to enter into a discussion of the opinion of their being a deposit from the constitution, and of the conclusion drawn from this opinion, that they ought not to be dispersed; for according to this theory, to disperse them would be to throw the venereal matter upon the constitution. But if this were really the case, then there would be no occasion for the use of mercury, provided that the bubo be allowed to proceed, as it would prove its own cure; but even those who were of this opinion were not satisfied with the cure which they supposed Nature had pointed out, but gave mercury, and in very large quantities. From the same history of a bubo I have also endeavoured to show that there are several buboes which are not in the least venereal, but scrofulous; and that there are also buboes which appear to be only in part venereal, or perhaps only a gland disposed to scrofula, brought into action by the venereal irritation, similar to what happens often from the matter of the smallpox in inoculation. Therefore, prior to the speaking of the method of cure the true venereal bubo is to be distinguished from the others, if possible. When it is well ascertained to be venereal, resolution is certainly to be attempted, if the bubo be in a state of inflammation only. The propriety of the attempt depends upon the progress which the disease has made. If it be very large, and suppuration appears to be near at hand, it is probable that resolution cannot be effected; and if suppuration has taken place, I should very much doubt the probability of success, and an attempt might now possibly only retard the suppuration, and protract the cure.

The resolution of these inflammations depends principally upon mercury, and almost absolutely upon the quantity that can be made to pass through them; and the cure of them, if allowed to come to suppuration, depends upon the same circumstances. The quantity of mercury that can be made to pass through a bubo depends principally upon the quantity of external surface for absorption beyond the bubo.

Mercury is to be applied in the most advantageous manner; that is, to those surfaces by an absorption from which it may pass through the diseased gland; for the disease there being destroyed, the constitution has less chance of being contaminated. The powers of mercury may often be increased from the manner in which it is applied. In the cure of buboes, it should always be made to pass into the constitution by the same way through which the habit received the poison; and therefore, to effect this it must be applied to the mouths of those lymphatics which pass through the diseased part, and which will always be placed on a surface beyond the disease.

But the situation of many buboes is such as not to have much surface beyond them, and thereby not to allow of a sufficient quantity of mercury being taken in in this way; as, for instance, those buboes on the body of the penis arising from chancres on the glans or prepuce.

These two surfaces are not sufficient to take in the necessary quantity to cure those buboes in its passage through them; therefore whenever the first symptoms of a bubo appear, its situation is well to be considered, with a view to determine if there be a sufficient surface to effect a cure, without our having recourse to other means. It is first to be observed, whether the absorbent vessels on the body of the penis are affected, or the glands in the groin. If the disease be in the groin, it must be observed in which of the three situations of the bubo, before taken notice of, it is; whether on the upper part of the thigh and groin, on the lower part of the belly before Poupart's ligament, or near to the pubes. If they are on the body of the penis, this shows that the absorbents leading directly from the surface of absorption are themselves diseased. If in the groin, and on the upper part of the thigh, or perhaps a little lower down than what is commonly called the groin, then we may suppose it is in the glands common to the penis and thigh. If high up, or on the lower part of the belly, before Poupart's ligament, then it is to be supposed that those absorbents that arise from about the groin, lower part of the belly, and pubes, pass through the bubo; and if far forwards, then it is most probable that only the absorbents of the penis and skin about the pubes pass that way. The knowledge of these situations is very necessary for the application of mercury for the cure by resolution, and for the cure after suppuration has taken place.

The propriety of this practice must appear at once when we consider that the medicine cannot pass to the common circulation without going through the diseased parts; and it must promote the cure in its passage through them; while at the same time it prevents the matter which has already passed, and is still continuing to pass, into the constitution from acting there, so that the bubo is cured and the constitution preserved.

But this practice alone is not always sufficient; there are many cases in which mercury by itself cannot cure. Mercury can only cure the specific disposition of the inflammation; and we know that this disease is often attended with other kinds of inflammation besides the venereal.

Sometimes the common inflammation is carried to a great height; at other times the inflammation is erysipelatous, and, I suspect, often scrofulous. We must therefore have recourse to other methods.

Where the inflammation rises very high, bleeding, purging, and fomenting are generally recommended. These will certainly lessen the active power of the vessels, and render the inflammation more languid; but they can never lessen the specific effects of this poison, which were the first cause, and are still in some degree the support of the inflammation. Their effects are only secondary, and if they reduce the inflammation within the bounds of the specific, it is all the service they can perform. If the inflammation be of the erysipelatous kind, perhaps bark is the best medicine that can be given; or if it be suspected to be scrofulous, hemlock, and poultices made with sea-water, may be of service.

Vomits have been of service in resolving buboes, even after matter has been formed in them, and after they have been nearly ready to burst; this acts upon the principle of one irritation destroying another; and sickness and the act of vomiting perhaps give a disposition for absorption. A remarkable instance of this kind happened in an officer who had a bubo at Lisbon. It came to fair suppuration, and was almost ready to burst. The skin was thin and inflamed, and a plain fluctuation felt. I intended to open it, but as he was going on board a ship for England on the day following, I thought it better to defer it. When he went on board he set sail immediately, and the wind blew so very hard that nothing could be done for some days, all which time he was very sick, and vomited a good deal; when the sickness went off he found the bubo had disappeared, and it never afterwards appeared. When he came to England he went through a regular course of mercury.

§. 1. *Of Resolution of the Inflammation of the Absorbents on the Penis.*

The surface beyond the seat of the disease in this case, that is, all that part of the penis before the bubo, is not large enough to take in a quantity of mercury sufficient to prevent the effects of absorption, and therefore recourse is to be had to other means; yet this application should by no means be neglected, and this surface, small as it is, should be constantly covered with mercurial ointment, which will assist in the cure of the local disease. It may be disputed whether any medicine can pass through diseased lymphatics, so as to have any effect upon them, but I judge from experience that it certainly can. As this surface is too small, and as it is necessary that a larger quantity should be taken in, it becomes proper to give it either by the mouth, or by friction on some larger surface; this is necessary, to prevent the lues venerea, as well as to cure the parts themselves. The quantity cannot be determined; that must be left to the surgeon, who must be directed by the appearances of the original complaint, and the readiness with which the disease gives way.

The same method is to be followed in women; but as there is a larger surface in this sex more mercury may possibly be absorbed; and there should be a constant application of ointment to the inside and outside of the labia.

§. 2. *Of the Resolution of Buboes in the Groin.*

The inflammation of the glands is to be treated exactly upon the same principle with the other; but we have in general a larger surface of absorption, so that we can make a greater quantity of mercury pass through the diseased parts.

It will be proper to apply the mercury according to the situation of the inflamed gland. If the bubo be in the groin, according to our first situation, then it is necessary to rub the mercurial ointment upon the thigh. This surface will in general absorb as much mercury as will be sufficient to resolve the bubo, and to preserve the constitution from being contaminated by the poison that may get into it; but if resolution does not readily take place, then we may increase the surface of friction, by rubbing the ointment upon the leg.

But if the bubo be on the lower part of the belly, that is, in the second situation, then the ointment should be rubbed also upon the penis, scrotum, and belly; and the same if the bubo should be still forwards; for probably those glands receive the lymphatics from all the surfaces mentioned, as well as from the thigh and leg.

The length of time for continuing the frictions must be determined by circumstances. If the bubo gives way, they must be continued till it has entirely subsided, and perhaps longer, on account of the cause of it, a chancre, which may not yield so soon as the bubo. If it still goes on to suppuration, the frictions may or may not be continued, for I do not know for certain if anything is to be gained by their continuance in this state.

The quantity here recommended may affect the mouth; and this effect must also be regulated according to circumstances.

§. 3. *Of the Resolution of Buboes in Women.*

When treating on the seat of buboes in women, I observed that two situations were peculiar to them, the others similar to those in men.

In the first and second situations, especially the first, the surface of absorption, beyond the bubo, is by much too small to be depended upon for receiving a sufficient quantity of mercury to produce resolution; but in the second, that is, between the labia and thigh, the mercury may be rubbed in all about the anus and buttock, as all the absorbents of those parts probably pass that way; we know at least that they do not pass into the pelvis by the anus, but go by the groin. Other means of introducing mercury must be recurred to, as is recommended in the case of men; but still it will be proper to rub in on these surfaces as much as possible.

In the situations common to both sexes we have a larger field; yet as they are divisible into three, the same observations hold good, and a similar mode of practice is to be followed in women as in men.

§. 4. *Of Buboes in other Parts.*

As venereal buboes arise from other modes of application of the poison besides coition, they are to be found in different parts of the body, but more frequently in the hands. They arise in the arm-pit from wounds in the hands or fingers being contaminated by venereal matter, and reduced to a chancre. In such cases it becomes necessary that the ointment should be rubbed on the arm and fore-arm; but this surface may not be sufficient, therefore we must apply it in another way, or to other parts, to produce its effects upon the constitution.

I have seen a true venereal chancre on the middle of the lower lip produce a bubo on each side of the neck under the lower jaw, just upon the maxillary gland. By applying strong mercurial ointment to the under lip, chin, and swellings, they have been resolved.

§. 5. *Of the Quantity of Mercury necessary for the Resolution of a Bubo.*

The quantity of mercury necessary for the resolution of a bubo must be proportioned to the obstinacy of the bubo, but care must be taken to stop short of certain effects upon the constitution. If it be in the first situation, and yields readily to the use of half a dram of mercurial ointment, made of equal parts of quicksilver and hog's lard, every night, and the mouth does not become sore, or at most only tender, then it will be sufficient to pursue this course till the gland is reduced to its natural size; and this probably will be a good security for the constitution, provided that the chancre, which may have been the cause of the bubo, heals at the same time. If the mouth is not affected in six or eight days, and the gland does not readily resolve, then two scruples or a dram may be applied every night; and if there be no amendment, then more must be rubbed in; in short, if the reduction is obstinate the mercury must be pushed as far as can be done without a salivation.

If there be a bubo on each side, then there cannot be so much mercury applied locally to each; for the constitution most probably could not bear double the quantity which is necessary for the resolution of one. But in such cases we must not so much attend to the soreness of the mouth as when there is but one; however, we must allow the buboes to go on to suppuration, rather than affect the constitution too much by the quantity of mercury; and therefore when there are two buboes they are more likely to suppurate than where there is only one.

In the second and third situation of buboes, if we find that most probably a sufficient quantity of mercury does not pass through them for their resolution, it may be continued to be thrown in by the leg and thigh to act upon the constitution, as has been already observed. The quantity admitted in this way must be greater than what would be necessary if the whole could be made to pass through the bubo. The mouth must be affected, and that in proportion to the state and progress of the bubo.

This method of resolving buboes occurred to me at Belleisle, in the year 1761, where I had good opportunities of trying it upon the soldiers: and I can say with truth that only three buboes have suppurated under my care since that time, and two of these were in one person, where a small quantity of mercury had considerable effects on the constitution, and therefore a sufficient quantity could not be sent through the two groins for their resolution; but in both cases the suppurations were small in comparison to what they threatened to be.

Many buboes, after every attempt, remain swelled without either coming to resolution or suppuration, but rather become hard and scirrhous. Such, I apprehend, were either scrofulous at first, or became so when the venereal disposition was removed. The cure of them should be attempted by hemlock, sea-water poultices, and sea-bathing, as will be further taken notice of.

§. 6. *Of the Treatment of Buboes when they suppurate.*

After every known method has been used, buboes cannot in all cases be resolved, but come to suppuration. They then become more an object of surgery, and are to be treated in some respects like any other abscess. If it be thought proper to open a bubo, it should be allowed to go on thinning the parts as much as possible. The great advantage arising from this is, that these parts, having become very thin, lose the disposition to heal, which gives the bottom of the abscess a better chance of healing along with the superficial parts; by this means too a large opening is avoided, and the different modes made use of for keeping the skin from healing till the bottom is healed become unnecessary.

It may admit of dispute whether the application of mercury should be continued or not through the whole suppuration. I should be inclined to continue it, but in a smaller quantity; for although the parts cannot set about a cure till opened, yet I do imagine that they may be better disposed to it; and I think that I have seen cases where suppuration has taken place, although under the above-mentioned practice, that were very large in their inflammation, but very small in their suppuration, which I imputed to the patient's having taken mercury in the before-mentioned way, both before and while suppuration was going on.

It has been disputed more in this kind of abscess than in others whether it should be opened or allowed to burst of itself; and likewise whether the opening should be made by incision or caustic.

There appears to be nothing in a venereal abscess different from any other to recommend one practice more than another. The surgeon should in some degree be guided by the patient. Some patients are afraid of caustics, others have a horror of cutting instruments; but when it is left wholly to the surgeon, and the bubo is but small, I suppose a slit with a lancet will be sufficient: in this way no skin is lost. But when a bubo is very large, in which case there is a large quantity of loose skin, perhaps the caustic will answer better, both on account of its destroying some skin, and because the destruction is attended with less inflammation than what attends incision. If done by a caustic, the lapis septicus is the best*; but it is not necessary to open every bubo, and perhaps it may be difficult to point out those where opening would be of service or necessary.

* I once opened two buboes in the same person, one immediately after the other. The first was with the lapis infernalis, which gave him considerable pain, and therefore he would have the other opened with a lancet, as the pain would only be momentary. But it was great, and the soreness continued long, while there was no pain in the other, deadened by the caustic, after it had done its business.

The bubo is to be dressed afterwards according to the nature of the disease, which, I have already observed, is often so complicated as to baffle all our skill. The constitution at the same time is to be attacked with mercury, either by applying it internally or externally: if externally, it should be applied to that side and beyond where the bubo is, as I before directed in treating of the resolution of buboes, for it may have some influence on the disease in its passing through the part.

Mercury, in these cases, answers two purposes: it assists the external applications to cure the buboes, and it prevents the effects of the constant absorption of the venereal matter from the sore.

How far it is necessary to pursue the mercurial course with a view to prevention, it is not possible to determine; but it may be supposed that it is necessary to give the same quantity to prevent a disease that would cure one that has already taken place. It will be necessary to continue the course till the bubo is healed, or till it has for some time lost its venereal appearance; but it may be difficult to ascertain this last fact; therefore we must have recourse to experience, not theory, and continue the course in general till the whole is healed, and even longer, especially if the bubo heals very readily; for we find in many cases that the constitution shall be still tainted after all. However, some restrictions are here necessary; for I have already observed that it often happens that buboes assume other dispositions besides the venereal, which mercury cannot cure, but will even make worse. It is therefore very necessary to ascertain the distinction, which will be taken notice of.

CHAPTER V.

OF SOME OF THE CONSEQUENCES OF BUBOES.

I formerly observed that the venereal disease is capable of bringing latent dispositions or susceptibilities into action. This is remarkably the case with buboes; and I believe the disposition is more of the scrofulous kind than any other. Whether this arises from the buboes being formed in lymphatic glands or not is probably not easily determined.

It sometimes happens that these sores, when losing or entirely deprived of the venereal disposition, form into a sore of another kind, and most probably of various kinds. How far it is a disease arising from a venereal taint and the effects of a mercurial course jointly is not certain ; but most probably these two have some share in forming the disease. If this idea of it were just, it would become a specific disease and be reducible to one method of cure ; but I should suspect that either the constitution or the part hath some, if not the principal, share in it ; that is, the parts fall into a peculiar disease independent cf the constitutional disease or method of cure ; for if it arose out of the two first entirely, we might expect to meet with it oftener. So far as the constitution or the part has a share in forming this disease, it becomes more uncertain what the disease is, because it must in some degree partake of the constitution or nature of the part.

Such diseases make the cure of the venereal affection much more uncertain, because when the sore becomes stationary, or the mercury begins to disagree, we are ready to suspect that the virus is gone ; but this is not always the case : the virus is perhaps only less powerful than the new-formed disease, and as it were lies dormant, or ceases to act ; and when the other becomes weaker, the venereal influence begins to show itself again.

The proper treatment in such cases is to attack the predominant disease ; but still the difficulty is to find out the disease, and to know when it is or is not venereal. The following case explains this difficulty very well.

A gentleman had a very large venereal bubo, which was opened. He took a great deal of mercury for about two months ; but, I suspect, not in sufficient doses, which produced a mercurial habit. The bubo had no disposition to heal, and I was consulted. From the account he gave me, I suspected that he had then too much of a mercurial habit to receive at this time any further good from that medicine. I therefore advised him to use a good nourishing diet for near a month ; after that I put him upon a brisk mercurial course by friction ; and the parts put on a better appearance. This course he continued for near two months, and then the sore, although much mended, began to be stationary. I did now conceive that the venereal action was destroyed, and therefore immediately left off the mercurial course, and put him upon a milk diet, and sent him into the country. But not gaining much ground, he had a strong decoction of the sarsaparilla with mezereon given him, which, although continued for above a month, produced little or no effect. I also gave him the cicuta as much as he could bear, with the bark almost the whole time, without effect : new sinuses formed, which were opened, and the sore became extremely irritable, with thickened lips. The dressings were poultices made with the juice of hemlock, sea-water, opium, and a gentle solution of lunar caustic; but nothing seemed to affect it. I suspected scrofula, and therefore proposed he should bathe in the sea; but this then could not be done. These different treatments, after mercury had been left off, took up about four months without the least benefit. Being doubtful whether there might not be still something venereal in the sore, especially as appearances were growing worse, and it was now four months since he had taken any mercury, I was inclined to try it once more, and sent him two portions of ointment, half an ounce each, to rub in in two nights. He had caught a little cold, and therefore did not rub in the mercury the two evenings as ordered; and called upon me the third day and told me he was much better. The sore now became easy, the watery or transparent inflammation began to subside, the lips became flatter and thinner, and the edges of the sore began to heal. I then desired him not to rub in the ointment, but wait a little. In eight or ten days the sore had contracted to three quarters of its former size, and had all the appearance of a healing sore.

Quære: What conclusions should be drawn from this case? I think the following: that the virus may be gone, although the sore may have no disposition to heal; therefore we are not to look upon the not healing of a bubo as a sign of the presence of the original disease. Secondly, that the sarsaparilla, mezereon, cicuta, and the bark will not succeed in all such cases: and thirdly, that some of these diseases are capable of wearing out the unhealthy disposition of themselves, and that we should not be too ready to attribute cures to our treatment; for if the mercury had been rubbed in, and the same effects had still taken place, I should then have certainly pursued the mercury with vigour, and attributed the cure to it: but I should not have rested here; I should have related the case, as an instance of the disease continuing after repeated courses of mercury, and should have contended that it is necessary in such cases, where the mercury appears to lose its power, and even do harm, to wait, and season the constitution to strength, and the loss of the mercurial habit; and that even four months are sometimes necessary for this purpose, after which we must begin again to give mercury.

A gentleman had a common gonorrhœa, which was severe. I gave him an injection of a grain of corrosive sublimate in eight ounces of water, with a few mercurial pills. After having continued the injection for ten or twelve days, without any visible benefit, I gave it as my opinion that it would be of no service to continue it any longer, and therefore desired he would be quiet for a little time. About this time a swelling in each groin took place, and supposing them to be venereal,

I ordered mercurial ointment to be rubbed into both the legs and thighs, to resolve them if possible. He appeared to be less uneasy about the buboes than he was about the gonorrhœa, but I told him that the cure of that complaint would be insensibly involved in the resolution of the buboes. I spoke too confidently of my power with respect to the resolution of the buboes, for they both suppurated, although the suppuration was small in comparison to the magnitude of the buboes when they first inflamed. The frictions were left off.

While we were attempting to resolve the buboes he got well of the gonorrhœa. The skin covering the buboes became thin; they were both opened, one with a caustic, the other with a lancet; he then was ordered to rub in mercury again on the thighs and legs for their cure. They began soon to look well, and to close fast; but when about half healed they became stationary. I suspected that a new disease was forming. On continuing the frictions a little longer they began to inflame and swell anew, and a suppuration took place about half an inch above each of the first suppurations, which broke into the first. I left off the mercury immediately upon their inflaming, and said that now a new disease had formed. I ordered poultices made with sea-water to be applied, and also a decoction of sarsaparilla to be taken; but this appeared not to be sufficient for the cure of this new disease. I then ordered him to go into the tepid sea-bath every evening, the heat of the water to be about ninety degrees. By the time he had been in the bath four times the inflammation and swelling had very much abated, and the first sores, or original buboes, were beginning to heal. He went on with the bathing every evening for about three weeks, when the sores rather began to look worse; I then suspected that the venereal disposition was become predominant, and I ordered the friction as before. In about a fortnight the first buboes healed, but the second suppurations were not yet healed; then I supposed it to be entirely the new-formed disease, and he went into the country, where I desired he might go into the open sea every day, as he then could have an opportunity, which he did, and got perfectly well, and has continued so.

This case plainly shows that there was another disposition formed besides the venereal, which was put into action by the venereal irritation.

I have seen some buboes most exceedingly painful and tender to almost everything that touched them, and the more mild that the dressings were, the more painful the parts became.

In some the skin seems only to admit the disease, ulceration going on in the surrounding skin, while a new skin forms in the centre, and keeps pace with the ulceration, forming an irregular sore like a wormeaten groove all round. This, like the erysipelatous inflammation, as also some others, appears to have only the power of contaminating the parts that have not yet come into action; and those that have already taken it seem to lose the diseased disposition, and heal readily.

In some they spread to an amazing extent, as the following case shows, the circumstances of which are very remarkable.

A young gentleman, aged eighteen years, in consequence of a venereal infection, had two buboes, which were both opened. They were treated in the usual manner, and at first put on a favourable appearance; but when they were nearly healed they began to ulcerate at their edges, and spread in all directions, rising above the pubes almost to the navel, and descending upon each thigh. His nights became restless, and his general health was affected. A great variety of medicines were tried, particularly mercury in different forms, with little or no effect. Extract of hemlock did more good than anything else, and was taken in unusual quantities. An ounce was swallowed in the course of the day for some time, which was afterwards increased to an ounce and a half, two ounces, and even two ounces and a half. It produced indistinct vision and blindness, loss of the voice, falling of the lower jaw, a temporary palsy of the extremities, and once or twice a loss of sensation; and notwithstanding he was almost every night in a state, as it were, of complete intoxication from the hemlock, his general health did not suffer, but, on the contrary, kept pace in his improvement with the ulcers. They could not, however, be healed by the hemlock; and among many other things, Æthiops mineral and Plummer's pill were liberally given, seemingly with advantage. Recourse was had to the hemlock from time to time. A great many different kinds of dressings were made trial of, none of which were found to exceed dry lint. The ulcers were nearly all healed, after having tormented him upwards of three years, when, committing some irregularities in diet, and the sores getting worse, he returned to the extract of hemlock, which he had for some time laid aside, and of himself swallowed in the course of the morning ten drams. This quantity was only the half of what he had formerly taken in twenty-four hours, but his constitution had been at that time gradually habituated to the medicine. The ten drams produced great restlessness and anxiety; he dropt insensible from his chair, fell into convulsions, and expired in two hours.

To return to the cure of buboes: where they only become stationary, and appear to have but little disposition to spread (which is most common), and where perhaps a sinus or two may be found running into them from some other gland, I have often seen them give way to hemlock sooner than to anything I am acquainted with, especially if joined to the bark.   If the hemlock is applied both internally and externally it answers better.

Sarsaparilla is often of singular service here, as well as in other cases arising seemingly from the same cause; and I have seen sea-bathing of great service, as also sea-water poultice.

At the Lock Hospital they use gold-refiners' water as an application, which is of service in some cases. Dr. Fordyce recommends the juice of oranges to be drunk in large quantities, which I have seen good effects from in some cases. The mezereon is in some instances of singular use.

PART VI.

CHAPTER I.

OF THE LUES VENEREA.

THE lues venerea, I have already observed, arises in consequence of the poisonous matter being absorbed and carried into the common circulation. This form of the disease, which I have called the constitutional*, would appear to be much more complicated, both in the different ways in which it may be caught, and in its effects when caught, than either a gonorrhœa or chancre. It generally arises from the local complaints before taken notice of, the matter being absorbed and carried into the constitution. The matter, however, appears to be capable of being taken into the constitution by simple application, without first having produced either of the before-mentioned local effects, as I observed in treating of the formation of the bubo; but this seems to be only when it is applied to some particular parts of our body, such as may be called a half-internal surface, as the glans penis. I think it is not capable of being received by the absorbents of the sound skin†; but this is matter only of opinion.

It may likewise be received into the constitution by being applied to common ulcers, although not necessarily rendering these ulcers themselves venereal; also by wounds, as has been observed; but, I believe, always previously producing ulceration in the wound.

Many other modes of infection have been supposed, but, I believe, erroneously, such suppositions most probably having taken their rise from ignorance or deceit, two great sources of error in this disease.

---

* The term *constitutional* is, perhaps, not strictly a proper term, for by constitutional disease strictly I would understand that in which every part of the body is acting in one way, as in fevers of all kinds, either sympathetic or original; but the venereal poison appears to be only diffused through the circulating fluids, and, as it were, to force certain parts of the body to assume the venereal action, which action is perfectly local, and takes place in different parts in regular succession of susceptibilities; there are but few parts therefore acting at the same time; and a person may be constitutionally affected in this way, and yet almost every function may be perfect.

† Added: "At least I know no instance of it."—*Home.*

It is most likely that contamination takes place about the beginning of the local complaints, especially when that is a chancre; for there is in most cases less chance of its happening afterwards, because the patient commonly flies to medicine, which generally becomes a prevention of contamination. For if it could take place through the whole time of the cure, we should have the parts contaminated at different periods, coming into action at different times, each according to its stated time, although in similar parts both in their nature and other circumstances; but as these similar parts do not vary much in the time of coming into action, it is reasonable to suppose that they were contaminated at or near the same time, and therefore that no contamination takes place in the time of the cure, although we may suppose that the power of absorption is equally strong then as at any other time.

In cases of contamination from a gonorrhœa, where no mercury has been taken, we might expect this irregularity in similar structures; but as contamination so seldom takes place in this way, we have not a chance of great variety from such; however, it would be worth while to ascertain the matter, which from a great many cases might be done.

Without being very exact in ascertaining the different proportions in those who have the lues venerea originating from the three several modes above described, I think we may venture to say, from general practice or experience, that where one contracts it from the first cause, that is, where no local effects have been produced, a hundred have it from the second, or gonorrhœa; and where one has it from the second, a hundred have it from the third, or chancre; and perhaps not one in five hundred who have connexion with venereal women have it in the first way, and not one in a hundred have it from the second; while not one in a hundred would escape it from the third, if the means of prevention were not made use of in the common method of cure of the chancre.

§. 1. *Of the Nature of the Sores or Ulcers proceeding from the Lues Venerea.*

In consequence of the blood being contaminated with real venereal pus, it might naturally be supposed that the local effects arising therefrom would be the same with the original which produced them; but from observation and experiment I have reason to believe that this is not so.

In considering this subject, we may first observe that local effects, from the constitution, are all of one species, that is, ulcers, let the surface upon which they appear be what it will, whether the throat or common skin, which is not the case in the local application of the mat-

ter in gonorrhœa and chancre; for there I observed that it produced
effects according to the nature of the surfaces. Now if the matter,
when in the constitution, were to act upon the same specific principles
with that which is applied, we should have gonorrhœas when it attacks
a canal, sores or chancres when it attacks other surfaces: but it has
never been yet known to produce a gonorrhœa from the constitution,
though this has indeed been suspected. For some gonorrhœas, the
origin of which has not been clear, and which have not easily given
way to the common methods of cure, have been supposed to have arisen
from the constitution. Whenever the disease affects the mouth and
nose, it has always been looked upon as producing a true chancre; yet
even here I find that such ulcers in their first appearance are very different from chancres. The true chancre, I observed, produces considerable inflammation, which of course brings on quickly suppuration,
attended often with a great deal of pain; but the local effects, from the
constitution, are slow in their progress, attended with little inflammation, and are seldom or never painful, except in particular parts. However, this sluggishness in the effects of the poison is more or less according to the nature of the parts which become diseased; for when the
tonsils, uvula, or nose are affected, its progress is rapid, and the sores
have more of the chancre in their appearance than when it affects the
skin; yet I do not think that the inflammation is so great in them as
in chancres that are ulcerating equally fast.

It has been supposed that even all the secretions from the contaminated blood could be affected so as to produce a like poison in them;
and as the parts of generation are thrown in the way of receiving it,
when fresh contracted, so they still lie under the censure of having it
returned upon them from the constitution. Hence it has been supposed that the testicles and vesiculæ seminales may be affected by the
disease; that the semen may become venereal, may communicate the
disease to others, and, after impregnation, may even grow into a pocky
child. But all this is without foundation: otherwise, when a person
has the lues venerea, no secreting surface could be free from the state
of a gonorrhœa, nor could any sore be other than venereal. Contrary
to all which, the secretions are the same as before; and if a sore is produced by any other means in a sound part, that sore is not venereal, nor
the matter poisonous, although formed from the same blood.

The saliva in the case of a mad dog, being a natural secretion rendered poisonous, may be brought as an argument in contradiction to
this theory; yet it is easily accounted for, and might be produced rather as an argument in support of it. In the dog there is an irritation
peculiar to the hydrophobia in the salivary glands; but the other and

natural secretions of the same dog are not capable of giving this infection, because they are not susceptible of the same specific irritation.

The breath and sweat are supposed to carry along with them contagion, the milk of the breast is supposed to be capable of containing venereal poison and of affecting the child who sucks it; but there are
several reasons which overturn these opinions.   First, we find that no
secretion is affected by this poison, excepting where the secreting organs have been previously affected by venereal inflammation or irrita-
tation, or its specific mode of action.   Again, if they were contaminated
so as to produce matter similar to that of an ulcer in the throat, such
matter would not be poisonous, nor possess a power of communicating
the disease, as will be explained more fully hereafter.   Further, true
venereal matter, even when taken into the stomach, does not affect either
the stomach or constitution, but is digested : as was evident in the two
following cases.

A gentleman, who had chancres which discharged largely, used to
wash the parts with milk in a teacup with some lint, and generally let
the lint lie in the cup with the milk.   A little boy in the house stole
the milk and drank it, but whether or not he swallowed the lint was
not known.   No notice was taken of this by the gentleman either to
the family or the boy ; and attention, unknown to the family, was paid
to the boy even for years, but nothing happened that could give the
least suspicion of his having been affected either locally in the stomach
or constitutionally.

A gentleman had a most violent gonorrhœa, in which both the inflammation and the discharge were remarkably great.   He had also a
chordee, which was very troublesome at night.   In order to cool the
parts, and keep them clean, he had a small bason of milk by the bedside, in which, when the chordee was troublesome, he got up and dipped
or washed the penis.   This operation he frequently repeated during the
night.   Under such complaints he allowed a young lady to sleep with
him.   Her custom was to have by the bedside a bason of tea to drink
in the morning before she got up ; but unfortunately for the lady, she
drank one morning the milk instead of the tea.   This was not known
till she got up, which was five or six hours afterwards.   I was sent for
directly, and in the mean time she endeavoured to vomit, but could not.
I ordered ipecacuanha, which proved slow in its operation.   She vomited, but it was more than eight hours after drinking the milk and
water, and what came up was nothing but slime, mucus, or water, the
milk being digested.   I was attentive to what might follow; but nothing uncommon happened, at least for many months.

It is also supposed that a fœtus in the womb of a pocky mother may be infected by her. This I should doubt very much, both from what may be observed of the secretions, and from finding that even the matter from such constitutional inflammation is not capable of communicating the disease. However, one can conceive the bare possibility of a child being affected in the womb of a pocky mother, not indeed from the disease of the mother, but from a part of the same matter which contaminated the mother, and was absorbed by her; and whether irritating her solids to action or not, may possibly be conveyed to the child, pure as absorbed; and if so it may affect the child exactly in the same way it did or might have done the mother. This idea has been carried still further; for it has been supposed that such a contaminated child could contaminate the breasts of a clean woman by sucking her; the possibility of which will be considered presently. We may observe that even the blood of a pocky person has no power of contaminating, and is not capable of giving the disease to another even by inoculation; for if it were capable of irritating a sound sore to a venereal inflammation, no person that has this matter circulating, or has the lues venerea, could escape having a venereal sore whenever he is bled or receives a scratch with a pin, the part so wounded turning into a chancre. For if venereal matter be on the point of the lancet, or on the point of the pin, the punctures must become chancres.

§ 2. Of the Matter from Sores in the Lues Venerea compared with that from Chancres and Buboes.

When the matter has affected the constitution, it from thence produces many local effects on different parts of the body, which are in general a kind of inflammation, or at least an increased action occasioning a suppuration of its own kind. It is supposed that the matter produced in consequence of these inflammations, similar to the matter from a gonorrhœa or chancre, is also venereal and poisonous. This I believe till now has never been denied: and, upon the first view of the subject, one would be inclined to suppose that it really should be venereal; for, first, the venereal matter is the cause; and again the same treatment cures both diseases; thus mercury cures both a chancre and a lues venerea; however, this is no decisive proof, as mercury cures many diseases besides the venereal. On the other hand, there are many strong reasons for believing that the matter is not venereal. There is one curious fact which shows it is either not venereal, or if it be, that it is not capable of acting in some respects on the same body or same state of constitution as that matter does which is produced from a

chancre or gonorrhœa. The pus from these latter, when absorbed, generally produces a bubo, as has been described; but we never find a
bubo from the absorption of matter from a pocky sore. For instance,
when there is a venereal ulcer in the throat, we have no buboes in the
glands of the neck; when there are venereal sores on the arms, or even
suppurating nodes on the ulna, there are no swellings of the glands of
the armpit; although such will take place if fresh venereal matter is
applied to a common sore on the arm, hand, or fingers. No swelling
takes place in the glands of the groin from either nodes or blotches on
the legs and thighs. It may be supposed that there is no absorption
from such sores; but I think we have no grounds for such supposition.
Its mode of irritation, or the action of the parts affected, is very different from what happens in the chancre, gonorrhœa, or bubo, being hardly
attended with inflammation, which in them is generally violent.

It might be supposed that a constitution truly and universally pocky
is not to be affected locally by the same species of matter; but from the
following experiments it would appear that matter from a gonorrhœa
or chancre is capable of affecting a man locally that is already poxed;
and that matter from pocky sores, arising from the constitution, has not
that power.

A man had been affected with the venereal disease a long time, and
had been several times salivated, but the disease still broke out anew.
He was taken into St. George's Hospital, affected with a number of
pocky sores; and before I put him under a mercurial course I made
the following experiment. I took some matter from one of the sores
upon the point of a lancet, and made three small wounds upon the back,
where the skin was smooth and sound, deep enough to draw blood. I
made a wound similar to the other three with a clean lancet, the four
wounds making a quadrangle; but all the wounds healed up, and none
of them ever appeared afterwards.

This experiment I have repeated more than once, and with the same
result. It shows that a pocky person cannot be affected locally with
the matter proceeding from the sores produced by the lues venerea.
But to see how far real venereal matter was capable of producing
chancres on a pocky person, I made the following experiment.

A man, who had venereal blotches on many parts of his skin, was
inoculated in sound parts with matter from a chancre, and also with
matter from his own sores. The wounds inoculated with the matter
from the chancres became chancres; but the others healed up. Here
then was a venereal constitution capable of being affected locally with
fresh venereal matter. This experiment I have likewise repeated more
than once, and always with the same effect.

OF THE LUES VENEREA.

I ordered a person, at St. George's Hospital, to be inoculated with the matter taken from a well-marked venereal ulcer on the tonsil, and also with matter from a gonorrhœa, which produced the same effects as in the preceding experiment; that is, the matter from a gonorrhœa produced a chancre, but that from the tonsil had no effect.

A woman, aged twenty-five, came into St. George's Hospital, August 21, 1782, with sores on her legs, and blotches over her body. Her husband gave her the venereal disease December 1781. Her symptoms then were a discharge from the vagina, and a small swelling of the glands of the groin, which were painful. She had taken some pills supposed to be mercurial. February 1782, about three months after being infected, the discharge stopped; but the swelling, which had been gradually increasing ever since its first appearance, had now suppurated. She applied some ointment to it, which was brought to her by her husband, and in two months it got well, that is, in April 1782. After the bubo got well a discharge from the vagina came on, for which she took more of the same pills she had taken before. After this time blotches came out over her whole body; some about her legs, under her arms, and upon her nipples, ulcerated.

Twins, which she brought forth at eight months, in March 1782, at the time the bubo was healing, had blotches upon them at their birth, and died soon after.

Another girl, about two years old, whom she suckled, was also covered with blotches when she came to the hospital.

To ascertain whether her secondary ulcers were infectious, that is, whether the matter of them would have the specific effects of venereal matter, she was inoculated with some matter from one of her own ulcers, and with some matter from a bubo of another person where mercury had not been used. This was done September 18, 1782. September 19, the puncture where she was inoculated with her own matter gave her pain three hours from the time of inoculation, and the day following inflamed a little. The other had not then inflamed at all.

September 20, both the punctures had suppurated, and had the appearance of a smallpox pustule; they spread considerably, and were attended with much inflammation. That from her own matter healed with common poultices, and ointments without mercury; but the other, although treated in a similar way, continued in the same state, attended with much pain and inflammation.

September 22, the child was inoculated with some matter from one of its own ulcers, and with some common pus. The punctures both inflamed in a small degree, but neither of them suppurated.

The mother and the child went into the ward appropriated to salivation October 21, 1782. The child took no mercury. It was supposed that its gums became a little sore ; and the blotches got well.

During the time that the mother was using mercury the ulcer from inoculation began to get well, and all her venereal symptoms disappeared. What shall we say to this case ? Were the blotches venereal ? There was every leading circumstance to make us think so, and our opinion was strengthened by the method of cure. If they were venereal, my opinion, that the constitutional appearances of the disease do not produce matter of the same species that produced them, is confirmed. If they were not venereal, then we have no absolute rule by which to judge in such cases.

It has been supposed, and asserted from observation, that ulcers in the mouths of children from a constitutional disease, which constitutional disease has been supposed to be derived from the parent, have produced the same disease upon the nipples of women who had been sucked by them ; that is, the children were contaminated either by their mothers or fathers having the disease in form of a lues venerea, of which I have endeavoured to show the impossibility. If, however, it were possible to contaminate once in this way, it would be possible to contaminate for ever[a].

How far the observations, upon which the before-mentioned opinion is founded, have been made with sufficient accuracy to overturn those which I made with a view to ascertain the truth, I know not. But, from a more accurate investigation of some of those cases, which were by most of the faculty called venereal, they appeared evidently not to be such. To say what they were would lead us into the consideration of other diseases. The following case may lessen our faith in the histories of such as have been supposed to be venereal.

Before I describe the case, I shall first mention some of the circumstances leading to it.

A child was supposed to have infected its nurse with the venereal disease. The parents had been married about twelve years when this child was born. The father was a very fond husband, and the mother a mild and most affectionate woman. The father had a venereal gonorrhœa two years before he married, that is, fourteen years before the birth of the child. About nine months after marriage they had a child, and afterwards a second, both of whom were extremely healthy at birth, and still continue so. The mother fell into a weakly state of health, and miscarried of her third child at the end of five months. The fourth child was born at seven months, but was puny, weak, and had hardly

---

[a] [See observations on this subject in notes to Part VII.]

any cuticle when born. It was immediately after birth attacked with
a violent dysentery. It died in a few days, and was opened by me. The
whole skin was almost one excoriated surface. The intestines were
much inflamed and thickened.

With her fifth child, from great care, she went eight months, and it
was now hoped that she might go the full time, and also that this child
might be more healthy than the former. When she was delivered the
child was very thin, but free from any visible disease.

Some days after birth it became blistered in a vast number of places
on its body, which blisters were filled with a kind of matter, and, when
they broke, discharged a thinnish pus. The inside of the mouth was in
the same condition. Bark was given to the nurse. Bark, in milk, was
given to the child by the mouth, and it was fomented with a decoction
of bark, but in about three weeks after birth it died.

Some weeks after the death of the child the nurse's nipple, and the
ring round the nipple, inflamed, and sores or ulcers were formed with a
circumscribed base*. They were poulticed, but without benefit. She
also complained of a sore throat, but the sensation she complained of
was so low in the throat that no disease could be seen. A swelling
took place in the glands of the armpit, but they did not suppurate. She
applied to a physician, and according to the account which she gave, he
pronounced that her disease was venereal, and that she had given suck
to a *foul* child; and he ordered ten boxes of mercurial ointment to be
rubbed in on her legs and thighs, eight of which had been used when I
saw her, and then her mouth was become extremely sore.

These circumstances came to the ears of the family, and an alarm took
place. The husband went from surgeon to surgeon, and from physician
to physician, to learn if it was possible for him to have the disease for
fourteen years, and never to have perceived a single symptom of it in all
that time; or if it was possible he could get children with the disease
now, when the two first were healthy. He also wanted to know if it
was possible for his wife to have caught the disease from him under such
circumstances, and also, if she could breed children with this disease,
although she herself never had a single symptom of it. If we take all
the above-mentioned circumstances as facts, the conclusion is, that it
was impossible there could be anything venereal in the case; but as they
could not be absolutely proved to be facts, there must remain a doubt
in the mind, a something still to be proved.

Now let us consider the result of the case. The nurse's mouth was
become extremely sore from the mercury when I first saw her. I de-

* She had but one breast that gave milk.

sired that Mr. Pott might see her along with me; and it was the opinion
of us both that the sores on the nipple and around it were not venereal;
but it was alleged, that as she had taken mercury, their not having a
venereal appearance now was owing to that cause. The bark was given,
as also the sarsaparilla, but the sores did not heal, nor did they become
worse; nor was the mouth better by leaving off the mercury. I ordered
the hemlock, but that appeared to have no effect. In the mean time
eruptions broke out on the skin. The skin of the hands and fingers
peeled off; the nails of both fingers and toes separated, and sores formed
about their roots, which were all supposed (by many) to be venereal.
But some of them appearing while the constitution was full of mercury,
and others disappearing without any further use of that medicine, I
judged that they were not venereal. We suspected that her mode of
living was such as contributed greatly to the continuance of her first
complaint, and gave rise to the new ones; for she looked dejected and
sallow. She was desired to go into an hospital, which she did. As
soon as she got into a warm bed, and had good wholesome food, she
began to mend, and in about five or six weeks she had become fat and
almost well; the sore only about the root of the nail of the great toe
had not healed; but that appeared now to be owing to the root of the
nail being detached, therefore acting as an extraneous body. She came
out of the hospital before this toe had got well, and, returning to her
old poor mode of living, she had a return of the soreness in the mouth;
however, she mended at last without the use of more mercury.

This case I shall further consider when on diseases resembling the
venereal.

The following case will further prove that we often suspect complaints to be venereal when they really are not.

A gentleman had for some time blotches on his skin. The face, arms,
legs, and thighs were in many places covered with them, and they were
in their different stages of violence. In this situation he applied to me,
and I must own they had a very suspicious appearance. I asked him
what he supposed these blotches were; he said he supposed them to be
venereal. I asked him when he had a recent venereal complaint; he
told me not for above twelve months. I then asked him how long he
had had the blotches; and the answer was, above six months. As this
was a sufficient time for making observations upon them that might ascertain better than the mere appearance what they were, I asked him if
any of the blotches that came first had disappeared in that time, and he
said many; I desired to see where those had been, and on examination
I found only a discoloured skin, common to the healing of superficial
sores. I then declared to him that they were not venereal, for if they

had arisen from that source none of them would have disappeared. He now informed me that he had been taking mercury; and this information obliged me to have recourse to further inquiries; and I therefore asked him whether, while he was taking mercury, many of the first got well? The answer was, yes. And was the cure of those imputed to mercury? The answer was again in the affirmative. I then asked him if, while he was taking the mercury, which appeared to have cured some, those that now remained arose? Yes. My next question was, how long had he taken mercury? He said for six months. I then declared they were not, nor ever had been venereal. I asked him, what was now the opinion of his surgeon? He said, that his opinion still was that they were venereal, and that he should go on with the mercury. I advised him to take no medicines whatever; to live well, avoiding excess, and to come to me in three weeks; which he did, and then he was perfectly well, only the skin was stained where the blotches had been. He now asked me what he was next to do? I told him he might go to the sea and bathe for a month. This he did, and returned well and healthy, and has continued so*.

§. 3. *Of the local Effects arising from the Constitution considered as critical.—Symptomatic Fever.*

How far the eruptions or local effects of this disease, arising from the constitution, are an effort of Nature to clear herself of this disease is not certain. I observed that a gonorrhœa might be produced by a general law in the animal œconomy, by which it endeavours to relieve itself of the irritation by producing a discharge; and that in chancres a breach is made in the solids for the same purpose, although this purpose is not answered in either; Nature not having a provision against this poison. But how far a similar attempt takes place in a lues venerea I do not know; and if it was upon the same principle, the same reason might be expected to be given why the constitution is not capable of relieving itself in the present instance that I gave when treating of the primary affections, because in this, as it was in the other, the matter formed might be supposed to be venereal; and therefore by being absorbed by the very surface which produced it as in a chancre, it might

* Added: "The impropriety of giving mercury where the case is not venereal, to indulge the wishes of the patient, is obvious, since it is confirming his suspicions, injuring his constitution, and, when the medicine fails, making him believe himself incurable, since the symptoms have not yielded to the only medicine capable in his opinion of removing them."—*Home.*

keep up the constitutional disease. If this were really the case, it would
be very different from many other specific diseases ; for the reason why
many specific diseases cure themselves is that the irritation cannot last
beyond a stated time ; and also that in many the patient is never susceptible of the same disease a second time, as in the smallpox. If this
was not the case, a person once having the smallpox would always have
them ; for according to one supposition, that absorption of its own pus
keeps up the disease ; and according to another, that the irritation never
wears itself out, the patient would either never be free, or have them
repeated for ever ; for his own matter would give the disease a second
time, a third time, and so on*.   But the venereal matter, when taken
into the constitution, produces an irritation which is capable of being
continued independent of a continuance of absorption ; and the constitution has no power of relief, therefore a lues venerea continues to increase.   This circumstance is perhaps one of the best distinguishing
marks of the lues venerea, for in its ulcers and blotches it is often imitated by other diseases, which not having this property will therefore
heal and break out again in some other part.   Diseases in which this
happens show themselves not to be venereal.   However, we are not to
conclude, because they do not heal of themselves and give way only to
mercury, that therefore they are not venereal, although this circumstance joined to others gives a strong suspicion of their being such.

When the parts are contaminated by the venereal poison, we commonly find fever, restlessness, or want of sleep, and often headache ; but
I believe that these symptoms are rather peculiar to the disease, when
the second order of parts, the periosteum and bones, are affected, although
they are sometimes found from the first.   Do these symptoms arise from
the local irritations affecting the constitution ?   And are they merely
sympathetic ?   Whatever the immediate cause may be, they never go
off till the local irritations are removed.   This fever at first has much
the appearance of the rheumatic fever ; and after a time it partakes a
good deal of the nature of the hectic.

These symptoms often take place independent of, or unattended by,
any local action ; and when that is the case it becomes very uncertain
what the disease is ; for in cases not admitting of clear proof we must
rest on the concurrence of circumstances.   Many of these symptoms
give way to mercury.   This is probably the only concurring circum-

---

* This circumstance alone is a strong proof that people cannot have the smallpox
twice, at least at any distance of time between, if they had fair eruptions the first time ;
for if the constitution was not so altered as not to be susceptible of this irritation a second time, a person would have them immediately upon the going off of the first.

stance attending this complaint that is any proof of its being venereal*. It rather, however, appears to militate against this idea that, for the most part, a much smaller quantity is sufficient for the cure of such symptoms than what is necessary for the cure of local complaints. But if mercury always cured them, it would not be very material what they are called. It is worthy of consideration, however, how far the venereal poison, when in the constitution, does or does not always produce local effects. That it in general does we are certain ; but whether it is ever a cause of constitutional symptoms simply, such as loss of appetite, wasting, debility, want of sleep, and fever, at last becoming hectic, is uncertain ; and it is also uncertain whether it is ever capable of producing local actions from irritations only, without an alteration of the structure of the parts irritated, as cough, secretion from the lungs, purging, headache, sickness, pains in different parts of the body, like rheumatic pains, but not from an alteration of the structure of the part taking place, as beginning nodes. If such effects take place, we must in such a case rely entirely on the history of the disease, and pronounce according to probability. Such complaints come oftener under the management of the physician than the surgeon, to whom I would recommend a particular attention to this.

The fever in consequence of the venereal irritation, like most other fevers, deranges the constitution, which thereupon suffers agreeably to its natural tendency. It is capable of producing glandular swellings in many parts of the body, and probably many of the nodes that arise in the time of this fever may proceed from the fever ; and similar to every such effect, from whatever cause, it does not partake of the disease which produced it, for it is not venereal : it only takes place in constitutions very susceptible of such action where the predisposing cause is strong, and probably at seasons most fitted to produce it, only waiting the immediate cause to put them into action. Such will and do go away of themselves when the predisposing cause ceases, such as season.

§. 4. *Of the local and constitutional forms of the Disease never interfering with one another.*

I observed, when treating of the gonorrhœa and chancre, that, when occurring in the same person, the one neither increases the symptoms nor retards the cure of the other. And it may also be observed that the chancre or gonorrhœa, and the constitutional form of the disease,

* Here it is to be understood that the circumstance of a previous gonorrhœa or chancre is not to be considered as strong evidence.

meeting in the same person, do not interfere with each other, either in their symptoms or cure.

To explain these effects more fully, let me observe, that if a man has a gonorrhœa, and a chancre appears some days after, the chancre does not either increase or diminish the gonorrhœa. Again, if a man has either a gonorrhœa, a chancre, or both, and a lues venerea ensue in consequence of either of these, neither the gonorrhœa nor chancre is affected by it. If a man has a lues venerea and gets either a gonorrhœa or chancre, or both, neither of them affects the lues venerea, nor are their symptoms the worse. Nor is the cure of either, singly, retarded by the presence of the other; for a gonorrhœa is as easily cured when there are chancres as when there are none, even although the chancres are not attempted to be cured; and a chancre may be cured locally independent of the gonorrhœa. Further, a gonorrhœa, chancre, or both, may be as easily cured when the constitution is poxed either by them, or previous to their appearance, as when the person is in perfect health; but the chancre has this advantage, that the constitution cannot be cured without its being likewise cured.

The gonorrhœa and chancre indeed so far influence one another as the one can be in some degree a cause of prevention of the other, as has been already observed; but I believe that this circumstance does not assist in the cure of either: yet I could conceive it might, each acting as a derivator to the other, without increasing its own specific mode of action.

§. 5. *Of the supposed Termination of the Lues Venerea in other Diseases.*

This disease seldom or never interferes with other disorders, or runs into, or terminates in any other, although it has been very much accused of doing so; for a termination of one disease in another, as I understand the expression, must always be a cure of the one terminated; but the venereal disease never terminates till the proper remedy is applied, and therefore never can run into any other disease.

That venereal complaints may be the cause of others I think is very probable. I have seen a chancre the immediate cause of an erysipelatous inflammation, but the venereal malady did not terminate in the erysipelatous inflammation; for if it had, the chancre would have been cured: nor was the erysipelatous inflammation venereal; the chancre only acted here as a common irritator, independently of the specific quality of the disease as a cause. I have known a venereal bubo become a scrofulous sore as soon as the venereal poison was destroyed by mercury : this was not a venereal terminating in a scrofulous affection, for in such a view the scrofula must have cured the venereal. The venereal disease would seem only to partake of the nature of such disorders as the constitution was previously disposed to, and may excite into action the causes of these disorders. The same observation and mode of reasoning holds equally good with respect to other diseases. The common symptoms, however, of the lues venerea, though in some degree according to the constitution, are not so much so as either in the chancre or the gonorrhœa; for the lues venerea is attended with very little inflammation, which in general partakes much more of the nature of the constitution than any other diseased action.

§. 6. *Of the specific Distance of the Venereal Inflammation.*

I have already observed that many specific diseases, as also those arising from poison, have their local effects confined to certain distances, which I have called their local specific distance ; and it would appear, from observation, that the venereal irritation and inflammation, of whatever kind it may be, is guided by this principle ; for it seldom extends far beyond the surface that receives it; the neighbouring part not having a tendency to sympathize or run easily into this kind of inflammation. This is the reason why we find a gonorrhœa for weeks confined to one spot in the urethra in men, and for months to the vagina in women, not extending further in either. In chancres also the inflammation is confined to the seat of the sore without becoming so diffused as when from common accidents. As a further proof of this fact, we find it is also confined to the glands of the groin, in cases of buboes, till matter is formed in them ; which matter acts as a common irritator, and the specific is in some degree lost, and then the inflammation becomes somewhat more diffused, as happens in common inflammation. We also see that the same thing happens in venereal ulcers when they arise from the constitution : their size is at first but small, and they are merely local; but as the disease increases the size increases, but still they remain circumscribed, not becoming diffused. Perhaps all poisons and specific diseases agree in this property of having their inflammation limited and circumscribed in a manner peculiar to themselves ; for we find that the inflammation of the smallpox, measles, and chickenpox is each circumscribed in its own way. From hence it must appear that the human body in general is not so susceptible of specific irritations as it is of the common, or what may be called the natural. But we must also consider that the common inflammation in very healthy constitutions has its specific distance, although not so determined or circumscribed as is that of the specific in such constitutions; therefore we may reasonably suppose that such healthy constitutions are the furthest in disposition from the inflammatory action; and we may also suppose still more so from the specific. What would appear to strengthen this idea is, that when the constitution is such as readily goes into inflammation, the more readily does the inflammation spread, every part being susceptible of such action; and we find that in many the specific also spreads, although not in so great a degree, from which we may suppose that the specific is always a more confined mode of action. I have suspected that when the body was disposed to increase the inflammation beyond the specific distance, it was of the erysipelatous kind, as was mentioned before, and which is to be attended to in the cure.

§. 7. *Of the Parts most susceptible of the Lues Venerea—of the time and manner in which they are affected.—What is meant by Contamination, Disposition, and Action.—Summary of the Doctrine.*

When I assigned the causes for so great a difference in the effects of the same poison upon two different surfaces, as forming the gonorrhœa and chancre, I then said I did not know whether similar surfaces in every part of the body were equally susceptible of this irritation, having but few comparative trials of the direct application of the poison to other parts besides those of generation. But it would appear that some parts of the body are much less susceptible of the lues venerea than others; and not only so, but many parts, so far as we know, are not susceptible of it at all. For we have not yet had every part of the body affected: we have not seen the brain affected, the heart, stomach, liver, kidneys, nor other viscera, although such cases are described in authors. But as there are different orders of parts respecting the times of the disease appearing, and as the person commonly flies to relief upon the first or second appearances, it may be supposed that the whole disease in the parts actually affected is cured before the other parts have had time to come into action, which will therefore be cured under the state of a disposition only, if we can conceive that a cure can take place before the parts have come into action. But if the parts visibly affected are cured, while those only disposed are not, and afterwards come into action, they would form a second order respecting time; and if these again are cured, and other parts under a disposition should come into action, such would form a third order of parts respecting time. The lungs have been believed to have been affected with the venereal disease, both from the circumstances preceding the complaint, and from the complaint itself being cured by mercury; and their being affected, when the other viscera are not, may arise from their being in some degree an external surface, as will be explained hereafter.

It is this form of the disease therefore that gives us the comparative susceptibility of parts both for disposition and action. For we must suppose that all parts are equally and at once exposed to the action of the poison; but though there may be various degrees of susceptibility, it will be sufficient for practice to divide them into two, under the following appellations of *first in order*, and *second in order*, to which we may add the intermediate.

Whether the parts that are really first affected are naturally more easily affected by this kind of irritation, or that some other circumstance which belongs to these parts is the cause, cannot be absolutely determined; but, the matter being attentively considered, it would appear to be owing to something foreign to the constitution, and also not depending on the nature of the parts themselves; for if we take a view of all the parts that are first affected by this disease, when arising from the constitution, which I shall suppose are the parts most susceptible of it, we shall see that in the recent state of the disease these parts are subject to one general affection, while there are similar parts of the body not affected by this disease, and not subject to this general affection. Probably the parts second in order may naturally be as susceptible of the irritation as those first in order; but not being under the influence of an irritating cause, they are later in coming into action; and there are also probably other causes in the nature of the parts themselves, such as being indolent in all their actions, and of course indolent in this, therefore later in coming into action. However, it is not universally the case that the parts which I have called first in order are always so; on the contrary, we find that this order is inverted in some cases, although but rarely. We cannot suppose that this difference arises from any active power in the poison, nor any particular direction of it, but from properties in the parts themselves; for it may be allowed us to suppose that when this matter has got into the circulation it acts on all parts of the body with equal force; that is, it is not determined to any one part more than another by any general or particular power in the animal machine; nor is the nature of the poison such as will fall more readily on one part of the body than another, when they are all in similar circumstances. That some parts therefore are more readily affected by it than others, owing to circumstances which are no part of the animal principle nor of the poison; and also that some parts of the body have a greater tendency to be irritated by it than others, must be allowed.

The parts that are affected by this form of the disease when in its early stage or appearance, which I have called first in order, are the skin, tonsils, nose, throat, inside of the mouth, and sometimes the tongue *. When in its later state, the periosteum, fasciæ, and bones come into action, and these I call *second in order of parts.* Perhaps the bones come into action from the membrane being affected.

That we may be able to account in some measure for these similar effects as to time in dissimilar parts, such as the skin and the tonsils, two very different kinds of parts, let us consider in what circumstance they agree, and why they are more susceptible of this irritation than those parts that probably are naturally as much so, although they do not receive it so readily, such as the periosteum, fasciæ, and bones.

The most remarkable circumstance perhaps to which the external surface is exposed, and to which the internal is not, is cold, or a succession of different degrees of cold. For we may observe in general that the atmosphere in which we live is colder than the human body† in its usual temperature, therefore the skin, &c. is continually exposed to a cold greater than what the internal parts are ; and we find that all those parts which are most exposed to this admit of being much more easily affected, or come more readily into action in this disease than the others.

It is certain that cold has very powerful effects on the animal œconomy. It would at least appear to have great powers of disposing the body for receiving the venereal irritation, and going readily on with it.

From this idea we may account for several circumstances respecting this disease, as the mouth, nose, and skin being the most frequently affected, since they are rendered most susceptible of it from the causes before mentioned, and for the same reason come very readily into action. If this be a true solution, it also accounts for those second in order being affected; for if the poison has contaminated parts which are both first in order of susceptibility and time of coming into action, it is natural to suppose that those parts which are most predisposed, as the external surfaces, shall come first into action; the parts exposed to cold, in the

---

* The tongue is very subject to have ulcers formed on it, especially on its edges. They are seldom very large, nor are they often either very foul or have a hard basis: these are commonly supposed to be venereal; but I believe they seldom are. I do not know whether I am or not acquainted with the distinguishing marks. I never saw but one that I suspected to be either venereal or cancerous from its foul look and its hard basis. It gave way readily to mercury, therefore I supposed it to be venereal.

† It is to be understood that this cannot hold good as an universal principle : it can only take place in the temperate and frigid zone ; for in the torrid the heat of the surrounding atmosphere is sometimes greater than that of the human body.

next degree, forming the second in order, come next into action, such as bones, periosteum, &c.; but even in them it is not in every bone alike, or every part alike of any one bone, for it appears first in those that are in some measure within the power of being affected by sympathy from application of cold to the skin : we find that when the deeper-seated parts, or the parts second in order, come into action, such as the periosteum or bones, it is first in these that are nearest the external surface of the body, such as the periosteum or bones of the head, the tibia, ulna, bones of the nose, &c., nor does it affect these bones on all sides equally, but first on that side next the external surface. However, it would appear that in the bones there is another cause, besides the vicissitudes of weather, why this disease should attack them ; for the periosteum of bones, or bones themselves, are not liable to be diseased on all parts in proportion to the distance from the skin, the periosteum which covers the ankles, or many of the joints, being as near the external surface as many other parts of the periosteum or bones that are affected. The nature of the bones themselves, which are covered by that periosteum, is somewhat different : they are softer in their texture, therefore they would seem to be affected in proportion to their nearness to the skin and hardness of the bones jointly; which would incline us to believe that the bones are more easily affected, and rather have some influence upon the periosteum in this disease than the periosteum upon them ; and this susceptibility in the hard bones would appear to be in proportion to their quantity of earth and exposure to cold combined.

It may be objected to this theory, that the fore part of the tibia, &c., cannot be really colder than the back part; but then it may be supposed that it is not necessary that the part should be actually cold, but only within the power of sympathy. For a part that is not actually cold is capable of being affected from its sympathizing with a cold part in the same manner as if actually cold, although perhaps not in so great a degree, and therefore requires a longer time to come into action than if it were actually cold. We find, for example, that when the skin is actually cold the muscles underneath are thrown into alternate action, so that we tremble, or our teeth chatter with cold, and yet it is possible that these muscles may not be colder at this time than any other; although it is most probable that they are really colder*, which will assist the power of sympathy. So far as cold can affect the actions of parts, so far also will the sympathizing part be affected in proportion as it is nearer to the parts actually cold; therefore the deeper-seated parts in the venereal disease are later in coming into action.

* See Philosophical Transactions, vol. 68, part i. page 7.

The actual cold parts come first into action, then those that are less so, and next those that are nearest in sympathy, and so on, except the parts first in order of susceptibility have been only partially cured, and then their recurrence may correspond with the action of those that are second in order of susceptibility, and all the parts will come into action together. What would seem to strengthen this opinion is the different effects that arise from different climates; in warm climates the disease seldom or never arises to such a height as in cold climates; it is more slow in its progress, and much more easy to cure, at least if we may give credit to the accounts we have received of the disease in such climates.

Whether the difference in the time of appearance between the superficial and deeper-seated parts in warm climates is the same as in cold ones, I do not know, but from the above theory it should not be so great in the warm as in the cold climates.

Besides the causes already mentioned, it would appear that there are others by which the lues venerea may be brought sooner into action than it otherwise would be if left entirely to the nature of the constitution; for I think I have seen cases where fever has brought it into action when the disposition had been previously formed. Like most other diseases to which there is a susceptibility or disposition, we find that any disturbance in the constitution shall call it forth: scrofula, gout, and rheumatism are often called forth in this way.

Having said that the deeper-seated parts of the body come into action later than those that are superficial, I shall now observe, that when the lues venerea has been cured so far as only to remove the first actions, but not to eradicate the disposition in the deeper-seated parts, as has been explained, under such circumstances of the disease it never attacks again the external, or the parts that were first affected, but only the deeper-seated parts which are second in order of time. The reason is, that the deeper-seated parts had not been affected at the time of the cure of the first. The following cases, selected from a great number of similar ones, will illustrate the doctrines we have laid down.

In January, 1781, A. B. had connexion with a woman, and two days after perceived an itching in the glans: at the end of four days he found chancres upon the prepuce. He took about twenty grains of calomel, and then applied to a surgeon, under whose care he remained three months, that is, till April. He thought himself nearly well, and went into the country, taking a few pills with him, and at the end of another month believed himself perfectly cured. Three months after, that is, in August, he caught cold, and had considerable fever, for which James's powders were given. Soon after this, spots of a copper colour appeared upon his legs, and he had violent pains in his shin bones. By the order of a country surgeon, he rubbed in about an ounce of mercurial ointment, and had a slight spitting; the pain ceased, the spots disappeared, and in a month he again conceived himself to be well. This was in October 1781. In June, 1782, he had the influenza; about a fortnight afterwards his left eye inflamed, and he had a pain in the head, and a noise in his ears. Five days afterwards his throat became sore. Three weeks after the inflammation of his eye several pustules made their appearance near the anus. These symptoms remained till the 21st of August, when he came into St. George's Hospital. He rubbed in strong mercurial ointment till his mouth became sore; he sweated very much; the pain in his head remained, but the complaint in his eye, and about the anus, together with the sore throat, were totally removed.

It appears that in this case some additional power was required to dispose the body more readily to exhibit venereal symptoms. That cold has a strong power of this kind we have allowed, which appears in this case to have been the first immediate cause; but a fever seems to have been equally effectual in producing the second return of the symptoms.

Here was the venereal disposition in the constitution from April, 1781, the time he was cured of the local complaint, till June 1782, fourteen months after; and then it reappeared eleven months after that, which periods might have been longer, if it had not been called forth by the two circumstances of cold and fever.

Let us consider how far this case corresponds with the opinion of the action being easier of cure than the disposition. The first action, that is, the chancres, were perfectly cured by the quantity of mercury he took at first, for they never recurred; but the venereal matter had produced the disposition in the constitution, which was not cured by the same quantity of mercury, for blotches appeared three months after; but all the parts that had taken on the disposition at that time had not then come into action, therefore only the parts which had come into action were cured by the second course of mercury, and the other parts which had not yet taken on the action went on with the disposition till the influenza (which happened eleven months after,) brought them into action. The first class of pocky appearances were perfectly cured by the second course of mercury, as the local had been cured by the first, for they never reappeared, not even with the second. The second set of pocky symptoms, we have observed, appeared to be perfectly cured by the third course of mercury. How far there may be a third set of pocky symptoms to come forth time can only tell.

This case further proves, that sometimes the second set of symptoms appear first, and the first second; and also shows the difference in times between the first pocky appearances after the healing of the local, and between the second appearance of the symptoms after the healing of the first.

A gentleman had a chancre in May 1781; in the same month of the next year, 1782, he had a gonorrhœa; and in May, 1783, he had a sore throat. He had no connexion with any woman from September, 1782, till May, 1783, which was about a fortnight before his throat became sore, and had had no immediate local complaints.

When I saw the throat first I said it was not venereal; and he being rather of a hectic habit, was desired to go to Bristol. When at Bristol an ulcer appeared at the root of the uvula, which made him immediately come back to London. When I saw this ulcer I said it was venereal. He now went through what I supposed was a sufficient course of mercury, and all the venereal symptoms appeared to be cured*. He went into the country about the month of August, and about the beginning of January, 1784, viz. four months after the supposed cure, he felt a pain, together with a swelling, in his shin bones, for which he went through a course of mercury, which removed both the pain and the swelling.

In this case we have every reason to suppose that the disposition had taken place in the bones or their coverings, from the same cause that affected the uvula; but the uvula suffered first, being of the first order of parts. Whether this was really the case or not, we must allow that in the parts second in order, the disposition, and not the action, did exist at the time when the disease in the uvula came into action, as also at the time when he went through a course of mercury sufficient to cure the uvula; we must also allow that the disposition was not removed by the quantity of mercury which was capable of removing the disease in the uvula. From all which I would draw the following inferences in confirmation of the preceding doctrine : first, that the parts about the throat are capable of assuming the action sooner than the bones; secondly, it is probable that mercury can cure the action only, and not the disposition; and thirdly, that the venereal pus is not present in the circulation while the secondary actions take place; for if it were, the parts first in order would stand an equal chance of being again contaminated, and of coming into action a second time. Supposing the venereal matter still to exist in the constitution after the parts first thrown into action are absolutely cured, so as to contaminate the parts that are second in order of action, we should certainly have the parts first in order take on

---

* I may remark here, that only the venereal ulcer got well by the mercury; for the former excoriation of the throat continued, but was afterwards cured by bark and sarsaparilla.

the disease a second and even a third time, and so on, while the second or third in order would be going on and only coming into their first action; and therefore we might have those that are first in order, and those that are second in order, in action at the same time. This might be carried still further, for as it is possible for the parts first in order of susceptibility to have the disease a second time, while the parts second in order are under the influence of the first infection, those first in order may be contaminated a second time from a new or fresh infection, which would be a lues venerea upon a lues venerea, a case which certainly may happen. If the matter does really continue in the constitution, it would be natural to suppose that the parts most easily affected by it would remain so long as the poison remained. It may indeed be alleged, that parts which have already been accustomed to this irritation, and cured, are rendered by that means less susceptible of it.

If the poison were still capable of circulating after its visible effects were cured, then mercury given in the time of a chancre can be of little service, as it can only assist in the cure of the chancre, but cannot preserve the constitution from infection, which does not agree with experience; for practice informs us, that not one in fifty would escape the lues venerea if the chancre were only cured locally; so that mercury has the power of preventing a disposition from forming, and therefore is necessary to be given while we suppose absorption going on, or while there is matter that may be absorbed.

Mercury, prior to the action, will not remove the disposition, and of course will not hinder the action coming on afterwards; however, it is possible, and most probable, that the medicine while it is present will hinder the action taking place; so that no venereal complaints will take place under the course of mercury, although the parts may be contaminated.

This is not peculiar to the venereal disease, but common to many others; and in some it may be reversed, for there are diseases whose disposition can be cured, and therefore the action prevented by such medicines as would rather increase the action if given in the time of it.

The parts first affected are more easily cured, according to our present method, than the parts second in order. A part once perfectly cured is never irritated again by the same stock of infection, though probably some other parts in the constitution are still under the venereal irritation. If the facts stated be just, the circumstance of the disease appearing to leave the parts first attacked, and attacking the secondary parts, is easily accounted for. It is no more than the first parts being cured while the secondary are not, and of course going on with the disease, the first remaining well.

If this mode of accounting for these circumstances be just, it proves two things; first, a former assertion, that this disease, in the form of lues venerea, has not the power of contaminating parts not already under its influence, even in the same constitution; secondly, that the venereal poison is not circulating in the blood all the time the disease is going on in the constitution; so that most probably the poison only irritates when just absorbed, and is soon expelled or thrown out in some of the secretions.

The above account of the lues venerea may be reduced to the following heads:

First, that most parts, if not all, that are affected in the lues venerea, are affected with the venereal irritation at the same time.

Secondly, the parts exposed to cold are the first that admit the venereal action; then the deeper-seated parts, according to their susceptibility for such action.

Thirdly, the venereal disposition, when once formed in a part, must necessarily go on to form the venereal action.

Fourthly, that all parts of the body, under such disposition, do not run into action equally fast, some requiring six or eight weeks, others as many months.

Fifthly, in the parts, that come first into action, the disease goes on increasing without wearing itself out, while those that are second in time follow the same course.

Sixthly, mercury hinders a disposition from forming, or, in other words, prevents contamination.

Seventhly, mercury does not destroy a disposition already formed.

Eighthly, mercury hinders the action from taking place, although the disposition be formed.

Ninthly, mercury cures the action.

These principles being established, the facts respecting the cure are easily accounted for.

CHAPTER II.

OF THE SYMPTOMS OF THE LUES VENEREA.

When the venereal matter has affected the constitution in any of the ways before mentioned, it has the whole body to work upon, and shows itself in a variety of shapes; many of which putting on the appearance of a different disease, we are often obliged to have recourse to the preceding history of the case before we can form any judgement of it. Probably the varieties in the appearances may be referred to the three following circumstances: the different kinds of constitutions, the different kinds of solids affected, and the different dispositions which the solids are in at the time; for I can easily conceive that a peculiarity of constitution may make a very material difference in the appearance of the same specific complaint, and I am certain that the solids, according to their different natures, produce a very different appearance when attacked with this disease; and I can also easily conceive that a different disposition from the common in the solids at the time may make a considerable difference in the appearances.

The difference of constitution, and of the same parts at different times, may have considerable effects in the disease with respect to its appearing sooner or later. This I am certain of, that the different parts of the body produce a very considerable difference in the times of appearance of this disease. That it appears much sooner in some parts than in others is best seen where different parts are affected in the same person; for I have already endeavoured to show that it is most probable that all the parts affected are contaminated nearly at the same time. This difference in the times is either owing to some parts being naturally put into action more easily by the poison than others, or they are naturally more active in themselves, and therefore probably will admit more quickly the action of every disease that is capable of affecting them.

When on the general history of the lues venerea, I divided the parts into two orders, according to the time of their appearance. I also observed that the first were commonly the external parts, as the skin, nose, tonsils; and that the second were more internal, as the bones, periosteum, fasciæ, and tendons.

The time necessary for its appearance, or for producing its local effects in the several parts of the body most readily affected, after it has got into the constitution, is uncertain, but in general it is about six weeks; in many cases, however, it is much later, and in others much sooner. In some cases it appears to produce its local effects within a fortnight after the possibility of the absorption of the matter. In one case a gentleman had a chancre, and a swelling in the groin came on, and within the before-mentioned time he had venereal eruptions all over the body. He could not impute this to any former complaint, yet there is a possibility of its having arisen from the first mode of catching the disease, by simple contact, at the time he got the local or chancre, which might extend the time to a week or more, although this is not probable. In another case, three weeks after the healing of a chancre, eruptions broke out all over the body, and this happened only a fortnight after leaving off the course of mercury that cured the chancre. The effects on other parts of the body, that are less susceptible of this irritation, or are slower in their action, are of course much later in appearing; and in those cases where both orders of parts are contaminated it is in general not till after the first has made its appearance for a considerable time, and even perhaps after it has been cured; for while the parts first in order of action were contaminated and under cure, the second in order are only in a state of contamination, and go on with the disease afterwards, although it may never again appear in the first.

From this circumstance of the parts second in order coming later into action, we can plainly see the reason why it shall appear in them, although the first in order may have been cured; for if the external parts, or first in order, have been cured, and the internal, or second, such as the tendons, bones, periosteum, &c., have not been cured, then it becomes confined solely to these parts. The order of parts may sometimes be inverted; for I have seen cases where the periosteum, or bone, was affected prior to any other part. Whether in the same case it might in the end have affected the skin or throat I will not pretend to say, as it was not allowed to go on; but it is possible that the second order of parts may be affected without the first having ever been contaminated.

Its effects on the deeper-seated parts are not like those produced in the external, and the difference is so remarkable as to give the appearance of another disease; and a person accustomed to see it in the first parts only would be entirely at a loss about the second.

The parts which come first into action go on with it, probably on the same principle, much quicker than the others; and this arises from the nature of the parts, as has already been observed.

Each succeeding part that becomes affected is slower and slower in its progress, and more fixed in its symptoms when produced; this arises also from the natural disposition of such parts, all their actions being slow, which indolent action may be assisted by the absence of the great

disposing cause, that is cold. I should, however, suspect that warmth
does not contribute much to their indolence of action; for if it did it
would assist in the cure, which it appears not to do, these parts being
as slow in their operations of restoration as they are in their actions of
disease. We may also observe that similar parts come sooner into action, and appear to go on more rapidly with it, as they are nearer the
source of the circulation. It appears earlier on the face, head, shoulders, and breast than on the legs, and the eruptions come sooner to suppuration in the before-mentioned parts *.

The circumstance of its being very late in appearing in some parts,
when it had been only cured in its first appearances, as mentioned, has
made many suppose that the poison lurked somewhere in the solids;
and others that it kept circulating in the blood for years.

It is not, however, easy to determine this point; but there can be no
good reason for the first hypothesis, as the lurking disposition never
takes place prior to its first appearance; for instance, we never find that
a man had a chancre a twelvemonth ago, and that it broke out after in
venereal scurfs upon the skin, or ulcers in the throat. The slowness
of its progress is only when the parts less susceptible of its irritation
have been affected by it.

§. 1. *Of the Symptoms of the first stage of the Lues Venerea.*

The first symptoms of the disease, after absorption, appear either on
the skin, throat, or mouth. These differ from one another according
to the nature of the parts affected. I shall therefore divide them into
two kinds, although there appears to be no difference in the nature of
the disease itself.

The appearance on the skin I shall call the first, although it is not
always the first appearance; for that in the throat is often as early a
symptom as any. The appearances upon the skin generally show
themselves in every part of the body, no part being more susceptible
than another, first in discolorations, making the skin appear mottled,
many of them disappearing, while others continue and increase with
the disease†.

In others it will come on in distinct blotches, often not observed till
scurfs are forming; at other times they appear in small distinct inflammations, containing matter and resembling pimples, but not so pyra-
midal, nor so red at the base.

Venereal blotches, at their first coming out, are often attended with

* See Introduction.
† This is not peculiar to this disease; it often takes place in the smallpox.

inflammation, which gives them a degree of transparency, which I think is generally greater in the summer than in the winter, especially if the patient be kept warm. In a little time this inflammation disappears, and the cuticle peels off in the form of a scurf. This sometimes misleads the patient and the surgeon, who look upon this dying away of the inflammation as a decay of the disease, till a succession of scurfs undeceives them.

These discolorations of the cuticle arise from the venereal irritation, and are seldom to be reckoned a true inflammation, for they seldom have any of its characteristics, such as tumefaction and pain; but this is true only on those parts most exposed, for in parts well covered, and in parts constantly in contact with other parts, there is more of the true inflammatory appearance, especially about the anus.

The appearance of the parts themselves next begins to alter, forming a copper-coloured dry inelastic cuticle, called a scurf; this is thrown off, and new ones are formed. These appearances spread to the breadth of a sixpence or shilling, but seldom broader, at least for a considerable time, every succeeding scurf becoming thicker and thicker, till at last it becomes a common scab, and the disposition for the formation of matter takes place in the cutis under the scab, so that at last it turns out a true ulcer, in which state it commonly spreads, although but slowly.

These appearances arise first from the gradual loss of the true sound cuticle, the diseased cutis having lost the disposition to form one; and, as a kind of substitute for this want of cuticle, an exudation takes place, forming a scale, and afterwards becoming thicker, and the matter acquiring more consistence, it at last forms a scab; but before it has arrived at this stage the cutis has given way, and ulcerated, after which the discharge becomes more of a true pus. When it attacks the palms of the hands and the soles of the feet, where the cuticle is thick, a separation of the cuticle takes place, and it peels off; a new one is immediately formed, which also separates, so that a series of new cuticles takes place, from its not so readily forming scurfs as on the common skin. If the disease is confined to those parts it becomes more difficult to determine whether or not it be venereal, for most diseases of the cutis of these parts produce a separation of the cuticle attended with the same appearances in all, and having nothing characteristic of the venereal disease.

Such appearances are peculiar to that part of the common skin of the body which is usually exposed; but when the skin is opposed by another skin which keeps it in some degree more moist, as between the nates, about the anus, or between the scrotum and the thigh, or in the angle between the two thighs, or upon the prolabium of the mouth, and in the armpits, the eruptions never acquire the above-described appearances, and instead of scurfs and scabs we have the skin elevated, or, as it were, tumefied by the extravasated lymph into a white, soft, moist, flat surface, which discharges a white matter. This may perhaps arise from there being more warmth, more perspiration, and less evaporation, as well as from the skin being thinner in such places. What strengthens this idea still more is, that in many venereal patients I have seen an approach towards such appearances on the common skin of the body; but this has been on such parts as were covered with the clothes, for on those parts of the skin that were not covered there was only the flat scurf; these, however, were redder than the above-described appearances, but hardly so high.

How far this is peculiar to the venereal disease I know not. It may take place in most scurfy eruptions of the skin. From a supposition of this not being venereal, I have destroyed them at the side of the anus with a caustic, and the patient has got well; however, from my idea of the disease, that every effect from the constitution is truly local, and therefore may be cured locally, a cure effected by this treatment does not determine the question.

This disease, on its first appearance, often attacks that part of the fingers upon which the nail is formed, making that surface red which is seen shining through the nail, and, if allowed to continue, a separation of the nail takes place, similar to the cuticle in the before-described symptoms; but here there cannot be that regular succession of nails as there is of cuticle.

It also attacks the superficies of the body which is covered with hair, producing a separation of the hair. A prevention of the growth of young hair is also the consequence while the disease lasts[a].

---

[a] [The variety of venereal eruptions is so great as almost to baffle description. Hence pathologists have usually contented themselves with fixing on some one characteristic which was generally applicable, and have neglected any attempt at distinct classification, or more accurate and detailed delineation. Thus the copper colour has been assigned by some, and the circular form by others, as the distinguishing character. Yet these general tests tend only to mislead, since the first is wanting in many species of venereal eruption, and the second is shared also by the great majority of eruptions which are not venereal.

It must be confessed that in the present state of our knowledge it would be impossible to produce a complete history of every form of venereal eruption. There are many sorts which are so indistinct and uncertain in their character that it would be difficult to find their proper place in any arrangement, and equally difficult to point out any constant and invariable signs by which they may be always identified. Yet the species of eruption which are of most frequent occurrence, and which are in practice of the greatest importance, are sufficiently distinct to admit of classification; and it is obvious that a clear history of the aspect and course of these more common forms of eruption

The second part in which it appears is most commonly the throat, sometimes the mouth and tongue.   In the throat, tonsils, and inside of

---

must greatly elucidate the whole subject, and ultimately facilitate the knowledge of those other varieties which are not included in the list.

The mottled state of the skin, to which allusion is made by the author, is certainly found in venereal cases.   Yet a similar appearance is often seen in cases where no venereal cause can be assigned; nor does there seem to be any peculiarity by which the one case can be distinguished from the other.   It may be doubted whether this mottled colour denotes more than an irritability of the skin, and a general disposition to eruptive disorders.

The more distinct sorts of venereal eruption may be divided into the following classes:

1. *Tubercles.*—The original seat of the tubercle is probably in the sebaceous glands, certainly in some structure which is below the surface of the cutis.   This is sufficiently evident from its aspect at the period of its commencement.   It appears in the first instance as a small hard substance like a pea, which may be felt by the finger before there is sufficient discoloration to attract the notice of the eye.   At this period the eruption is scarcely discernible if the light falls directly on the part, though if it is viewed by a side light the prominence is sufficient to cast a distinct shadow.   However, this stage is of short duration: the inflammation soon reaches the surface, and the spot then wears the appearance of a small red elevation, evenly rounded on the surface.   In the next place the cuticle dies, and becomes detached from the cutis; but it usually remains for a time, forming a horny cap, which covers the surface, and protects the formation of a new cuticle beneath.   In this state it frequently resembles a large vesicle, but the appearance is deceptive.   If the dead cuticle be removed by a probe, not a particle of fluid will be found under it.

The tubercle may remain in this state with little change, except that it slightly enlarges, and that successive layers of cuticle desquamate from the surface.   But it often happens that it goes on to ulceration.   In such cases the ulcer always commences at a central point, which is slightly depressed, and may be distinctly seen on the first removal of the cuticle, and which appears to be the orifice of the sebaceous duct.   As the ulcer proceeds it usually destroys the centre of the tubercle only, and leaves an indurated and elevated portion, by which it is encircled and separated from the sound skin.   In the progress of the ulcer this tubercular thickening continues to precede it, so that there is always a margin of red induration, more or less marked, as the powers of the system are greater or less; frequently of considerable breadth in those who are strong and vigorous, but in the feeble often so slight as to be scarcely distinguishable; yet in all cases leaving, as it subsides, the peculiar brown stain, which is the chief characteristic of the tubercle.

It is from this stain that the tubercle has received the appellation of the copper blotch. The hue varies with the age and the progress of the eruption.   In the earliest stages it differs in nothing from that of common inflammation, and is effaceable, or nearly so, on pressure.   But in a short time a yellow or copper tinge is blended with the florid red, and gives it a peculiar brightness, the cause of which is made evident by passing the finger over the spot.   The vessels are thus emptied for the moment, and the florid arterial colour disappears, but the yellow or copper stain remains unchanged, and is shown to depend on something which has been effused on the surface, and which cannot be removed by pressure.   While the tubercle is stationary the colour becomes deeper, and more yellow, but retains much of its brightness; but as the disease is subdued, and as the tubercular thickening subsides under treatment, the copper tinge gradually fades

the mouth, the disease generally shows itself at once, in the form of an ulcer, without much previous tumefaction, so that the tonsils are not

---

away, and gives place to a dirty brown. Though the hue is changed, the stain remains equally indelible, even at a time when all elevation has disappeared, and the spot is on the same level with the surrounding skin. There is still a later stage, at which this brown stain gradually fades away, and the seat of the spot is altogether undistinguishable.

This peculiar stain is not found in all forms of venereal eruption; it seems to be confined to the varieties of the tubercle; and there is reason to think that its exact nature and cause might be ascertained if we had a fuller acquaintance with the causes of the general colour of the skin, and with the functions of the sebaceous glands.

2. *Lichens.*—This eruption consists of small acuminated pimples, of a red colour, which are sometimes evenly scattered over the surface, at other times arranged in patches. It is not correct to characterize this eruption, as has been sometimes done, by the absence of suppuration. Many of the papulæ imperfectly suppurate; that is, a small quantity of opake serum is effused under the cuticle at the apex, and this serum soon becomes purulent: but the pus never accumulates; in a few days the greater part is absorbed; the rest dries into a small scab; and when this scab falls off, no ulcer, or depression, or cicatrix, is left behind. The pus is effused from the surface of the cutis, and is altogether unattended by ulceration.

Lichens differ much in the size of the papula and the depth of the colour; but they have one character which is very generally present, and which is shared by no other venereal eruption. They tend to pass spontaneously through their successive stages, and then spontaneously to subside. In other venereal eruptions the course of the disease in the skin is a test of the course of the disease in the general system. A diminution in the eruption argues an improvement in the affection of the constitution. In lichen, on the contrary, the colour may fade, and the elevation diminish, at a time when other symptoms are continuing to increase, and even when a fresh crop of lichen is appearing. Hence the same case frequently presents specimens of every stage of this eruption, from the first rise of the small papula, before maturation has taken place, to the period when all elevation has subsided, and the seat of the spot is marked only by a a pale or purple discoloration of the skin, which is effaceable by the pressure of the finger. This progress towards recovery, which often occurs spontaneously, may be very readily produced by remedies, which are altogether inadequate to cure the disease, especially if they are exhibited when the eruption has run through its natural periods, or about a fortnight or three weeks from the date of its appearance.

Yet this natural tendency to pass off is subject to exceptions. It sometimes happens that the small papula continues slowly but steadily to enlarge, and at length attains the size, and assumes the copper stain, and all the other characters of the tubercle. A close examination shows the mode in which this change takes place. The lichenous papula is situated on one of those small elevations on the surface of the cutis, which mark the orifices of the ducts that perforate the cutis, and proceed to the glands which are situated beneath it. The inflammation, which began on the surface, gradually extends down the duct, and involves the sebaceous gland which is at the bottom. This tubercular lichen is not so much a peculiar form of lichen, as an eruption of lichen passing into an eruption of tubercles, by a process which is very easily understood. In such cases the subsequent course and the treatment are exactly those of the tubercle.

Most forms of lichen present no indelible stain. But where the eruption has been unusually lasting there will be seen, after the subsidence of the papula, a brown stigma, occupying a central point, and commonly presenting an appearance of depression or

much enlarged ; for when the venereal inflammation attacks these parts, it appears to be always upon the surface, and it very soon terminates in an ulcer.

These ulcers in the throat are to be carefully distinguished from all others of the same parts.   It is to be remarked, that this disease, when it attacks the throat, always, I believe, produces an ulcer, although this is not commonly understood ; for I have seen cases where no ulceration had taken place called, by mistake, venereal.   It is therefore only this ulcer that is to be distinguished from other ulcers of these parts.   This species of ulcer is generally tolerably well marked, yet it is perhaps in all cases not to be distinguished from others that attack this part, for some have the appearance of being venereal, and what are really venereal resemble those that are not.   We have several diseases of this part which do not produce ulceration on the surface, one of which is common inflammation of the tonsils, which often suppurates in the centre, forming an abscess, which bursts by a small opening, but never looks like an ulcer begun upon the surface, as in the true venereal ; this case is

---

pitting.   This appearance is, however, in almost all cases delusive.   It arises from the stain being situated deep in the substance of the cutis, and shining through the more superficial parts, which are transparent.   These stigmata seem to characterize an earlier and more imperfect form of the preceding variety.   There has been an attempt to form a tubercle, but the complaint has been arrested before the sebaceous gland has been fully involved.

3. *Psoriasis and lepra.*—Scaly eruptions are very common in venereal cases, but they differ little from those which occur from other causes.   They appear generally in small circular spots, but they vary much in the degree of elevation, the size of the spot, and the depth of the colour; yet they never assume the copper tinge of the tubercle.   The colour is rather sandy, and is in almost all instances nearly effaceable by pressure. The difference of colour, the superficial origin of these eruptions, and the total absence of ulceration in all forms and stages, sufficiently distinguish them from tubercles.

4. *Rupia.*—This eruption shows itself at first by a slight blush on the surface.   Generally in a few hours, sometimes at a longer period, the cuticle at this part is elevated into a small blister, by the effusion of opake serum, which soon becomes purulent, and shortly afterwards concretes into a scab.   The disease spreads by a process in all respects similar.   Effusion takes place under the cuticle at the edge, and the concretion of this effusion enlarges the diameter of the scab, and elevates it from the surface of the cutis.   Hence the scab as it grows consists of a series of concentric layers, those towards the apex having been formed at the commencement of the disease, and being consequently small in size; those at the base, which have been formed by the latest effusion, being commensurate with the present size of the sore.   The accumulation of the whole forms a cone, which projects like a horn when the extension of the ulcer has been slow, but has a wide base and comparatively a slight projection where the ulcer has rapidly enlarged.

That rupia begins on the surface of the cutis is manifest, not only from the course of the ulcer, but also from the aspect of the cicatrix which it leaves.   The sore most frequently heals first at the centre, an island of skin forming there while the edges are still

always attended with too much inflammation, pain, and tumefaction of the parts to be venereal; and if it suppurates and bursts it subsides directly, and it is generally attended with other inflammatory symptoms in the constitution.

There is another disease of these parts, which is an indolent tumefaction of the tonsils, and is peculiar to many people whose constitutions have something of the scrofula in them, producing a thickness in the speech. Sometimes the coagulable lymph is thrown out on the surface, and called by some ulcers, by others sloughs, and such are often called putrid sore throats. Those commonly swell to too large a size for the venereal; and this appearance is easily distinguished from an ulcer or loss of substance : however, where it is not plain at first sight it will be right to endeavour to remove some of it; and if the surface of the tonsil is not ulcerated, then we may be sure it is not venereal. I have seen a chink filled with this, appearing very much like an ulcer, but upon removing the coagulable lymph the tonsil has appeared perfectly sound. I have seen cases of a swelled tonsil where a slough formed in its centre, and that slough has opened a passage out for itself,

---

stationary, or even spreading; and this is an occurrence which is known to be extremely rare in ulcers which have destroyed the whole substance of the cutis. Again, after the sore has healed, the surface of the cicatrix, especially near the edges, often presents distinctly to the eye the minute points that mark the ducts which perforate the cutis, and which must have been destroyed if the whole thickness of the cutis had been involved.

Some cases of ulcerating tubercles closely resemble rupia; but in rupia there is neither tubercular thickening nor copper stain. When these exist at the edges of the sore the eruption is not rupia, but tubercle, passing rapidly into ulceration. In such cases the spots which resemble rupia will generally be found intermixed with distinct tubercles, and the treatment required will be that which is adapted to the tubercle.

All pustular venereal eruptions seem to partake of the characters which belong to rupia, as far as the superficial origin, the mode of extension, and the accumulation of the crust are concerned; but they differ much in the degree of inflammation which precedes the formation of matter, and the size of the original pustule. In genuine rupia the vesicle is preceded only by a slight blush of inflammation, and at its first appearance is nearly of the size of a silver penny. But it often happens that the inflamed spot is smaller, and somewhat more elevated, and that the fluid effused is purulent from the first, and forms immediately a small scab at the top of the eminence. Such a spot resembles a common pustule, and the small size of the scab, and the slowness of its progress, give it an appearance which is not readily recognised as that of rupia. Yet it is difficult to point out any essential difference; and if the ulcer be allowed to increase, the aspect in the more advanced stages will be precisely similar. The description, therefore, which has been given may be taken as applicable to pustular venereal eruptions in general, if not in all the minuter details, at least in the prominent and essential characters.

It must not be forgotten that this classification of venereal eruptions is intended to include the principal varieties only, and that other forms of eruption occur which are less frequent and less distinctly marked, but which yet, from the history of the case, and the accompanying symptoms, must be referred to a venereal origin.]

and when it has been, as it were, sticking in this passage, it has appeared like a foul ulcer.

The most puzzling stage of the complaint is when the slough is come out, for then it has most of the characters of the venereal ulcer; but when I have seen the disease in its first stages I have always treated it as of the erysipelatous kind, or as something of the nature of a carbuncle.

When I have seen them in their second stage only I have been apt to suppose them venereal: however, no man will be so rash as to pronounce what a disease is from the eye only, but will make inquiries into all the circumstances before he forms a judgment. If there have been no preceding local symptoms within the proper date he will suspend his judgment, and wait a little to see how far Nature is able to relieve herself. If there has been any preceding fever, it will be still less probable that it is venereal. However, I will not say of what nature such cases are, but only that they are not venereal as they are often believed to be. I have seen a sore throat of this kind mistaken for venereal, and mercury given till it affected the mouth, which when it did, it brought on a mortification on all the parts concerned in the first disease. It would therefore appear that this species of the sore throat is aggravated by mercury.

There is another complaint of those parts which is often taken for venereal, which is an ulcerous excoriation, where the ulceration or excoriations run along the surface of the parts, becoming very broad, and sometimes foul, having a regular termination, but never going deep into the substance of the parts, as the venereal ulcer does. There is no part of the inside of the mouth exempted from this ulcerous excoriation, but I think it is most frequent about the root of the uvula, and spreads forwards along the palatum molle. That such are not venereal is evident, from their not giving way in general to mercury; and I have seen them continue for weeks without altering, and a true venereal ulcer appear upon the centre of the excoriated part.

The difference between the two is so strong that there can be no mistake; patients have gone through a course of mercury which has perfectly cured the venereal ulcers, but has had no effect upon the others, which have afterwards been cured by bark.

The true venereal ulcer in the throat is perhaps the least liable to be mistaken of any of the forms of the disease. It is a fair loss of substance, part being dug out, as it were, from the body of the tonsil, with a determined edge, and is commonly very foul, having thick white matter adhering to it like a slough, which cannot be washed away.

Ulcers in such situations are always kept moist, the matter not being allowed to dry and form scabs, as in those upon the skin; the matter is carried off the ulcers by deglutition, or the motion of the parts, so that no succession of scurfs or scabs can take place, as on the skin.

Their progress is also much more rapid than on the common skin, ulceration taking place very fast.

Like most other spreading ulcers, they are generally very foul, and for the most part have thickened or bordered edges, which is very common to venereal or cancerous sores, and indeed to most sores which have no disposition to heal, whatever the specific disease may be[a].

---

[a] [There is as great a variety in venereal sore throats as in venereal eruptions, and, from the situation of the part, the distinguishing characters are, on the whole, less easily observed. Yet some of the principal species are sufficiently distinct to be noticed.

1. The most genuine form of venereal sore throat appears to begin in the centre of the tonsil. In the early stages it is attended with very little pain or swelling, and is seldom observed until it has formed a distinct ulcer. But if attention is from any cause directed to the throat, an earlier appearance may sometimes be discovered. The tonsil may be found slightly swelled, and a yellow appearance may be seen occupying the substance of that part, and shining through the membrane on the surface which is yet entire. In a day or two ulceration takes place, and discloses a yellow or whitish slough, penetrating deep into the centre of the tonsil. There is little enlargement, and the surrounding parts are not violently inflamed. There is some sense of pricking, especially at the time of swallowing; but there is on the whole less difficulty of deglutition, and less uneasiness than might be expected from the magnitude and appearance of the ulcer. As it spreads, however, the surrounding parts become involved, and then it occasions more distress. The voice is altered, the hearing is rendered dull, and the inflammation of the soft palate impedes deglutition. Yet on the whole the progress is slow, and there is little accompanying disorder of the general system.

This species of sore throat often attends tubercular eruptions on the skin. There is reason to suppose that the secretion of the tonsils is analogous to that of the sebaceous glands of the skin, and hence it naturally happens that both parts are attacked simultaneously.

2. Venereal sores often commence on the surface of the mucous membrane, by a small foul ulceration, which passes at an early period into rapid and extensive sloughing. These ulcers are not limited to the membrane covering the tonsils, but may arise on the soft palate, the arches of the palate, or any part of the pharynx, and are most frequently found immediately behind one of the posterior arches, or at the upper and back part of the pharynx, where the early appearance is concealed by the velum pendulum and uvula. They are sometimes preceded and always accompanied by much pain and inflammation. The soft palate is swelled and very pendulous, and the attempt to raise it in swallowing is attended with excruciating pain. In speaking it seems to be absolutely quiescent. The irritation of the tumid velum and the slough excites a profuse secretion of saliva, and frequently much cough. The great distress which is thus occasioned produces a remarkable anxiety of countenance, which, conjoined with rapid emaciation, an accelerated pulse, and expectoration of a puriform character, gives the patient the aspect of considerable danger, and often suggests the idea that he is labouring under phthisis. The ravages committed by these ulcers are very extensive. The bone at the back part of the nares is frequently laid bare, and the disease proceeds to the destruction of the nose: and it occasionally occurs that the bodies of the vertebræ are exposed, and affected with fatal caries.

At other times, especially in cases of long standing, these sores shall extend not by

When it attacks the tongue it sometimes produces a thickening and hardness in the part; but this is not always the case, for it very often ulcerates, as in the other parts of the mouth.

They are generally more painful than those of the skin, although not so much so as common sore throats arising from inflamed tonsils.

They oblige the person to speak thick, or as if his tongue was too large for his mouth, with a small degree of snuffling.

These are the most common symptoms of this stage of the disease,

sloughing, but by rapid ulceration. The aspect is less formidable, but the progress is scarcely less destructive. This variety is most commonly seen on the soft palate. The surface is foul, but the slough which occupies it is of little depth. The sore is edged by a very narrow fringe of yellow slough, and beyond this, for the extent of a quarter of an inch, there is an inflamed margin of a deep crimson colour; but there is not much general swelling of the surrounding parts. Yet the sore extends daily with extraordinary rapidity. The substance of the part seems to melt away under the ulceration, and the greater part or the whole of the soft palate is often destroyed before it can be arrested, though no distinct slough can be seen to separate through the whole of its course.

These ulcers frequently accompany rupia.

3. A third appearance, which is shortly described by John Hunter under the name of an ulcerous excoriation, is of very common occurrence. It is distinguished by the opake white colour of the surface. This appearance sometimes supervenes at the edges of an ulcer on the tonsil. More frequently there is no ulceration, but simply this change of the surface, accompanied by more or less of redness, and, as it were, of excoriation of the neighbourhood, more or less swelling of the membrane, much soreness, but very little pain. This superficial affection may attack any part of the tonsils, arches of the palate, velum pendulum, and uvula, and even the tongue or the inside of the cheeks. It is very frequently to be seen at the angles of the mouth. It often occupies the soft palate, spreading upwards in a semicircular form towards the roof of the mouth. The white appearance may be removed by slightly touching it with caustic, and then the surface beneath looks as if excoriated.

This complaint very often accompanies psoriasis of the skin, and it is reasonable to suppose that the white colour which peculiarly characterizes it implies a change analogous to that which shows itself on the surface of the body in thickening of the cuticle and scaliness.

The author seems to be of opinion that this affection is never venereal; but cases occur where it exists in union with other venereal symptoms, and where it is only ultimately cured by the use of mercury. Yet it cannot be denied, that in the majority of cases it is not venereal; that very often mercury aggravates instead of removing it; that it may take place where there is no suspicion of syphilis, in patients labouring under psoriasis or lepra; and that in general the presumption is so far against its venereal origin that the treatment should be rather directed to the regulation of the diet, and to the prevention of acid secretions in the stomach, than to the extirpation of the venereal virus. The complaint is in this respect also analogous to scaly diseases of the skin. Both affections depend most usually on causes which are not syphilitic; nor do there appear to be any signs in the aspect of either by which the syphilitic can be distinguished from the non-syphilitic cases.

There are other forms of sore throat which are less important, and of which it is less easy to convey an idea by description.]

but it is perhaps impossible to know all the symptoms this poison produces when in the constitution. I knew a gentleman who had a teasing cough which he imputed to it; for it came on with the symptomatic fever, and continued with it, and by using mercury both disappeared.

There are inflammations of the eyes which are supposed to be venereal; for after the usual remedies against inflammation have been tried in vain, mercury has been given, on the supposition of the case being venereal, and sometimes with success, which has tended to establish this opinion. But if such cases are venereal, the disease is very different from what it is when attacking other parts from the constitution, for the inflammation is more painful than in venereal inflammation proceeding from the constitution; and I have never seen such cases attended with ulceration, as in the mouth, throat, and tongue, which makes me doubt much of their being venereal[a].

§. 2. *Experiments made to ascertain the Progress and Effects of the Venereal Poison.*

To ascertain several facts relative to the venereal disease, the following experiments were made. They were begun in May 1767.

Two punctures were made on the penis with a lancet dipped in venereal matter from a gonorrhœa; one puncture was on the glans, the other on the prepuce.

This was on a Friday; on the Sunday following there was a teasing itching in those parts, which lasted till the Tuesday following. In the mean time, these parts being often examined, there seemed to be a greater redness and moisture than usual, which was imputed to the parts being rubbed. Upon the Tuesday morning the parts of the prepuce where the puncture had been made were redder, thickened, and had formed a speck; by the Tuesday following the speck had increased, and discharged some matter, and there seemed to be a little pouting of

---

[a] [The author has here been misled, either by the general principle which he imagined he had discovered, and which may be shown to be in many instances erroneous, or by the want of opportunity for a more extended observation of diseases of the eye. It is established beyond the possibility of doubt, that iritis is frequently a secondary symptom of the venereal disease. The general symptoms of iritis are well known. The distinctive signs of syphilitic iritis have been supposed to be chiefly the deposit of masses of lymph, of a reddish or brownish colour, on the surface of the iris, and the nocturnal exacerbation of pain. However, the accuracy of the diagnosis may be questioned, since it is certain that in venereal cases many instances of iritis occur where these peculiar symptoms are wanting, and where the appearance differs in nothing from the idiopathic forms of the disorder.]

the lips of the urethra, also a sensation in it in making water, so that a discharge was expected from it. The speck was now touched with lunar caustic, and afterwards dressed with calomel ointment. On Saturday morning the slough came off, and it was again touched, and another slough came off on the Monday following. The preceding night the glans had itched a good deal, and on Tuesday a white speck was observed where the puncture had been made; this speck, when examined, was found to be a pimple full of yellowish matter. This was now touched with the caustic, and dressed as the former. On the Wednesday the sore on the prepuce was yellow, and therefore was again touched with caustic. On the Friday both sloughs came off, and the sore on the prepuce looked red, and its basis not so hard; but on the Saturday it did not look quite so well, and was touched again, and when that went off it was allowed to heal, as also the other, which left a dent in the glans. This dent on the glans was filled up in some months, but for a considerable time it had a bluish cast.

Four months afterwards the chancre on the prepuce broke out again, and very stimulating applications were tried; but these seemed not to agree with it, and nothing being applied, it healed up. This it did several times afterwards, but always healed up without any application to it. That on the glans never did break out, and herein also it differed from the other.

While the sores remained on the prepuce and glans a swelling took place in one of the glands of the right groin. I had for some time conceived an idea that the most effectual way to put back a bubo was to rub in mercury on that leg and thigh; that thus a current of mercury would pass through the inflamed gland. Here was a good opportunity of making the experiment. I had often succeeded in this way, but now wanted to put it more critically to the test*. The sores upon the penis were healed before the reduction of the bubo was attempted. A few days after beginning the mercury in this method the gland subsided considerably. It was then left off, for the intention was not to cure it completely at present. The gland some time after began to swell again, and as much mercury was rubbed in as appeared to be sufficient for the entire reduction of the gland; but it was meant to do no more than to cure the gland locally, without giving enough to prevent the constitution from being contaminated.

About two months after the last attack of the bubo, a little sharp pricking pain was felt in one of the tonsils in swallowing anything, and

---

* The practice in 1767 was to apply a mercurial plaster on the part, or to rub in mercurial ointment on the part, which could hardly act by any other power than sympathy.

on inspection a small ulcer was found, which was allowed to go on till the nature of it was ascertained, and then recourse was had to mercury. The mercury was thrown in by the same leg and thigh as before, to secure the gland more effectually, although that was not now probably necessary.

As soon as the ulcer was skinned over the mercury was left off, it not being intended to destroy the poison, but to observe what parts it would next affect. About three months after, copper-coloured blotches broke out on the skin, and the former ulcer returned in the tonsil. Mercury was now applied the second time for those effects of the poison upon the constitution, but still only with a view to palliate.

It was left off a second time, and the attention was given to mark where it would break out next; but it returned again in the same parts. It not appearing that any further knowledge was to be procured by only palliating the disease a fourth time in the tonsil, and a third time in the skin, mercury was now taken in a sufficient quantity, and for a proper time, to complete the cure.

The time the experiments took up, from the first insertion to the complete cure, was about three years.

The above case is only uncommon in the mode of contracting the disease, and the particular views with which some parts of the treatment were directed; but as it was meant to prove many things which, though not uncommon, are yet not attended to, attention was paid to all the circumstances. It proves many things, and opens a field for further conjectures.

It proves, first, that matter from a gonorrhœa will produce chancres.

It makes it probable that the glans does not admit the venereal irritation so quickly as the prepuce. The chancre on the prepuce inflamed and suppurated in somewhat more than three days, and that on the glans in about ten. This is probably the reason why the glans did not throw off its sloughs so soon.

It renders it highly probable that to apply mercury to the legs and thighs is the best method of resolving a bubo; and therefore also the best method of applying mercury to assist in the cure, even when the bubo suppurates.

It also shows that buboes may be resolved in this way, and yet the constitution not be safe; and therefore that more mercury should be thrown in, especially in cases of easy resolution, than what simply resolves the bubo.

It shows that parts may be contaminated, and may have the poison kept dormant in them while under a course of mercury for other symptoms, but break out afterwards.

It also shows that the poison having originally only contaminated certain parts, when not completely cured, can break out again only in those parts[a].

§.3. *Of the Symptoms of the Second Stage of the Lues Venerea.*

This stage of the disease is not so well marked as the former; and, as it is of more importance, it requires all our discernment to determine what the disease is.

The parts less susceptible of this irritation are such as are more out of the way of the great exciting cause, which is the external air, as has been before related. And they begin to take on the venereal action whether it may or it may not have produced its local effects upon the external or exposed surfaces; and they even go on with the action, in many cases, after these surfaces first affected have taken on the action and have been cured, as has been already observed. These deeper-seated parts are the periosteum, tendons, fasciæ, and ligaments; however, what the parts affected may be when the disease is in this stage is not always certain: I have known it produce total deafness, and some of those cases to end in suppuration, attended with great pain in the ear and side of the head. Such cases are generally supposed to arise from some other cause; and nothing but some particular circumstance in the history of the case, or some symptom attending it, can lead the surgeon to the nature of the complaint.

When these deeper-seated parts become irritated by this poison the progress is more gradual than in the first: they have very much the character of scrofulous swellings or chronic rheumatism, only in this disease the joints are not so subject to it as they are in the rheumatism. We shall find a swelling come upon a bone when there has been no possible means of catching the infection for many months, and it will be of some size before it is taken notice of, from having given but little pain. On the other hand, there shall be great pain, and probably no swelling to be observed till some time after. The same observations are applicable to the swelling of tendons, and fasciæ.

As these swellings increase by slow degrees, they show but little signs of inflammation. When they attack the periosteum the swelling

---

[a] [See the note at p. 146. If the experiment had been made by one less practised and less accurate than John Hunter, the history of the case would lead to the suspicion that the venereal virus had been conveyed to the punctures by means of the caustic with which they were repeatedly touched. Certainly the course which they held was very different from that which is usually observed in common chancre.]

has all the appearance of a swelling of the bone, by being firm and closely connected with it.

The inflammation produced in these later stages of the disease can hardly get beyond the adhesive, in which state it continues growing worse and worse, and when matter is formed it is not true pus but a slimy matter. This may arise in some degree from the nature of the parts not being in themselves easily made to suppurate; and when they do suppurate the same languidness still continues, insomuch that this matter is not capable of giving the extraneous stimulus, so as to excite true suppuration or ulceration, even after the constitution is cleared of the original cause, and then the disease is probably scrofulous. Some nodes, either in the tendons or bones, last for years before they form any matter at all; and in this case it is doubtful whether they are venereal or not, although commonly supposed to be so.

I have already observed that the pain in the first stages of this disease is much less than might be expected, considering the effects produced by the poison. The disease being very slow and gradual in its progress, its giving little pain may be accounted for. An ulcer in the throat causes no great pain; and the same may be said of blotches on the skin, even when they become large sores.

When the periosteum and bones become affected the pain is sometimes very considerable, and at other times there is hardly any. It is not perhaps easy to account for this. We know also that the tendinous parts, when inflamed, give in some cases very considerable pain, and that of the heavy kind, while in others they will swell considerably without giving any pain.

These pains are commonly periodical, or have their exacerbations, being commonly worst in the night. This is common to other aches or pains, especially of the rheumatic kind, which the venereal pains resemble very much.

When the pain is the first symptom, it affords no distinguishing mark of the disease; it is therefore often taken for the rheumatism [a].

---

[a] [Venereal affections of the bones are of different kinds.

1. Simple inflammation of the periosteum, which is marked by thickening of the periosteum, with much pain and tenderness, and usually terminates in the deposit of osseous matter beneath it, and the permanent enlargement of the bone. Sometimes, though more rarely, the periosteum suppurates, and then it often happens that a portion of the bone beneath it dies and exfoliates. This constitutes the most common venereal node, and is frequent on the tibia, the ulna, and the cranium.

2. Caries of the bone, which commences in the cancellous structure and gradually perforates the external plate; and then appears as a soft tumour, which may be seen and felt externally. If this tumour is laid open, a glairy fluid is evacuated; the periosteum is found to be somewhat thickened and the bone beneath is denuded, and in

§ 4. *Of the Effects of the Poison on the Constitution.*

The poisonous matter, simply as extraneous matter, produces no change whatever upon the constitution, and whatever effects it has depend wholly upon its specific quality as a poison. The general effects of this poison on the constitution are similar to other irritations, either local or constitutional. It produces fever, which is of the slow kind; and when it continues a considerable time it produces what is called a hectic disposition, which is no more than an habitual slow fever arising from a cause which the constitution cannot overcome. While this exists it is impossible that anything salutary can go on in such a constitution. The patient loses his appetite, or even if his appetite is good, loses his flesh, becomes restless, loses his sleep, and looks sallow*.

In the first stage of this disease, before it begins to show itself externally, the patient has generally rigors, hot fits, headaches, and all the symptoms of an approaching fever.

These symptoms continuing for some days, and often for weeks, show that there is some irritating cause which works slowly upon the constitution. It is then supposed to be whatever the invention or ingenuity of the practitioner shall call it; but the venereal eruptions

---

* This kind of look, although arising entirely from a harassed constitution, is always supposed to be peculiar to a venereal one. This idea, however, does not arise from the look only, but from the leading symptoms.

---

the centre of the denuded part is found a small hole, which perforates the cortical plate, and communicates with the interior of the bone. This affection is very common in the skull, and may be occasionally seen in the tibia, the jaw, and the ulna. It constitutes in its aggravated forms the worm-eaten caries, which is sometimes seen to pervade extensively the bones of the cranium.

3. There is, less frequently, a third form of disease, which seems to be originally simple inflammation of the bone, and which is most commonly seen in the skull. The thickness of the bone is greatly increased, and the structure becomes dense and ponderous. The periosteum is for the most part unaltered; but during the course of the disease it is often attacked by inflammation at particular points, and then it rises into small nodes. These nodes generally subside again in a week or two, when similar enlargements occur elsewhere, and usually in like manner disappear in their turn. Sometimes, however, instead of subsiding, they suppurate, and the surface of the bone becomes carious. Yet no considerable portion dies and separates: the ulcer does not spread, but after a certain lapse of time heals again, leaving the surface of the bone uneven, and the cicatrix closely adhering to it. The enlargement of the bone subsides on the cure of the disease, except in cases where the disease has been of very long continuance.]

or nodes upon either the periosteum, bones, tendons, or other parts appearing, show the cause, and in some degree carry off the symptoms of fever and relieve the constitution for a little time, but they soon recur.

These constitutional complaints, however, are not always to be found, the poison stimulating so slowly as hardly to affect the constitution, unless it be allowed to remain in it a long time.

There are a number of local appearances, mentioned by authors, which I never saw, such as the fissures about the anus, &c. There are also a number of diseases described by authors as venereal, especially by Astruc and his followers, which are almost endless. The cancer, scrofula, rheumatism, and gout have been considered as arising from it, which may be in some measure true; but they are with them the disease itself, and all their consequences, as consumption, wasting from want of nourishment, jaundice, and a thousand other diseases, which happened many years before the existence of the lues venerea, are all attributed to it.

There is even at this day hardly any disease the practitioner is puzzled about, but the venereal comes immediately into his mind; and if this became the cause of careful investigation it would be productive of good, but with many the idea alone satisfies the mind.

CHAPTER III.

GENERAL OBSERVATIONS ON THE CURE OF LUES VENEREA.

It has been observed before, that there are three forms of the venereal infection, gonorrhœa, chancre, and the lues venerea, which various forms I have endeavoured to account for. As they all three arise from the same poison, and as the two first depend only on a difference in the nature of the parts, and the lues venerea on another circumstance which has been explained, it would be natural to suppose that one medicine, whatever it be, would cure all the forms of this disease. But we find from experience that this does not hold good; for one medicine, that is mercury, cures only the chancre and the lues venerea, and the gonorrhœa is not in the least affected by it; and what is still more remarkable is, that the two which it cures are in no respect similar, while the gonorrhœa, which it does not cure, is similar in some respects to the chancre, which it does cure.

It may be remarked in general, that there is not only a difference in the form of the disease, but also in the modes of cure, and in the times necessary for the cure of the different forms of the disease, even when the same medicines cure. The gonorrhœa, in its cure, is the most uncertain of the three, the chancre next, and the lues venerea the most certain, although cured by the same medicine which cures the chancre.

A gonorrhœa in some cases shall be cured in six days, and in others require as many months, which, with regard to time, is about the proportion of thirty to one. A chancre may be sometimes cured in two weeks, and often requires as many months, which is in the proportion of four to one. The lues venerea in general may be cured in one or two months, which is only two to one. This calculation shows the regularity and irregularity, as to time, in the cure of each form of the disease.

I have formerly observed, that indispositions of the body often affect this disease very considerably, more especially the gonorrhœa and the chancre.

When an increase of symptoms takes place in a gonorrhœa, from an indisposition of body, nothing should be done for the gonorrhœa, the indisposition of body being only to be attended to; because we have no specific for the gonorrhœa, and in time it cures itself. But this practice is perhaps not to be followed in a chancre or lues venerea. It may be necessary in those to continue the mercury, although perhaps more gently; for the mercury is a specific that cannot be dispensed with, because neither the chancre nor lues venerea are cured by themselves, but always increase.

This form of the venereal disease I have divided into two stages. When in the parts most susceptible of the disease, which I have called the first order of parts, and which appear to be the superficies only, the lues venerea is perhaps subject to less variety than either the gonorrhœa or chancre, and its mode of cure is of course more uniform, although the disease be less easily ascertained, at least for some time. In the second order of parts the lues venerea becomes more complicated, and its cure still less to be depended upon.

The cure of this form is much more difficultly ascertained than either of the two former: they, being always local, and their effects visible, become more the object of our senses, so that we are seldom or never deceived in the cure, although at the same time the cure is often more tedious and difficult; for whenever the symptoms of the gonorrhœa or

chancre have entirely disappeared, in general the patient may look upon himself as cured of them; but this is not the case in the lues venerea.
: A lues venerea is the effects of the poison having circulated in the blood till it has irritated parts so as to give them a venereal disposition, which parts sooner or later assume the venereal action, according to the order of their susceptibility.

When the venereal matter is circulating I have supposed that certain parts are irritated by it, and that a vast number of other parts escape, as is evidently the case with the chancre; for in the case of a chancre the whole glans, prepuce, and skin of the penis have had the matter applied to them, yet only one or more points are contaminated or irritated by it, all the others escaping; and we often see in the lues venerea, that when the parts contaminated assume the action, it is confined to them without affecting other parts, although the disease be allowed to go on for a considerable time without any attempt to a cure; and also, if these parts are imperfectly cured, the disease returns only in them; therefore these effects, although arising from the constitution, are in themselves entirely local, similar to the gonorrhœa and chancre, and like them may be cured locally; and the person may still continue to have the lues venerea, although not in these, yet in other parts, because there may be many other parts in the same body that are under the venereal disposition, although they may not yet have assumed the venereal action.   To cure the local and visible effects of the disease we must attack it through that medium by which it was communicated, that is, the blood; without, however, considering the blood itself as diseased, or containing the poison, but as the vehicle of our medicine which will be carried by it to every part of the body where the poison was carried, and in its course it will act upon the diseased solids.   This practice must be continued some time after all symptoms have disappeared; for the venereal action may to appearance be stopped, and symptoms disappear, and yet all return again, the venereal action not being completely destroyed.   If the medicine were also a cure for the disposition in the parts second in order, and could prevent their coming into action, it would be necessary to continue it somewhat longer on their account; but this is not the case, for the visible effects, symptoms, or appearances in the first order of parts, give way to the treatment, while the parts that have only acquired the disposition, and are still inactive, afterwards assume the action and continue the disease.   This deceives the surgeon, and leaves the groundwork for a second set of local effects in the parts second in order; but I have asserted that what will cure an action will not cure a disposition; if so, we should push our medicine no further than the cure of the visible effects of the poison,

and allow whatever parts may be contaminated to come into action afterwards.

The parts that first assume the venereal action are easiest of cure;
and I have suspected that those effects of the disease being external,
were in some degree assisted in their cure by the local action of the
medicine, which evidently passes off through those parts.

When the disease has attacked the parts second in order of susceptibility, it generally happens that they are more difficult of cure than the
former; therefore when they are affected at the same time with the
former, and are cured, we may be sure that the first will be also cured.
From hence, as it would appear that the parts most susceptible of the
disease are also easiest of cure, it follows that the parts least susceptible
of the disease are also most difficult of cure; and I believe that this is
seldom or never reversed; therefore those second in order of susceptibility have this advantage, that we have the local complaints for our guide
to judge of the whole; and in such we have only to continue the treatment till they all vanish, being certain that the cure of the first, if there
are any, will be involved in those of the second.

As the second are attended with more tumefaction or swelling than
the first, it becomes a question whether the mercurial course should be
continued till the whole has subsided. But I believe it is not necessary
to continue the method of cure till the whole tumefaction disappears,
for as those local complaints cannot contaminate the constitution by re-
absorption, and as the venereal disposition and action from the constitution can be cured while the local effects still remain, even where the
tumefaction forming nodes on the bones, fasciæ, &c. is carried the length
of suppuration, there can be no occasion for continuing the course longer
than the destruction of the venereal action. But this effect of our medicine is not easily known; therefore it will be necessary to pursue the
method of cure till the appearances become stationary, and probably a
little longer to destroy the whole action of the disease. From these
circumstances it would appear that the venereal irritation, when in this
stage of the disease, is easier of cure than the effects of that irritation,
such as the tumefaction.

§. 1. *Of the Use of Mercury in the Cure of the Lues Venerea.*

Mercury in the lues venerea, as in the chancre, is the great specific,
and hardly anything else is to be depended upon. It is necessary that
we should always consider well the effects of this medicine, both on the
constitution at large and the disease for which it is given. The effects

of mercury on a constitution will always be as the quantity of mercury in that constitution; and when the same quantity affects one constitution more than another, it is in the proportion of the irritability of that constitution to the powers of mercury, entirely independent of any particular preparation, or any particular mode of giving it.

With regard to the preparations of the medicine, and the modes of applying it, we are to consider two things; first, the preparation and mode that is attended with the least trouble or inconvenience to the patient; and second, the preparation and mode of administering it that most readily conveys the necessary quantity into the constitution.

Nothing can show more the ungrateful or unsettled mind of man than his treatment of this medicine. If there is such a thing as a specific, mercury is one for the venereal disease in two of its forms; yet mankind are in pursuit of other specifics for the disease, as if specifics were more common than diseases; while at the same time they are too often contented with the common mode of treating many other diseases for which they have no specific; and these prejudices are supported by the public, who have in their minds a dread of this medicine, arising from the want of knowledge of our predecessors in administering it; and many of the present age, who are equally ignorant, take advantage of this weakness.

Mercury in the constitution acts on all parts of the machine, cures those which are diseased, affecting but little those that are sound. Mercury is carried into the constitution in the same way as other substances, either externally by the skin, or internally by the mouth: it cannot, however in all cases, be taken into the constitution in both ways, for sometimes it happens that the absorbents on the skin will not readily receive it, at least no effect will be produced, either on the disease or constitution, from such application; when this is the case it is to be considered as a misfortune, for then it must be given internally by the mouth, although possibly this mode may be very improper in other respects, and often inconvenient. On the other hand, it sometimes happens that the internal absorbents will not take up this medicine, or at least no effect is produced either upon the disease or constitution; in such cases it is right to try all the different preparations of the medicine, for it will sometimes happen that one preparation will succeed when another will not. I have never seen a case where neither external nor internal applications of mercury were absorbed; such a case must be miserable indeed.

I may just observe here, that many surfaces appear to absorb this medicine better than others, and most probably all internal surfaces and sores are of this kind; for when we find that thirty grains of calomel rubbed in on the skin has no more effect than three or four taken by the mouth, it becomes a kind of proof that the bowels absorb it best; also, when dressing a small sore with red precipitate produces a saliva-tion, it shows that sores are good absorbing surfaces, especially too when we know that the lues venerea generally arises from a chancre.

A patient with a stump which produced too much granulation was dressed with ointment containing a large proportion of red precipitate; the sore was about the size of a crown piece. It very nearly brought on a salivation, and the patient was obliged to leave it off.

A mulatto woman had upon her leg a very bad ulcer, which was about the breadth of two palms; it was dressed with red precipitate mixed with common ointment, which soon threw her into a violent salivation.

A lady, in the month of December 1782, was burnt over the whole breast, neck, and shoulders, as also between her shoulders, on which parts deep sloughs were formed. The sores at first healed nearly up, and tolerably well for burns; but they broke out anew and then became more obstinate. Seven months after the accident she came to London, with very large sores extending across the breast and upon each side to the shoulders; they were extremely tender and painful. They con-tinued to heal for some time after she came to London; but she became ill, having been affected with extreme irritability, loss of appetite, sick-ness, and throwing up of her food and medicines. At this time the sores again began to spread, and became very large. After having been two months in town with little advantage, I tried warmer dressings, as basilicon, to some parts, to see if any advantage would arise from such treatment, and it was found that these parts healed rather faster than the others; but the soreness was so great, even from the mildest dress-ings, that they could only be used in part. I next tried red precipitate mixed with the ointment; and, that it might increase the pain as little as possible, I ordered only ten grains to two ounces of the ointment. This appeared to agree better with the sores than the ointment alone; and we were happy in having found a dressing which both hastened on the cure, and was easier than the former. But about the fourth or fifth dressing from beginning the use of the precipitate, she began to com-plain of her gums; the next day began to spit, and by the seventh or eighth day the mouth was so sore, and the spitting so considerable that, upon considering the case, we began to suspect that it might proceed from the red precipitate in the dressing. The gums, inside of the cheeks, and the breath were truly mercurial. We immediately left off this dressing, except to a small corner, and had recourse to the former dress-ings. In a few days the effects of the mercury abated, and the sores looked more healthy than ever, and we again began to dress part of the sores with the ointment containing precipitate, which still agreed with them. When the mouth first became affected she had not used much above one half of the ointment; and by the time we had discovered the cause about three fourths of it had been expended in dressings, so that there was not quite ten grains of precipitate applied; and although this took up seven or eight days, and the ointment must have been soon removed from the sore by the discharge, yet a considerable spitting was produced, which lasted above a month. It is hardly to be conceived that above a grain or two could really be taken into the constitution; for when we consider the particles of precipitate were covered with ointment, and a vast discharge of matter, so as soon to remove this small quantity from the sore, we can hardly admit the possibility of more being absorbed; and if this idea of the quantity taken in is just, to what must we attribute the great susceptibility to the effects of the medicine? Was it the irritable state of the patient at the time? For the state of the constitution appeared to me to be that in which the locked jaw often takes place; and I often had this disease in my mind. The patient afterwards got well by the use of an ointment in which pitch was an ingredient *. All this tends to show that sores and internal surfaces absorb better than the skin.

Besides the practicability of getting the medicine into the constitution in either way, it is proper to consider the easiest for the patient, each mode having its convenience and inconvenience, which arises from the nature of the constitution or of the parts to which it is applied, or from certain situations of life of the patient at the time. It is therefore proper to give it in that way which suits these circumstances best.

To explain this further, we find that in many patients the bowels can hardly bear mercury at all, therefore it is be given in the mildest form possible; also joined with such other medicines as will lessen or correct its violent local effects, although not its specific ones on the constitution at large.

When it can be thrown into the constitution with propriety by the external method it is preferable to the internal, because the skin is not nearly so essential to life as the stomach, and therefore is capable in itself of bearing much more than the stomach; it also affects the constitution much less; many courses of mercury, which are absolutely necessary, would kill the patient if taken by the stomach, proving hurtful both to the stomach and intestines, even when given in any form, and joined with the greatest correctors: on the other hand, the way of life will often not allow it to be applied externally. It is not every one

---

* Added: "A gentleman introduced a bougie into the urethra smeared with mercurial ointment, and rubbed in a little on the fraenum three times, and his mouth became affected."—*Home*.

that can find convenience to rub in mercury, therefore they must take it by the mouth if possible. To obviate the inconvenience often arising from the visible effects of mercury, many preparations have been invented ; but any preparation of mercury producing an effect different from the simple effects of mercury in that constitution, such as sweating, or an increased discharge of urine, must be supposed either not to act as mercury, or the substance with which it is compounded produces this effect ; but if its peculiar effects are less than usual, I should very much suspect that the mercury is acting in part as a compound, and not entirely as mercury.

Mercury, like many other medicines, has two effects, one upon the constitution and particular parts, which is according to its mode of irritation, independent of any disease whatever. The other is its specific effects upon a diseased action of the whole body, or of parts, whatever the disease be, and which effects are only known by the disease gradually disappearing. The first becomes an object of consideration for the surgeon, as it is in some measure by them he is to be guided in giving this medicine so as to have its specific effects sufficient for the cure of the disease.

Whatever injury mercury may do to the constitution it is by its visible effects, and thence the pretended art in avoiding those visible effects has been too much the cause of great imposition. The part upon which its effects are most likely to fall is the part that is in most cases attempted to be avoided, or guarded against, and that is the mouth. I believe that we are not possessed of any means of either driving the mercury to the mouth, or of preventing it from attacking that part. Cold and warmth are the two great agents mentioned by authors : we find them recommending the avoiding of cold, for fear the mercury should fly to the mouth, as if warmth was a prevention ; while others, and even the same authors, when talking of bringing the mercury to the mouth, recommend warmth, as if cold were a preventive. This being the case, we may reasonably suppose that neither the one nor the other has any material effect*

In giving mercury in the venereal disease the first attention should be to the quantity, and its visible effects in a given time ; which when brought to a pitch are only to be kept up, and the decline of the disease to be watched ; for by this we judge of the invisible or specific effects of the medicine, which will often inform us that some variation in the quantity may be necessary.

The visible effects of mercury are of two kinds, the one on the constitution, the other on some parts capable of secretion. In the first it

* The whole of this paragraph omitted.—*Home.*

appears to produce universal irritability, making it more susceptible of all impressions ; it quickens the pulse, also increases its hardness, producing a kind of temporary fever ; but in many constitutions it exceeds this, acting as it were as a poison. In some it produces a kind of hectic fever, that is, a small quick pulse, loss of appetite, restlessness, want of sleep, and a sallow complexion, with a number of consequent symptoms ; but by the patient being a little accustomed to the use of it these constitutional effects commonly become less, of which the following cases are strong instances.

A gentleman rubbed in mercurial ointment for the reduction of two buboes. He had only rubbed in a few times when it affected his constitution so much that it was necessary to leave it off. He was seized with feverish complaints of the hectic kind, a small quick pulse, debility, loss of appetite, no sleep, and night sweats. He took the bark, with James's powder, and asses' milk, and got gradually rid of these complaints. As the buboes were advancing, it was necessary to have recourse to mercury again ; and I told him that now it would not produce the same effects so quickly nor so violently as before. He rubbed in a considerable quantity without his constitution or mouth being affected ; but the buboes suppurating, I ordered it to be left off a second time ; and when they were opened he had recourse to the ointment again for the third time, and without producing any disagreeable effects. The buboes put on a healing disposition for a while, and then became stationary, showing that a new disposition was forming. He was directed to leave off the ointment and to bathe in the sea, which he did, and the buboes began to heal. In about three weeks, however, it was thought necessary to use more friction, and when he began, which was the fourth time, it had almost an immediate and violent effect upon his mouth ; he left off again till his mouth became a little better, and then returned to the mercury a fifth time, and was able to go on with it.

A stout healthy man used mercurial friction for a bubo till it affected his mouth ; it further brought on very disagreeable constitutional complaints, such as loss of appetite, watchfulness, sallow complexion, lassitude from the least exercise, and swelled legs ; and although various means were used to reconcile the constitution to it, yet it continued to act as a poison.

Mercury often produces pains like those of the rheumatism, and also nodes which are of a scrofulous nature : from thence it has been accused of affecting the bones, " lurking in them," as authors have expressed it*.

* The following paragraphs are added.
" Mercury often produces an itching of the skin, so much so in some that they can hardly bear it.
" Although mercury does not always affect the mouth, yet it sometimes affects the

It may be supposed to be unnecessary to mention, in the present state of our knowledge, that it never gets into the bones in the form of a metal, although this has been asserted by men of eminence and authority in the profession, and even the dissections of dead bodies have been brought in proof of it; but my experience in anatomy has convinced me that such appearances never occur. Those authors have been quoted by others, imaginary cases of disease have been increased, the credulous and ignorant practitioner misled, and patients rendered miserable[a].

constitution of the person whose mouth cannot be affected, producing loss of appetite, pains of the rheumatic kind, and all the constitutional symptoms of hectic fever; and at the same time shall be curing the venereal disease effectually.

" A person had pains in his shoulders and blotches on the skin, supposed to be venereal. He never could be affected with mercury. I made him rub in two drams of strong mercurial ointment every night, and the symptoms entirely disappeared, without any effects being produced by the mercury on the mouth, skin, or kidneys."—*Home.*

---

[a] [The symptoms which mark what the author has denominated the poisonous effects of mercury are of such importance as to require a more particular description. They assume two different forms, the one having an acute, the other a chronic character.

The former constitutes what has been denominated mercurial erethismus. The effect of the poison is here chiefly felt on the heart. The pulse becomes hurried, small, and irregular; the action of the heart violent, but at the same time irregular, and fluttering; and the weakness and imperfection of the circulation are further testified by paleness of the countenance, by frequent sighing, and anxiety about the præcordia, and by unsteadiness of the limbs. In very severe cases the countenance becomes contracted, and the extremities cold. Nevertheless the stomach and bowels show no signs of derangement, and the tongue, though unsteady and tremulous, is clean. Under these circumstances muscular exertion is often suddenly fatal. Syncope ensues, from which the heart is too weak to recover.

If mercury is discontinued, and proper remedies are used, the action of the heart will be restored to its natural tone and regularity, and the affection will entirely disappear, leaving no consequences behind it.

In the second form the derangement may be less immediately dangerous, but it more extensively pervades the whole system, and is more permanent. There shall be no palpitation of the heart, but the pulse shall be small and accelerated; there shall be loss of sleep and of appetite, a sallow paleness of the countenance, often a loaded tongue, and always great debility and emaciation. The general aspect shall be that of extreme ill-health. If this state be allowed to continue, other symptoms indicative of general cachenia will supervene. There will be scrofulous enlargements of the glands, rheumatic pains in the limbs, or languid inflammation of the joints, having something of a scrofulous character. The ulcerative will everywhere supersede the adhesive process. Slight wounds will form sores, and when fractured bones have been recently united the union will give way.

This state of constitution, if once fully established, is not easily corrected. Years frequently pass before all traces of it are removed. It is the result not so often of an inordinate dose of mercury continued only for a short period, as of a long and obstinate perseverance in the exhibition of moderate doses, notwithstanding evident signs of deteriorated health and diminished powers.

The expression of the author, added in a subsequent edition, that mercury " at the same time shall be curing the venereal disease effectually," must be understood as referring to the absence of ptyalism, and not to the existence of the poisonous effects of

§. 2. *Of the Quantity of Mercury necessary to be given.*

The quantity of mercury to be thrown into the constitution for the cure of any venereal complaint must be proportioned to the violence of the disease. Two circumstances are, however, to be strictly attended to in the administration of this medicine; which are, the time in which any given quantity is to be thrown in, and the effects it has on some parts of the body, as the salivary glands, skin, or intestines. These two circumstances, taken together, are to guide us in the cure of the disease; for mercury may be thrown into the same constitution in very different quantities so as to produce the same ultimate effect; but the two very different quantities must be also in different times. For instance, one ounce of mercurial ointment, used in two days, will have more effect upon the constitution than two ounces used in ten; and to produce the same effect in the ten days, it may perhaps be necessary to use three ounces or more.

The effects on the constitution of one ounce used in two days are considerable, and also its effects upon the diseased parts; therefore a much less quantity in such a way will have greater effects. But if these effects are principally local, that is, upon the glands of the mouth, the constitution at large not being equally stimulated, the effect upon the diseased parts must also be less, which is to be determined by the local disease not giving way in proportion to the effects of the mercury on some particular part.

If it is given in very small quantities, and increased gradually so as to steal insensibly on the constitution, its visible effects are less, and it is hardly conceivable how much may at last be thrown in without having any visible effect at all*.

These circumstances being known, it makes mercury a much more efficacious, manageable, and safe medicine than formerly it was thought to be; but unluckily its visible effects upon some particular parts, such

---

* To give an idea of this, ten grains of the ointment used every day, during ten days, affected a gentleman's mouth. The ointment was of equal parts of mercury and hogs-lard. But, by means of omitting the ointment occasionally, and returning to the use of it, he at last rubbed in eighty grains every night for a month, without having his mouth, or any of the secretions, visibly affected.

---

the remedy. Experience fully proves that these poisonous effects are altogether inconsistent with its action as an anti-venereal; and that perseverance in its use, after they have shown themselves, while it exposes the patient to imminent danger, at the same time in no degree answers the object of the surgeon in the removal of the disease for which it is given.]

as the mouth and the intestines, are sometimes much more violent than
its general effect upon the constitution at large; therefore a certain
degree of caution is necessary not to stimulate these parts too quickly,
as that will prevent the necessary quantity being given.

The constitution, or parts, are more susceptible of mercury at first
than afterwards: if the mouth is made sore, and allowed to recover, a
much greater quantity may be thrown in a second time, before the same
soreness is produced; and indeed I have seen cases where it could not
be reproduced by as much mercury as possibly could be thrown in.
Upon a renewal of the course of mercury therefore the same precautions are not necessary as at first. We are, however, every now and
then deceived by this medicine, it being hardly possible to produce
visible effects at one time; and afterwards the mouth and intestines
shall all at once be affected.

Mercury, when it falls on the mouth, produces in many constitutions
violent inflammation, which sometimes terminates in mortification. The
constitutions in which this happens I suspect are of the erysipelatous
kind, or what are called the putrid; therefore in such greater caution
is necessary. Mercury in general, that is, where it only produces its
common effects, seldom or never does any injury to the constitution;
it should seem only to act for the time, and to leave the constitution in
a healthy state. But this is not always the case, for probably mercury
can be made to affect every constitution very materially, being capable
of producing local diseases, as has been mentioned, and also capable of
retarding the cure of chancres, buboes, and certain effects of the lues
venerea, after the poison has been destroyed.

§. 3. *Of the sensible Effects of Mercury upon Parts.*

The sensible effects of mercury are generally an increase of some of
the secretions, a swelling in the salivary glands, and increase of saliva;
an increase of the secretion of the bowels, which produces purging, and
an increase of the secretion of the skin producing sweat, also often an
increase of the secretion of urine. Sometimes one of these secretions
only is affected, sometimes more, and sometimes all of them together;
but the effects upon the mouth are the most frequent.

Mercury often produces headaches, and also costiveness, when its action on other parts becomes sensible, especially upon the glands of the
mouth.

When the mercury falls upon the mouth, it does not affect all parts
of it equally, sometimes attacking the gums, at other times the cheeks,

which become thickened and ulcerate, while the gums are not in the least affected, as appears by the patient being capable of biting any-thing hard.

Mercury, when it falls upon the mouth, and parts belonging to the mouth, not only increases the discharge of those parts, but it brings on great tumefaction, which is not of the true inflammatory kind, where coagulable lymph is thrown out, but rather resembling erysipelatous tumefaction. The tongue, cheeks, and gums swell, and the teeth be-come loose ; all which effects are in proportion to the quantity of mer-cury given, and susceptibility of the parts for such irritation. It pro-duces great weakness in the parts, in which ulceration easily takes place, especially if they are in the least irritated, which is often done by the teeth, and even mortification sometimes ensues. How far it produces similar effects when it falls on other parts, I do not know. The saliva, in such cases, is generally ropy, as if principally from the glands affected. The breath acquires a particular smell *.

As mercury generally produces evacuations, it was naturally imagined that it was by this means that it effected a cure of the venereal disease; but experience has taught us that, in curing the venereal disease by this medicine, evacuations of any kind produced by it are not at all neces-sary. And this might have been supposed, as similar evacuations, pro-duced by other medicines, are of no service ; therefore it was reason-able to imagine that these evacuations, when produced by mercury, were also of no service, except we could suppose that the evacuation produced by the mercury was not the same with that produced by other medicines, but that it was a specific evacuation; that is to say, a discharge carry-ing off the venereal poison by its union with the mercury, and therefore the faster the mercury went off the sooner would the poison be carried out of the constitution. But this is not found to be the case in prac-tice : on the contrary, evacuations produced by the medicine retard the cure, especially if the secretory organs are too susceptible of this sti-mulus; for then the quantity which is necessary or sufficient for the cure of the disease cannot be taken in, the effects of the medicine upon particular parts being greater than the patient can bear ; and the quan-tity of mercury to be thrown into the constitution must be limited and regulated according to the quantity of evacuation, and not according to the extent of the disease. On the other hand, if it is given with care,

* Added : " A person could not have mercury applied externally without its occa-sioning violent inflammation. He could take ten or twelve grains of the mercurius calcinatus every day without affecting his bowels or mouth, but it affected his head, so that he could hardly walk; and, to use his own expression, he did not know ' whether his head was off or on.' "—*Home.*

so as to avoid violent evacuation, any quantity may be thrown in sufficient for the cure of the disease.

Certain evacuations may be supposed to be a mark of the constitutional effects of mercury, but they are not to be entirely depended upon,
the secretions being only a proof of the susceptibility of some parts to
such a stimulus; however, it is probable that in general they are a good
gauge of its constitutional effects. Some have gone so far as to suppose that quantity of mercury alone, without any sensible effects, is
sufficient for the cure of the disease; and this is in some degree the case,
but not completely so, for we have no good proof of its affecting the
constitution but by its producing an increase of some of the secretions.

§. 4. Of the Action of Mercury.

Mercury can have but two modes of action, one on the poison, the
other on the constitution: we can hardly suppose it to act both ways.
If mercury acted upon the poison only, it might be supposed to be in
two ways, either by destroying its qualities by decomposing it, or by
attracting it and carrying it out of the constitution. If the first were
the action of mercury, then we might reasonably suppose that quantity
alone would be the thing to be depended upon; if the second, that the
quantity of evacuation would be the principal circumstance.

But if it act upon the principle of destroying the diseased action of
the living parts, counteracting the venereal irritation by producing
another of a different kind, then neither quantity alone, nor evacuation,
will avail much; but it will be quantity joined with sensible effects that
will produce the quickest cure, which from experience we find to be the
case. But although the effects that mercury has upon the venereal disease are in some degree in proportion to its local effects on some of the
glands, or some particular part of the body, as the mouth, skin, kidneys and
intestines, yet it is not exactly in this proportion, as has been mentioned.
When mercury disagrees as it were constitutionally, producing great
irritability and hectic symptoms, this action or irritation is not a coun-
ter-irritation to the venereal disease, but is a constitutional irritation
having no effect on the disease, which continues to increase. Mercury,
losing its effects upon the disease by use, gives a proof that it neither
acts chemically, nor by carrying off the poison by evacuation, but by its
stimulating power.

The effects will always be in proportion to the quantity in a given
time, joined with the susceptibility of the constitution to the mercurial
irritation. These circumstances require the minutest attention; and in

order to procure its greatest action with safety, and to procure this in the most effectual way, it must be given till it produces local effects somewhere, but not too quickly, that we may be able to throw in a proper quantity ; for local effects produced too quickly prevent the sufficient quantity being thrown in for counteracting the venereal irritation at large. I have seen cases where the mercury very readily acted locally, and yet the constitution was hardly affected by it, for the disease did not give way.

A gentleman had a chancre which he destroyed with caustic, and dressed the sore with mercurial ointment. He had also a slight uneasiness in one of his groins, which went no further, but which showed an absorption of the poison. The chancre soon healed, and he rubbed in about two ounces of mercurial ointment. He began this course with small quantities, that is, a scruple at each rubbing, and increased it; however, it soon affected his mouth, and he spit for about a month. Two months after he had a venereal ulcer in one of his tonsils. Here was a considerable sensible effect from a small quantity of mercury, which proved ineffectual, because its specific effects, as I apprehend, were not in proportion to its sensible effects, the salivary glands being too susceptible of the mercurial irritation.

On the other hand, I have seen cases where quantity did not answer, till it was given so quickly as to affect the constitution in such a manner as to produce local irritation, and consequently sensible evacuations, which is a proof that the local effects are often the sign of its specific effects on the constitution at large, and shows that the susceptibility of the diseased parts to be affected by the medicine is in proportion to the effects of it upon the mouth. Its effects are not to be imputed to evacuation, but to its irritation ; therefore mercury should be given, if possible, so as to produce sensible effects upon some parts of the body, and in the largest quantity of mercury that can be given to produce these effects within certain bounds; and these sensible effects should be the means of determining how far the medicine may be pushed, in order to have its best effects upon the disease without endangering the constitution. The practice here must vary according to circumstances ; and if the disease is in a violent degree, less regard must be had to the constitution, and the mercury is to be thrown in in larger quantities; but if the disease be mild it is not necessary to go beyond that rule, although it is better to keep up to it on purpose to cure the disease the sooner.

If the disease is in the first order of parts, a less quantity of mercury is necessary than if it were in the second order of parts, and had been of long standing, with its first appearances only cured, and the venereal disposition still remaining in the secondary parts. To cure the disease, whether in the form of chancre, bubo, or lues venerea, probably the same quantity of mercury is necessary, for one sore requires as much mercury as fifty sores in the same person, and a small sore as much as a large one; the only difference, if there is any, must depend upon the nature of the parts affected, whether naturally active or indolent. If there be any material difference between the recent and constitutional, which, I apprehend, there is, it may make a difference in the quantity. I do conceive that the recent are upon the whole more difficult to cure; at least they commonly require longer time, although not always.

Having thus far premised these general rules and observations, I shall now give the different methods of administering mercury.

§. 5. Of the different methods of giving Mercury—externally—internally.

Previously to the giving of mercury it is very proper to understand, as much as possible, the constitution of the patient with regard to this medicine, which can only be known in those who have already gone through a mercurial course; but as many of our patients are obliged to undergo this treatment more than once, it becomes no vague inquiry; for as there are many who can bear this medicine much better than others, it is very proper that this should be known, as it will be a direction for our present practice. I think that few constitutions alter in this disposition, although I knew one case which admitted of a considerable quantity at one time without being visibly affected; but about a twelvemonth after the patient was affected with a very little.

When mercury is given to cure the lues venerea, whatever length we mean to go in the sensible effects of it, we should get to that length if possible, and we should keep up to it. For we shall find it difficult to bring its effects to that standard again if we allow it to get below it. If the mercury should get beyond what we intended, we should be very much upon our guard in lowering it, and should probably begin to give it again before its effects are reduced to the intended standard: for the same quantity now will not operate so powerfully as before, insomuch that what at first produced greater effects than was intended will not be sufficient afterwards.

Mercury is best applied externally in form of an ointment. Unctuous substances keep it divided, attach it to surfaces, and do not dry; it may also be supposed that they become a vehicle for the mercury, and carry it through the absorbents to the general circulation; for it is probable that oil is as easy of absorption as watery substances.

If the symptoms are mild in the first order of parts, and the patient not accustomed to mercury, or it is known that he cannot bear the medicine in great quantity, and it is intended to conduct the cure by almost insensible means, it is proper to begin with small quantities. One scruple, or half a drachm, of an ointment made of equal parts of quicksilver and hog's lard, rubbed in every night for four or six nights, will be sufficient to begin with. If the mouth is not affected the quantity may be gradually increased, till two or three drachms are rubbed in at each time; but if the first quantity has affected the mouth, we may be almost certain that the glands of the mouth are very susceptible of the mercurial stimulus; therefore it will be proper to wait two or three days till that effect begins to go off.

When we begin the second time, the quantity may be gradually increased, at least a scruple every time, till two drachms or more are rubbed in each night, which may be done without affecting the patient very considerably a second time, as has been already observed.

If all the symptoms gradually disappear, there is no more to be done but to continue this practice for a fortnight longer by way of security.

This method, steadily pursued, will cure most recent cases of lues venerea, but it is not sufficient if the disease has been merely kept under by slight courses of mercury; a greater quantity becomes necessary, from a kind of habit the constitution has acquired, by which it is rendered less susceptible of the mercurial stimulus.

If the disease should return in the second order of parts, we may be certain the same quantity of mercury will not be sufficient to cure them, their action being slow under the venereal irritation, therefore requiring more than what had been first given.

I may be allowed to remark, that where the venereal symptoms have been ulcers in the mouth or throat, I have suspected that the mercury being brought to the mouth, and the saliva being impregnated with it, and acting as a mercurial gargle, cured those parts locally, and that the constitution has remained still tainted, the mercurial action in it having been much inferior to what it was in the mouth. Perhaps something similar may take place in eruptions of the skin where the mercury passes off by sweat: for we know that sulphur will cure the itch by passing off in perspiration. If these are facts, then it may in some degree account for the local symptoms in the first order of parts being easier of cure than those in the second*.

---

* Added: "After venereal blotches on the skin have been removed by mercury they sometimes recur afterwards, which has led many to have recourse to mercury again; but the proper practice is to desist some time, to see what becomes of them, as they often disappear again spontaneously; but as in some they may be a recurrence of the disease, in such mercury must be given."—*Home.*

The manner of living under a mercurial course need not be altered from the common, because mercury has no action upon the disease which is more favoured by one way of life than another.   Let me ask any one what effect eating a hearty dinner and drinking a bottle of wine can have over the action of mercury upon a venereal sore, either to make it affect any part sensibly, as falling upon the glands of the mouth, or prevent its effect upon the venereal irritation ?   In short, I do not see why mercury should not cure the venereal disease under any mode whatever of regimen or diet*.

I own, however, that I can conceive cold affecting the operations of mercury upon the venereal disease ; it is possible that cold may be favourable to the venereal irritation, and therefore contrary to that produced by mercury ; and there is some show of reason for supposing this, for I have before asserted that cold was an encourager of the venereal irritation ; and therefore keeping the patient warm may diminish the powers of the disease while under the cure.

Mercury given internally is in many cases sufficient, although in general it is not so much to be depended on as the external application ; therefore I would not recommend it, or give it in cases where the disease has not been sufficiently cured by former courses of mercury†. It is the most convenient way of giving this medicine, for many will swallow a pill who do not choose to rub the body with the ointment ; indeed there are many circumstances in life which make this mode of introducing it into the constitution the most convenient; but, on the other hand, there are many constitutions that cannot bear mercury given internally.   When these two circumstances meet in the same patient it is unfortunate.

Mercury taken internally often produces very disagreeable effects upon the stomach and intestines, causing sickness in the one, and griping and purging in the other.

If it be found necessary to give it internally, and it disagrees either with the stomach or intestines, or both, even in the most simple preparation, its effects, whatever they are, must be corrected or prevented, by joining with the mercury other medicines.   If it affect the stomach only, the mercury may be joined with small quantities of the essential oils, as the essential oil of cloves, or camomile flowers, which will in many cases take off that effect.   If it disagree both with the stomach and bowels, I believe it arises either from the mercury meeting with an acid in the stomach, by which part of it is dissolved, forming a salt, or from being given in the form of a salt, both of which will generally

* The last sentence omitted.—*Home.*
† The last part of the preceding sentence, beginning at "although," omitted.—*Home.*

purge, and become the cause of their own expulsion. There are two ways of obviating these effects; the first is by preventing the salt from forming; the second, by mitigating its effects on the intestines if formed, by taking off their irritability. To prevent the salt from forming, the best way is to join the mercury with alkaline substances, either salts, or earths; and when given in a saline state it may be joined with opium, or some of the essential oils.

To prevent the formation of the salt, take of the preparations of mercury, such as mercurius calcinatus, mercurius fuscus, or calomel, forming them into pills, with the addition of a small quantity of soft soap, or any of the alkaline salts; the alkaline salt also prevents the pill from drying: or instead of these a calcareous earth may be joined with the mercury, such as chalk or crabs'-eyes: upon this principle is the mercurius alkalizatus, which is crude mercury rubbed down with crabs'-eyes. But these substances add considerably to the bulk of the medicine, no less than twenty grains being necessary for a dose, which contains seven grains and a half of crude mercury. The mercurius calcinatus, rubbed with a small portion of opium, makes an efficacious pill, and in general agrees well both with the stomach and bowels. Opium has long been joined with mercury to cure the venereal disease. By some as much has been attributed to the opium as the mercury; however, opium should be given with care, for it is not every constitution with which it agrees, often producing irritability, in some lassitude and debility, in others spasms.

If the mercury is not given in the above manner, but in the form of a salt, or the salts are allowed to form, then it should be joined with one third of opium, and a drop of the oil of cloves, or camomile, which will make it agree with the stomach, and prevent its purging; or, if it is found still to disagree both with the stomach and bowels, compound it still further, by joining with the mercury the alkaline salts, the opium, and some essential oil.

A grain of mercurius calcinatus made into a pill, with the addition of such medicines as the stomach or bowels may require, may be given every night for a week, and if in that time it has not affected the mouth, it may be repeated evening and morning; and after the patient has been accustomed to the medicine, and it is found not to fall much upon the mouth, it may be increased to two grains in the evening, and one in the morning.

The same directions hold equally good either with the mercurius fuscus, or calomel; but it requires more of these last preparations of mercury to have the same medicinal effect upon the disease than of the before-mentioned; perhaps the proportion of their effects are about two

or three to one.   Why this should be the case is probably not easily
accounted for, the quantity of mercury being very nearly the same in a
given weight in both, for in eight grains of calomel there are seven
grains of crude mercury.   Three grains of these preparations appear
only equal to one of the mercurius calcinatus.   The crude mercury
given in the same quantities with either of the former appears the least
efficacious of all; for fifteen grains of crude mercury rubbed down with
any mucilage, seems only equal to one or two of the mercurius calcinatus.

The corrosive sublimate, which is a salt capable of stimulating violently, is generally given in solution in common water, brandy, or some
of the simple waters, and has been used with the appearance of considerable success.   It would appear that it removes ulcers in the mouth
as soon, if not sooner, than any of the other preparations; but this I
suspect arises from its application to these parts in its passage to the
stomach, acting upon them locally as a gargle.   However, from experience, it appears not to have sufficient powers over the venereal irritation; in recent cases only removing the visible local effects, without
entirely destroying the venereal action : for many more have been found
to relapse after having taken this preparation than from many of the
others, which is owing to its passing very readily off by the skin.   Besides, it disagrees much more with the stomach and intestines than any
of the other preparations.

A grain of this medicine, dissolved in about an ounce of some fluid,
is generally the dose, and increased according as it agrees with the
bowels, and according to its effects upon the mouth and disease[a].

---

[a] [The passage stands thus in every edition, and yet there must be some error, for
the dose is larger than has ever been recommended by practitioners deserving of credit,
and could not be taken without danger.   The usual quantity is from a quarter of a
grain to half a grain in the course of the day, and even this is generally divided into
at least two doses.

But larger quantities of corrosive sublimate may be given with safety, if proper precautions are used.   The object is that it should be introduced into the system, without
producing any irritation on the surfaces which immediately absorb it.   And this object
is best answered by administering it in the form of a pill, and by giving it at the time
of meals, so that it may mix with the food, and its acrid qualities may be corrected by
dilution.   It will be found that corrosive sublimate may be given in this way, in the
dose of one third of a grain, three times in the day, or of one grain daily, without more
inconvenience, or more risk of derangement of the stomach or bowels, than is incurred
from the ordinary doses, given without these precautions.

An opinion prevails that a course of corrosive sublimate gives the patient little security against a relapse.   The observation applies chiefly to the smaller doses of the remedy, which scarcely admit of the introduction of a sufficient quantity of the mercury,
unless the course be very greatly prolonged.   If it be given in the dose which is men-

As corrosive sublimate contains an acid, and as you must be guided by the effects of the acid on the bowels, the quantity of mercury you can give in this form is necessarily smaller than in the other preparations. Ward's drop, containing less acid, can be given in larger quantity, and is more efficacious on that account. Perhaps any of these preparations united with a scruple of gum guaiacum may have more effect than when given alone, since guaiacum is found to have considerable effects on the venereal disease *.

This practice, continued for two months, will in general cure a common lues venerea; but here it is not meant that any time should be specified. After all the symptoms of the disease have disappeared, this course should be continued at least a fortnight longer; but if the symptoms disappear very suddenly, as they often do, perhaps within eight or ten days, probably from the medicine going off by those surfaces where the disease appears, the medicine should be continued three weeks, or perhaps a month, longer, and the dose increased. In such cases the visible local effects appear to be cured, while a venereal disposition remains in the parts.

Various are the preparations of mercury recommended for internal use, while practitioners have generally been satisfied with but one for external application. Every practitioner finds some one of the preparations answering better to appearance in some one case than another, which casts the balance in favour of that medicine in his mind; or others, finding the bad effects of a particular preparation at one time, have generally condemned that preparation; not to mention that deceit is often practised in the cure of this disease. One would naturally suppose that the simplest preparation is the best, that which is easiest dissolved in the animal juices, does least mischief to the stomach or general health, and is least disturbed or hindered in its operations; for we can hardly suppose that any substance joined with mercury, which alters either its chemical or mechanical properties out of the body, can add to its power in the body, except a substance which had a similar power when acting alone. The preference generally given to the ointment shows this; and if we could find a preparation still more simple than the ointment, that preparation should be used in preference to the crude mercury.

* See pages 456, 457.

---

tioned above, and if the course can be continued for the usual period, without interruption from its effects on the bowels, or the mouth, it may be doubted whether relapses are more frequent than after the exhibition of other preparations of mercury.]

§. 6. *Of the Cure of the Disease in the second or third Stage.*

In the more advanced stages of the disease the mercurial course must be pushed further. The greatest quantity of that medicine that the patient can bear at a time is to be thrown in, and continued with steadiness till there is great reason to suppose the disease is destroyed. It will not be possible in such cases to prevent the mouth from being considerably affected, the quantity of mercury necessary to be used for the cure of these stages of the disease being such as will in most cases produce that effect.

Before the disease has advanced so far the patient most probably has taken mercury, and it is proper to inquire how he has been affected by it, and what quantity of it he can bear, which will in some degree direct us in the quantity now to be begun with. If the patient has not taken mercury for a considerable time, and is easily affected by it, which is the case that admits of the least quantity, it will be necessary to begin cautiously, regulating the quantity according to circumstances; but if the person has taken mercury lately, although easily affected by it, more freedom may be used on returning to it, because it will have less power on his mouth, as also on the disease. Again, if the person has been taking mercury very lately, and is with difficulty affected by it, which is the case that admits of the greatest quantity, then it may be administered freely so as to affect the constitution in the proper time. If the mercury is brought to the mouth in six or eight days, and a considerable soreness is produced in twelve, it will in general be a good beginning. In such cases the constitution is, if possible, to be surprised by the medicine so as to produce its greatest effects, but with such caution as to be able to keep up these effects by quantity.

Mercurial friction will answer better than mercury given internally; for in this way we are surer of throwing in a larger quantity in a given time than could be taken internally without hurting the stomach.

The quantity of mercury applied in this way should be, under certain circumstances, in proportion to the surface on which it is applied, and the surface should be completely covered with the ointment; for half an ounce of mercurial ointment, rubbed in upon a given surface, will have nearly the same effect as one ounce rubbed in on the same surface; therefore one ounce to have double the effect should have double the surface. The quantity of ointment must therefore be adapted to the quantity of surface, for on a certain extent of surface no more than a determined quantity of ointment can be applied so as to be absorbed, and applying a greater quantity would be useless; and if the quantity of surface is greater, the same portion of ointment cannot be diffused so as to employ fully all the absorbents. Every surface which is used may therefore have its full quantity of ointment, but certainly should not have more, if we are to attribute the effects of the mercury to the quantity.

It has most probably been always the practice to rub the mercury well in, as it is termed; but I suspect that this arose rather from an idea of the surface being porous like a sponge than of absorption being performed by the action of vessels; and it is probable that this action in the vessels producing absorption may be rather disturbed than excited by friction.

How long the course is to be followed is not to be exactly ascertained : it may be thought proper to continue it till the local appearances, as nodes, have subsided; but I suspect that this is hardly necessary, except they give way readily, for in such cases the local complaints, or tumefaction, &c., generally require a longer time to be removed than. the venereal action; and local applications must be of service, especially if such tumefactions are obstinate.

The manner of living under such a severe course, which is in every respect weakening, is to be particularly attended to. The patient must be supported; and the local effects of the medicine, in the mouth, preventing his taking many kinds of nourishment, especially such as are of a solid form, fluids must form his only nourishment, and these should be such as will become solid after they are swallowed : milk is of this kind. An egg beat up with a little sugar, and a little wine, sago, salep, &c. form a proper diet. In many cases wine and bark must be given through the whole course. Sugar is perhaps one of the best restoratives of any kind we are acquainted with, when a constitution has been very much debilitated by long fasting, from whatever cause, whether from the want of food when in health, or in the time of disease, or where the food has not been allowed to answer the constitutional waste, as in a course of mercury; and when the disease or course of mercury. is gone, then sugar will restore such constitution, probably better than anything else.

Although it is not a common opinion, and therefore not a common practice, to give sugar entirely with this view, yet there are sufficient proofs of its nutritive quality over almost every other substance. It is a well-known fact that all the negroes in the sugar islands become extremely lusty and fat in the sugar-cane season; and they hardly live upon anything else. The horses and cattle that are allowed to feed upon them all become fat; the hair of the horse becomes fine. Birds which feed upon fruit never eat it till it becomes very ripe, when it has formed the greatest quantity of sugar, and even then only such as furnish the largest quantity of sugar. Insects do the same; but we cannot have a stronger instance of this fact than in the bee. Honey is composed of sugar, with some other juices of plants, with a little essential oil; but sugar is the principal ingredient. When we consider that a swarm of bees will live a whole winter on a few pounds of honey, keep up a constant heat about ninety-five or ninety-six degrees, and the actions of the animal œconomy equal to that heat, we must allow that sugar contains perhaps more real nourishment than any other known substance.

We see too that whey is extremely fattening, which is the watery part of the milk, containing neither the oil nor the coagulable matter : this arises principally from the sugar it contains, for being composed of the watery part it holds all the sugar of the milk in solution. If the milk is allowed to become sour it is not so fattening, because it is the sugar which is become sour.

Although the nutritive qualities of sugar have not been so generally known as to introduce it into universal practice, yet they have not entirely escaped the notice of practitioners. Mr. Vaux, from observing the negroes in the West Indies growing fat in the sugar season, has been induced to give it in very large quantities to many of his patients, and with very good effects. Honey is perhaps as good a mode of taking this substance as any. Sweetening everything that is either eat or drunk, whether by sugar in honey or sugar alone, is probably immaterial. Yet it is probable that the other ingredients in honey may add to its nutritive quality.

§. 7. *Of Local Treatment.*

If the local effects have gone no further than inflammation and swelling, either of the soft or hard parts, most probably no local treatment will be necessary, for the treatment of the constitution will in general remove them entirely.

It sometimes, however, happens that the local complaints will not give way, but the parts remain swelled in an indolent and inactive state, even after there is every reason for supposing the constitution is perfectly cured. In such cases the constitutional treatment is to be assisted by local applications of mercury to the part, either in the form of a plaster or ointment. The latter is by much the best mode. If these are not sufficient, as often happens, we must endeavour to destroy this disposition by producing an inflammation of another kind. I have seen a venereal node which gave excruciating pain cured by an incision only being made down to the bone the whole length of the node; the pain has ceased, the swelling has decreased, and the sore healed up kindly,

without the assistance of a grain of mercury. Blisters have been applied to nodes with success; they have removed the pains and diminished
the swellings; so far furnishing a proof that local treatment may assist
mercury in many cases.

This treatment has not only been used to assist mercury in those cases
where the medicine did not appear to be equal to the disease, but it has
been used at the commencement of the cure, and even before mercury
had been applied; but it was still thought necessary to go through the
same mercurial course as if nothing had been done to the local complaints.

It may be asked, What advantage arises from the incision or application of the blister? The advantage is immediate relief from violent
pains; and as there are two powers acting, it is natural to suppose the
cure will be more speedy.

After all the above-mentioned trials, it may happen that the local effects shall still remain, forming as it were a new disease, which mercury
may increase, and therefore other methods of cure may be tried, as will
be described hereafter.

§. 8. *Of Abscesses—Exfoliation.*

When an abscess forms in a node in the periosteum the bones are generally affected, and make part of the abscess. Great attention should
be paid to them, for suppurations in them are not like suppurations in
common abscesses; they are seldom produced from the true suppurative
inflammation, and therefore are slow in their progress, rarely producing
true matter, but a mucus, something resembling slime, which lies flat
upon the bone. This circumstance makes it difficult to determine when
suppuration has taken place, and in many cases to detect matter, even
where it is formed. Another circumstance, which renders the presence
of matter in such cases doubtful, is, that the progress of the disease is
generally checked very early by the use of mercury. This matter is
often reabsorbed during a mercurial course, and it is proper, particularly
in an early state of the complaint, to give it this chance; but if the absorption does not take place, and the complaint is in an advanced state,
it must be opened.

The surgical treatment of the parts under such circumstances is the
same as in other diseases of these parts; opening with great freedom is
absolutely necessary; for the more parts are exposed, the more inclin-
able they are in general to heal, and still more so here; for violence assists in destroying the venereal disposition. No skin covering a bone
should be removed from an abscess, especially in the lower extremities.

If the abscess is opened freely, and an exfoliation takes place, which is generally the case, it is to be treated as any other exfoliation. Exfoliations succeed much better here than in many other cases, because the disease from which they proceed can generally be corrected, which is not the case in many diseases of bones where exfoliation takes place. Cases, however, sometimes occur in which, after the venereal disposition has been corrected, another disease takes place in the bone, the nature of which will be explained when we shall consider the effects remaining after the disease is cured, and the diseases sometimes produced by the cure.

§. 9. *Of Nodes on Tendons, Ligaments, and Fasciæ.*

The observations made on the nodes of the periosteum and bones are applicable to swellings and suppurations of the ligaments and fasciæ; but it is still more difficult to ascertain the presence of matter in them than in the former.

When a thickening only of the ligaments or fasciæ is the consequence of the disease, it is very obstinate, as in many cases the diseased part may be cleared of all venereal taint and still the swellings remain. Blisters may often be applied here with success; but if they fail, then it will be absolutely necessary to make an incision into the part, to excite a more vigorous action; for although the complaint has nothing venereal in it, nor is any contamination to be feared from it in future, yet as it leaves often very obstinate and disagreeable swellings, which neither give way to medicine nor time, it is proper to use every means for their removal.

§. 10. *Of Correcting some of the Effects of Mercury.*

Formerly, when the management of mercury was not so well understood, nor its effects in this disease so well known as they are at present, it was generally supposed to act by evacuation from the salivary glands, and was therefore always given till that evacuation took place; and, as its effects in the cure were imagined to be in proportion to the quantity of this evacuation, it was pushed as far as possible without endangering suffocation. From this treatment it often happened in those constitutions which were very susceptible of the mercurial irritation, and in which the medicine produced much more violent effects on some particular secretions than could be wished, that recourse was obliged to be had to medicines correcting the effects of mercury, as these effects were often an hindrance to its being given in sufficient quantities for the cure of the disease.

I mentioned, when treating of the effects of mercury, that the sensible increase of the secretions produced by it were in the following order : first of saliva, then sweat, then urine, and often of the mucus of the intestines, producing purging; I also observed, that when any of those secretions became too violent, the hand of the surgeon was tied up till they were moderated. Attempts have been made to lessen those effects in two ways, either by the destruction of its power on the body in general, or by its removal, but neither of these means has succeeded. It never has once been thought necessary to attempt to lessen its powers on the organs of secretion, so as still to retain the same quantity in the constitution, or even to throw in more, which, if it could be effected, would be sometimes of great service; but as we are not yet acquainted with powers sufficient for these purposes, we are obliged to observe great caution in our mode of giving the medicine.

I have endeavoured to show that this medicine need not be given with a view to procure those evacuations, and that it may be given in any quantity without increasing either of those secretions in any evident degree; however, after every precaution we may still be deceived, and the medicine will every now and then produce greater effects than were intended. It is very necessary therefore to seek for a preventive of the effects of mercury, when likely to be too violent; or to remedy those effects when they have already taken place.

The common practice, when mercury produced violent effects upon the intestines, was to counteract these effects; but this was not done with a view to retain the mercury in the constitution, but to relieve the bowels that were suffering by the action of the medicine; whereas the proper practice would be to stop its progress here, as in every other outlet, that more mercury may be retained in the constitution.

Although these increased secretions arise from the constitution's being loaded with mercury, yet there is no danger in stopping them, for they do not arise from an universal disposition becoming a local or critical one; and therefore if such an action be checked or stopped in one place, it must necessarily fall upon some other; but it is from the part being more susceptible of this irritation than any other, and the quantity now in the constitution being equal to the susceptibility of the part; and therefore, though its effects are stopped here, it does not break out anywhere else, every other part being capable of supporting this quantity, and of remaining unaffected till more is thrown in.

When the mercury attacked the salivary glands, it increased that secretion so much as in some cases to oblige practitioners to administer such medicines as were thought likely to remove this new complaint. This susceptibility of the glands of the mouth, and the mouth in general, to be easily put into action by this medicine, was generally supposed to arise from a scorbutic constitution, to which most complaints of the mouth are attributed. I am of opinion that scrofulous people, and those of a lax and delicate habit, are more subject to have it fall on the mouth than those of a contrary temperament.

Purges were given upon a supposition that mercury could be carried off by the evacuation produced by them, and they were repeated according to the violence of the effects of the medicine and the strength of the patient; but I can hardly say that I ever have seen the effects of mercury upon the mouth lessened by purging, whether it arose spontaneously, was produced by purging medicines, or even when arising from the mercury itself. As this method was not found sufficient for the removal of the complaint, other medicines were tried; sulphur was supposed to be a specific for the removal of the effect of mercury. Whether this idea arose from practice or reasoning is not material*, but I think I have seen good effects from it in some cases. If we can suppose purging of any service, purging with sulphur would answer best, as it would exert its effects both as a purge and a specific.

Sulphur certainly enters the circulation as sulphur, because our sweat and urine smell of it; if it does not combine with the mercury, and destroy its properties as mercury, it is possible, agreeably to the opinion of those who first thought of giving it with this intention, that it may so combine as to form æthiops mineral, or something similar, for we know that the æthiops mineral, however formed, does not in general salivate. It is possible, too, that sulphur may act as a contrary stimulus to mercury, by counteracting the effects of it in the constitution. Sulphur has even been supposed to hinder the mercury from entering the circulation. Upon the whole, as these preparations of sulphur and mercury are still supposed to have good effects, and as I think I have seen good effects in other cases, we must either allow that they enter the circulation, or that their whole effects are on the stomach and intestines, with which the rest of the body sympathizes. The good effects from sulphur in lessening or altering the immediate effects of mercury, can only take place when that medicine is really in the constitution; therefore a distinction is to be made between such as arise immediately from mercury, and one continued from habit, after the mercury has been eva-

---

* Sulphur, united with any of the metals, probably destroys their solubility in the juices, or at least their effects in the circulation: none of the cinnabars act either as sulphur or mercury. Crude antimony, which is regulus and sulphur, has no effect. Arsenic, when joined with sulphur, has no effect; nor has iron.

cuated from the constitution ; a case that sometimes happens, and which will be taken notice of in its proper place[a].

The taste in the mouth, from the use of mercury, has been known to go off, and not be perceived for a fortnight, and the same taste has recurred : this I am informed has happened twice to one gentleman, from the first quantity of mercury taken.   To account for this is not easy ; in whatever way it happens, it is a curious fact.

When the mercury has fallen upon the mouth and throat, washing those parts with opium has often good effects ; for opium takes off irritability, and of course the soreness, which is one means of lessening the secretion.   A drachm of tinctura thebaica to an ounce of water makes a good wash or gargle*.

When the mercury falls upon the skin, it is neither so disagreeable nor so dangerous as when it falls upon the mouth ; however, it may often happen that it will be proper to check such a discharge, both upon account of its being troublesome, and of its lessening the effects of the medicine in the constitution, by carrying it off.   The bark is, perhaps, one of the best correctors of this increased secretion.

When the medicine attacks the kidneys and increases the secretion of those glands, it is not so troublesome as when it produces sweating, though it is possible that it may carry off the mercury too soon ; but as we have but few medicines that can lessen that secretion, in most cases it must be allowed to go on.   The bark may in such cases be given with advantage.

When the mercury falls upon the bowels, it proves often more dangerous and troublesome than in any of the former cases, especially the two last ; but it is, perhaps, most in our power to prevent or palliate. Opium should be given in such quantities as to overcome the complaint, and I believe will seldom fail of removing all the symptoms[b].

* My using opium in this way was from analogy. Finding that opium quieted the bowels when a purging came on in consequence of mercury, I tried it by way of gargle to the mouth, and found good effects from it, but not equal to those which it produced in the bowels.

---

[a] [Nitric acid has far more power than any other medicine in checking and curing soreness of the gums and ptyalism.]

[b] [Opium will often prevent the occurrence of disorder of the bowels from mercury ; but when dysenterical symptoms are actually present, it will seldom remove them unless it be preceded by a purgative.]

§. 11. *Of the Form of the different Preparations of Mercury when in the Circulation.*

It would appear from reason, and many circumstances, that mercury must be in the state of solution in the juices of the body before it can act upon the venereal disease, and indeed before it can act upon any other disease. That mercury is in a state of solution in our juices, and not in the state of any preparation of mercury that we know of, is very probable from the following facts.

First, crude mercury, every salt of mercury, and calx of mercury, is soluble in the spittle, when taken into the mouth, by which means it is rendered sensible to the taste; from thence it must appear that it is capable of solution in some of our juices.

Secondly, crude mercury, when divided into small parts by gum arabic, &c., so as to be easier of solution when taken into the stomach, generally purges; but crude mercury taken without such division has no such powers, not being so readily dissolved in the juices of the stomach. The simple calx of mercury has the same effects, purging, and much more violently, from being, I suppose, readier of solution in the animal juices; for if it only purged from its union with the acid which happened to be in the stomach, it most probably would not purge more than crude mercury; although it is very probable that the calx is easier of solution in a weak acid than even the crude mercury.

Thirdly, every preparation of mercury producing the same effect in the mouth, and also having one and the same effect in the constitution, shows that they must all undergo a change by which they are reduced to one particular form. We cannot say what that form is, whether it is the calx, the metal, or any other that we are acquainted with; but it is probable that it is not any of them, but a new solution in the animal juices peculiar to the animal itself. This is rendered still more probable by this circumstance, that every preparation of mercury put into the mouth undergoes the same change, and the spittle has the same taste from every one of them. If every different preparation of mercury had the same properties in the constitution that it possesses out of it, which we must suppose if it enters and continues in the same form, in that case the venereal poison must be eradicated in as many different ways as there are preparations. Crude mercury would act mechanically, by increasing the weight and momentum of the blood; the calx would act like brickdust, or any other powder that is heavy; the red precipitate would stimulate by chemical properties in one way, while the corrosive sublimate would act in another, and the mercurius flavus in a third;

this last would most probably vomit, as ipecacuanha does, which vomits whether thrown into the stomach or circulation.

Fourthly, all the preparations of mercury, when locally applied, act always in one way, that is, as mercury; but some have also another mode of action, which is chemical, and which is according to the specific nature of the preparation. The red precipitate is a preparation of this kind, and acts in both these ways: it is either a stimulant or an escharotic.

To ascertain whether this opinion of mercury being in solution in our juices was just, I made the following experiments upon myself. I put some crude mercury into my mouth, as a standard, and let it stay there, working it about, so as to render it easier of solution, till I tasted it sensibly; I then put into my mouth the mercurius calcinatus, and let it remain till I perceived the taste of it, which was exactly the same; but I observed that it was easier of solution than the crude mercury. I tried calomel in the same way, and also corrosive sublimate, after being diluted with water, and the taste was still the same. It was some time before I perceived the taste of the crude mercury in my mouth. I tasted the calx and calomel much sooner. The corrosive sublimate had at first a mixed taste, but when the acid was diluted it had exactly the same taste with the former: all these different preparations producing the same sensation or taste in the mouth.

From the effects of these experiments it would appear that the mercury in every one of them was dissolved in the spittle, and reduced to the same preparation or solution.

To try whether mercury in the constitution would produce the same taste in the mouth, I rubbed in mercurial ointment upon my thighs till my mouth was affected, and I could plainly taste the mercury; and, as far as I could rely upon my memory, the taste was exactly the same as in the former experiments.

I allowed some time for my mouth to get perfectly well and free from the taste; I then took calomel in pills till it was affected again in the same way. I afterwards took mercurius calcinatus, and also corrosive sublimate. All these experiments were attended with the same result; the mercury in every form producing the same taste, which was also exactly the same as when the several preparations were put into the mouth.

From the above experiments it must appear, that when mercury produces evacuation by the mouth it certainly goes off in that discharge; and from thence we may reasonably conclude, that when other evacuations are produced from the medicine when in the constitution, as purging, sweating, or an increased flow of urine, that it also goes off by these evacuations, which become outlets to the mercury.

From the above experiments it appears to be immaterial what preparation of mercury is used in the cure of this disease, provided it is of easy solution in our juices, the preparations easiest of solution being always the best.

§. 12. *Of the Operation of Mercury on the Poison.*

Mercury may be supposed to act in three different ways in curing the venereal disease. First, it may unite with the poison chemically, and decompose it, by which means its powers of irritation may be destroyed; secondly, it may carry it out of the constitution by evacuation; or, thirdly, it may produce an irritation in the constitution which counteracts the venereal and entirely destroys it.

It has been supposed that mercury acts simply by its weight in the circulating fluids, but of this we can form no adequate idea; and if it were so, other substances should act on this disease in proportion to their weight, and of course many of them should cure it. But from experience we find that such bodies as have considerable weight, as most of the metals, have no effect on this disease. We have no proof of mercury acting by a decomposition of the poison from any of the concomitant circumstances.

Mercury certainly does not cure the venereal disease by uniting with the poison and producing an evacuation. For in those cases where mercury is given in such a way as to produce considerable evacuations, or in those constitutions where evacuations are easily excited by mercury, its effects upon the diseased action are the least; and the same evacuations produced by any other means have not the least effect on the disease.

Whether the mercury be supposed to carry off the circulating poison or to decompose it, in neither way could it produce, when locally applied, any effect on a venereal inflammation or sore arising from the constitution; for as long as any of the poison existed in the circulation, none of them could be healed by local applications, the circulation constantly carrying the poison to them; but we find the contrary of this to be true, for a venereal sore arising from the constitution may be cured locally.

The last or third of our modes of action of mercury seems to me the most probable, and for many reasons. First, because the disease can in many cases be cured by raising a violent stimulus of another kind; and perhaps if we could raise such a constitutional irritation without danger, as we often can in local cases, we might cure the venereal disease in the same manner, and in one quarter of the usual time. Secondly, we find that mercury acts as an universal stimulus, causing great irritability in the constitution, making the heart beat faster, and rendering the arteries more rigid, so as to produce a hard pulse, as has been already observed. It may further be said to produce a disease, or a peculiar or unnatural mode of action, in a certain degree. The following case will illustrate this. A gentleman had electricity recommended to him for some complaint he had. The electricity was applied, but without any visible effect. Besides the complaint for which he used electricity, he had a venereal one, for which he was first put under a course of mercury, and while under it the electricity was applied for the former complaint; but he had become so irritable that he could not bear the shocks of one half their former strength. But the most curious part of the case was that the shocks had a much greater effect on the disease than what they had before when twice as strong, and he now got cured. This gave the surgeon a hint; and having another occasion to use electricity, also without effect, he put the patient under a gentle course of mercury, and then found the same effects from the electricity as in the former case, and the patient also got well.

The powers of mercury upon the constitution appear to be as the quantity of mercury and the susceptibility of the constitution to be affected with it, without any relation to the disease itself; and we find that the power of mercury upon the disease is nearly in the same proportion. This fact gives us an idea of the irritation of mercury upon the constitution, and consequently an idea of administering it, and of the cure of any disease for which it is a remedy.

As we find that a given quantity of mercury produces double effects in some constitutions to what it does in others; also, that in those cases it produces its effects upon the disease, we are led to believe that it is this effect upon the constitution which cures the disease; and therefore if it did not produce this effect it would also not have performed a cure. I have already observed that the cure does not go on exactly in proportion to the visible effects upon the constitution, except quantity in the medicine is joined with it, which, if true, would incline us to believe that there was something more than simply a constitutional stimulus, which most probably is a peculiar specific effect which is not regulated entirely by its visible effects, either constitutional or local, although they appear to have some connexion.

This fact being known, obliges us to be more liberal in giving mercury in those constitutions where it makes but little impression, than in those which it easily irritates; although in these last we must not be entirely regulated by its local effects, nor depend upon a commonly sufficient quantity, but be ruled by the sensibility of the constitution and quantity joined; for in those where the constitution appears to be very susceptible of the mercurial irritation, where small quantities pro- duce considerable local effects, it is still necessary to have quantity, al- though it is not so necessary to take the quantity in general that is sup- posed to be sufficient. We must be guided by the three following cir- cumstances, the disappearance of the disease, the quantity of irritation produced, and the quantity of the medicine taken.

§. 13. Of Gum Guaiacum and Radix Sarsaparillæ in the Ve- nereal Disease.

I have hitherto only recommended mercury in the cure of the vene- real disease, and indeed it is the only medicine to be depended upon. However, as both the guaiacum and sarsaparilla have been recommended as powerful remedies in this complaint, I took a favourable opportunity of trying their comparative powers in the venereal disease upon the same person.

The guaiacum* I found had considerable specific power over the dis- ease, consequently it may be of service in slight cases where it may be inconvenient or improper to give mercury on account of some other dis- ease. These cases, however, I have not yet ascertained: or it may be given in those cases where it is apprehended that the quantity of mer- cury necessary to subdue the disease would be too much for the consti- tution to bear, cases which sometimes occur. The sarsaparilla appeared to have no effect at all.

I shall relate exactly the case in which their comparative powers were tried. A man came into St. George's Hospital with venereal sores over almost his whole body: there were many excrescent sores in the arm- pits, some of which were about the size of a halfpenny; there were the same appearances about the anus, between the buttocks, along the pe- rinæum, between the scrotum and thigh, where those parts come in contact with one another. Those upon the skin in general had the common appearance. I ordered a poultice of the gum guaiacum to be applied to the sores in the right armpit; also a poultice of a strong de- coction of sarsaparilla and oatmeal, mixed, to be applied to the left armpit. These poultices were changed every day for a fortnight; the

* The lignum guaiaci was imported by the Spaniards from Hispaniola, as a cure for the venereal disease, in the year 1517, having been given to one of them by a native.

excrescent sores in the right armpit were entirely healed, and become even with the skin, and covered with a natural skin, although somewhat discoloured; the sores in the left armpit, which were poulticed with sarsaparilla, were rather worse than when the poultice was first applied, as indeed were all the sores, except those in the right armpit. I then ordered the poultice of guaiacum to be applied to the left armpit, which was done, and the sores there also got well in a fortnight. I was now perfectly convinced that the gum guaiacum had cured these eruptions locally.

I next wished to see what effect the gum guaiacum would have upon the remaining sores when given internally, that is, those about the anus, scrotum, and on the skin in general. The patient began with half a drachm three times every day, which purged him; but this was prevented by joining it with opium. In about four weeks all the eruptions were cured, and he was allowed to stay in the hospital some time longer, to see if he would continue well; but about a fortnight after he began to break out anew, and in a very short time was almost as bad as ever. I began a second time the gum guaiacum internally, but it had lost all its powers, or rather the constitution was no longer affected by it. He was put under a course of mercury. and cured[a].

CHAPTER IV.

OF THE EFFECTS REMAINING AFTER THE DISEASE IS CURED, AND OF THE DISEASES SOMETIMES PRODUCED BY THE CURE.

In treating of the local effects of the venereal disease, the gonorrhœa, and chancre, as also the bubo, I observed, that after the virus was destroyed there remained in many cases some of the same symptoms, and

---

[a] [For a detailed examination into the use of these and other remedies in the venereal disease, the reader is referred to "Observations on the effects of various articles of the Materia Medica in the cure of Lues Venerea," by John Pearson, a work which contains the result of a long and extensive experience, chiefly devoted to the investigation of this particular subject, and is in every part replete with excellent practical remarks.]

particularly after the gonorrhœa.　It was also observed, that though all the symptoms were entirely cured, yet they were liable to break out again.　A gleet will appear, sometimes attended with pain, so as to resemble a gonorrhœa; after chancres there will be sores resembling them; and buboes after the virus is gone, will not heal, but spread.　In the lues venerea the same thing often happens, especially if the inflammation and suppuration have been violent in the parts.　These cases puzzle considerably; for it is difficult to say when the venereal virus is absolutely gone.　In such doubtful cases the treatment to be followed becomes more undetermined.

Such complaints are more common in the tonsils than in any other part, for we often find that while a mercurial course is going on, and the ulcer on the tonsils healing, or even healed, they shall swell, become excoriated, and the excoriations shall sometimes spread over the whole palatum molle, which renders the nature of the disease doubtful.　I believe these excoriations, as well as such other appearances of disease as come on during the use of mercury, are seldom or never venereal.　In all such cases I would recommend not to continue the mercury longer than what appears sufficient for overcoming the original venereal complaints, not considering those changes in the case as venereal.　The bark is often of service here, and may be given either with the mercury, or after the mercurial course is over.

It often happens that venereal abscesses will not heal up, although they have gone a certain length towards it, for while the venereal action remained in the part, the mercury disposed that part to heal; but under that course the constitution and part had acquired another disposition, proceeding from a venereal and mercurial irritation affecting a particular habit of body or part, at the time, which new disposition differs from the venereal, mercurial, and natural, being a fourth disposition arising out of all the three.　I suspect, however, that it depends chiefly on the constitution, because if it was owing to the other two, we should always have the same disease; and what makes this opinion more probable is, that it differs in different people, at least it is not cured in all by the same means.　The constitution being predisposed, the other two become the immediate causes of action.　As soon as the venereal irritation is destroyed by the mercury, or becomes weaker than the other two, then the effects of the others take place.　While the venereal action prevails the mercury is of service, and the sore continues healing; but when it is lessened to a certain degree, or destroyed, the mercury not only loses its powers, but becomes a poison to the new disposition that is formed; for if mercury is continued, the sore spreads; it should therefore be immediately left off.

Some of the sores formed in this way not only resist all means of cure, but often inflame, ulcerate, and form hard callous bases, so as to put on the appearance of a cancer, and are often supposed really to be so.

We find also that new diseases arise from the mercury alone. The tonsils shall swell where no venereal disease has been before; the periosteum shall thicken, and also probably the bones, and the parts over them shall become œdematous and sore to the touch; but as these complaints arise while under a mercurial course, they are not to be reckoned venereal, but a new disease, although they are too often supposed to be venereal, and on that account the mercury is pushed as far as possible. In such cases, if the complaints for which the mercury was given are nearly cured, and the medicine has been continued a sufficient time after to complete the cure of those complaints, then of course it should be left off; and if there be any doubt, it should be left off rather sooner than if no such complaint had taken place, because it is probably producing a worse disease than the venereal; and if, after the cure of these complaints from the mercury, the venereal disease begins again to come into action, mercury must be given a second time; and now the constitution will be better able to bear it, especially if attention has been paid to the restoring the strength of it. Those diseases of the tonsils and periosteum I suspect to be of scrofulous origin.

Besides local complaints, arising from the combined action of the mercury, the disease, and the constitution, there is sometimes a constitutional effect, which is a weakness or debility, a languor, want of appetite, frequent sweats threatening hectic; but these happen mostly in those constitutions with which mercury disagrees. These complaints, local as well as constitutional, arise in some measure from weakness. They are difficult of cure, whether arising from a venereal chancre, bubo, or the lues venerea. Strengthening medicines are of most service : the bark is of great use, though in general not sufficient, as it can only more or less remove the weakness, the specific qualities still remaining. What these are is, I believe, not yet known; but I suspect that many partake of the scrofula, and this opinion is strengthened by their frequently giving way to sea-bathing*.

---

* In a case of an ulcerated rib from a venereal cause, and five nodes on the shin-bone, of twelve months' standing, a deep salivation of six months was undergone, after fruitless attempts by gentle friction. None of the sores were healed by the mercury, and the patient was ordered to bathe in the sea, and take the bark. In three or four months the sores all healed up very kindly, but the side the last of all.

§. 1. *General Observations on the Medicines usually given for the Cure.*

A decoction of the woods, among which are commonly included guaiacum and sarsaparilla, is one of the first medicines in the cure, and many of the cases yield to it, which gives them the credit of curing the venereal disease, while such diseases were supposed to be venereal. The sarsaparilla was often given alone, and was found to produce nearly the same effect. The good effects of it in one case gave it some reputation*. A diet-drink discovered at Lisbon was also of considerable service, and as it cured cases similar to those cured by the sarsaparilla, it was imagined that the diet-drink consisted principally of a decoction of this root. This was still on the supposition that all those cases were venereal; but it was observed at last that those medicines did not cure this disease till mercury had been given, and in tolerably large quantity. This was sufficient to lead some thinking minds to doubt whether they were venereal or not; and their being cured by different medicines ought to produce a conviction of their being different from the venereal disease, and that they are themselves of different kinds.

The mezereon has also been found to be of service in some symptoms of the lues venerea, such as nodes of the bones; but their being venereal was taken for granted. The mezereon is seldom given in venereal ulcers in the throat, or blotches on the skin, which, of all the venereal symptoms, are the most certain, and the most easy of cure; yet it was conceived that it removed such symptoms as are the most difficult of cure; but all those cases in which the mezereon has been given with success plainly appear not to have been venereal.

When the hemlock came into fashion in this country, it was given in almost every disease, and of course was tried in some of those complaints consequent to the venereal disease, and some of these it was found to cure, so that it now stands upon the list of remedies. Velno's vegetable syrup has had similar effects in some of these cases, and opium appears also to have many advocates. Opium, like the sarsaparilla and mezereon, was supposed by its first introducers to cure the lues venerea†, but, like the sarsaparilla, it appears to have no effect till mercury has done its best or its worst‡. It has certainly considerable effects in many

---

* See London Medical Essays, a case published by Mr. Fordyce, now Sir William Fordyce.

† See Medical Communications, vol. i. page 307.

‡ See a pamphlet published by Mr. Grant.

diseases, both in such as are consequent to the venereal disease, and others arising from other causes.

It has been long a favourite medicine of mine, not only as relieving pain, for that is its common effect, but as a medicine capable of altering diseased actions, and producing healthy ones. In all sores attended with irritability, a decoction of poppy heads, made into a poultice, is an excellent application. Bleeding sores that do not arise from weakness, but from irritability, have the bleeding stopped immediately by this application. Mr. Pott is, I believe, the first who showed the world its use in mortifications. My first mode of applying it for the cure of diseases was locally, in which I found it had most salutary effects in some cases, and it was ordered afterwards internally upon the same principle; and it was also found to have salutary effects in this mode. In two cases that had been long suspected to be venereal, its effects were very remarkable, and, by its having cured them, it confirmed me in my opinion that they were not. But when I was informed that they cured the venereal disease in the army in America by opium, I then began to question myself, whether I had formed a right judgment of the nature of those two cases which were cured by opium. To ascertain whether opium would cure the lues venerea or not, I made the following trial at St. George's Hospital.

A woman was taken into the hospital with blotches on her skin, which had arrived to the state of scabs, and with well-marked venereal ulcers on both tonsils. A grain of opium was ordered to be taken the first night, two the second, and so on, increasing a grain every night, unless something should arise to forbid it. This was closely followed till the nineteenth night, when she was ordered a dose of physic, as she had become costive, and the opium was omitted. On the 20th she began again, and continued increasing the dose, as before, till it amounted to thirty grains, no alteration being produced in the sores, except what arose from the loss of time, whereby they were rather worse. I concluded, that if she had taken mercury to affect the constitution as much as the opium did, the venereal disease must have been nearly cured, or at least much lessened; but as that was not the case, it convinced me that the opium had no effect whatever on the venereal disease. I then put her under a course of mercury, by friction, and in a short time it affected her mouth; the sores soon began to look better, and they went on healing without interruption, till the disease was cured. I may just observe, the inconvenience from the opium was not considerable, for although it kept her quiet, she was not constantly dosing.

Luke Ward was admitted into St. Bartholomew's Hospital, January 12, 1785; his complaint was an ulcer in the throat of three months' standing, which, both from its appearance, and the symptoms which preceded it, seemed to be venereal. He was ordered two grains of opium twice a day, which he took a few days without any other effect than that of sleeping better at night than usual, when the dose was increased to two grains three times a day. His throat now gave him less pain, but upon inspection was not found to be at all mended. After two days the dose was increased to three grains thrice a day ; from this quantity he felt little or no inconvenience : he complained of being a little drowsy ; his eyes were rather inflamed, and his face rather flushed. He continued to take this quantity for five days, and then it was increased to three grains four times a day. Next morning the redness and heat of his face were much increased, and had extended over his whole skin ; he complained of pain in his head. His pulse was full and strong; he was bound in his body, and his belly was tense and painful. The opium was omitted, and such remedies as the present symptoms seem to require were given, but without effect, all his symptoms continuing to increase till he died, which was on the fourth day after ; during this time the ulcer increased much, and the discharge of saliva was so great as to resemble a slight salivation.

This case proves, in the first place, that the opium had no effect upon the ulcer in the throat ; and, in the next, that it is a medicine capable of producing very violent effects on the skin, requiring therefore great caution in the mode of administering it.

John Morgan was admitted into St. Bartholomew's Hospital with an ulcerated leg. The common applications were tried for seven weeks, at the end of which time he was in every respect worse, having no sleep from constant pain, and he was sinking very fast. Two grains of opium were given every two hours for twenty-three days ; it made him hot and costive, and his pulse became strong and full, but without sleep or abatement of pain. The dose was increased to four grains every two hours in the day, and eight grains every two hours during the night. The effects were costiveness, retention of urine, loss of appetite, an inflammatory disposition, no sleep, without any amendment of the ulcer. On the third day of taking the last-mentioned quantities he awoke from a short sleep, delirious, and continued so for twelve hours, when it left him very weak, sick at his stomach, and with a low pulse. In three or four hours the delirium returned, and continued forty-eight hours ; the pulse, on its return, immediately rose, and his strength returned to a very great degree. When it went off he fell into a sound sleep for about eight hours, and awoke very tranquil, though weak ; no more opium was given, and the leg in the space of a month healed.

In the first twenty-three days he took twenty-four grains a day ; for the last three days he took seventy-two grains a day. In twenty-six days he took seven hundred and sixty-eight, which is nearly two ounces of opium.

Sarsaparilla, from the comparative experiment made with it and the guaiacum, would appear to have no effect upon the venereal irritation itself, and therefore can be of no service till that irritation is destroyed; and as mercury is the antidote to that poison, and becomes one of the causes of the complaints in which sarsaparilla is useful, therefore mercury is not only necessary to destroy the poison, but also assists in forming the diseases we are now treating of.

It is easy to conceive it in many cases to be of use in preventing the formation of the disease arising from mercury. When given along with the mercury it is often joined with the gum guaiacum, or the wood of the guaiacum, which we know will have some effect.

The sarsaparilla is generally given in form of a decoction, three ounces to three pints of water, boiled down slowly to a quart, and the half or whole is drunk every day, generally at three different times, often at meals. It is sometimes ground to a powder and taken every day with the same effect; but I should prefer the extract made into pills, as the easiest way of taking this medicine.

In many of these cases I have seen good effects from the hemlock, of which the following is an instance; and I would further refer the reader back to my observations on this medicine, which I gave when treating of the disease produced in consequence of a bubo, p. 380.

A poor woman had undergone repeated salivations, which had always relieved the most pressing symptoms; but after that she was afflicted more or less for three or four years, ulcers broke out in her nose, and all over her face, with what is called a true cancerous appearance. The sores became soon very deep, and gave very considerable pain. Mercury, sarsaparilla, and bark were given, without effect; the sores getting daily worse, the parts affected were ordered to be held over the steam of a decoction of hemlock every four hours, and as much extract to be taken internally as the patient could bear. She had sleep, and was free from pain the first night; and in a few days the sores put on a healing appearance. She lost her nose and one side of her mouth; but in six weeks' time every part was skinned over. She remained well for three months, when the disease returned with redoubled violence, and soon destroyed her.

§. 2. *Of the Continuance of the Spitting.*

It sometimes happens that the spitting continues after there is every reason for supposing the mercury to be entirely out of the constitution. As it is only a continuation of an action, or an effect of mercury having been in the constitution, it is necessary to distinguish it from the original, or from the immediate effect of mercury ; since on this distinction rests the method of cure. Such constitutions have been generally supposed scorbutic ; and where there is a great susceptibility of the mercurial stimulus in these parts, the salivation will continue for months after the mercury has been completely removed ; but this medicine not being given now in quantity sufficient to produce such violent effects on the salivary glands, these cases seldom occur.

In such cases I would recommend strengthening diet and strengthening medicines. Sea-bathing is one of the best restoratives of relaxed habits, especially after mercury. Mead's tincture of cantharides is supposed to be of service in those cases.

The alveolar processes have sometimes become dead, and exfoliations have taken place ; and this alone has kept up a discharge of saliva. When this happens we must wait till separation takes place, and extract the loose pieces, after which the salivation will subside.

I have seen part of the jaw exfoliate from this cause. In most cases the teeth become loose, and in many they drop out.

CHAPTER V.

OF PREVENTING THE VENEREAL DISEASE.

As diseases in general should not only be cured, but, when it is possible, prevented, it will not be improper to show, as far as we know, how that may be done ; for in this disease we can with more certainty prevent infection, its origin being known.

Preventives are previous or immediate applications, and may be divided into various kinds ; as those that will not allow the venereal matter to come in contact with the parts, those which wash it off before it stimulates, and those which will act chemically and destroy the poison.

Oils, rubbed on a dry part, stick to it and prevent anything that is watery from coming in contact with it; and, as the venereal poison is mixed with a watery fluid, it is not allowed to touch the part.

Everything which has a power of mixing with the venereal matter, and removing it from the part to which it is applied, may prove a prevention. Caustic alkali is the best for this purpose : it unites with the matter, forming a soap, and is then easily washed off.

It is possible this union with the alkali may destroy the poison : the alkali must be much diluted, or it will excoriate.

Lime-water would make a good wash.

If both these methods were put in practice there would be still more security.

Corrosive sublimate in water, about a grain or two to eight ounces, has been known to prevent the catching of the disease.

PART VII.

CHAPTER I.

OF DISEASES RESEMBLING THE LUES VENEREA, WHICH HAVE BEEN MISTAKEN FOR IT.

THERE is probably no one disease to which some other may not bear a strong resemblance in some of its appearances or symptoms, whereby they may be mistaken for each other. The situation of a complaint also may mislead the judgment. A lump, for instance, in the breast of a woman, may resemble a cancer so much as to be mistaken for one, if all the distinguishing marks of cancer are not well attended to. An ulcer on the glans penis, or in the throat and nose, creates a suspicion of the venereal disease. Even the way in which a disease is caught becomes a cause of suspicion. The fluor albus in women sometimes produces a simple gonorrhœa in men. Drinking out of the same cup with a venereal patient was formerly supposed to be capable of communicating the lues venerea, but this notion is I believe now exploded. Of late years a new mode of producing the venereal disease is supposed to have arisen; this is by the transplanting of a tooth from the mouth of one person into the mouth of another. That such practice has produced diseases is undoubted, but how far it has been venereal remains to be considered.

Diseases which resemble others seldom do it in more than one or two of the symptoms; therefore, whenever the nature of the disease is suspected, the whole of the symptoms should be well investigated, to see whether it agrees in all of them with the disease it is suspected to be, or only in part. This observation seems to be more applicable to the venereal disease than any other, for there is hardly any disorder that has more diseases resembling it in all its different forms than the venereal disease; and when a disease resembles the venereal in some of its symptoms, but not at all in others, then those other symptoms are to be set down as the specific or leading ones of the disease to which it belongs, the resembling symptoms to the venereal being only the common ones. But if a disease is suspected to be venereal, though it is not perfectly marked, yet if it resembles the venereal in most of its symptoms, it must be supposed to be venereal, that being the most probable, although it is by no means certain ; for probably the venereal can hardly be demonstrated in any case, especially in the form of the lues venerea, from its not having the power of contamination[a].

---

[a] [There has been much confusion respecting syphilitic and pseudo-syphilitic diseases, which would have been in a great measure avoided had due attention been paid to the obvious principles which should determine the identity or diversity of diseases. This confusion is in a very slight degree chargeable on Mr. Hunter. Yet there are a few instances where he seems to have been misled by preconceived opinions respecting the venereal disease, which a longer observation would have shown him were more than doubtful.

Diseases may be confounded with syphilis which have no connexion with any virus whatever. This is frequent in sores on the genitals, where superficial excoriations, which by proper treatment may be healed in three days, and herpetic vesicles, which exactly resemble in their appearance and course those which so frequently occur on the lips, have been often erroneously treated as venereal. The same observation applies with equal force to some forms of sore throat and cutaneous eruptions.

The existence of a morbid poison as the cause of lues venerea is inferred from two facts. In the first place the primary symptoms have been ascertained by long observation to be the consequence of communication with infected persons, and to be capable in the same way of infecting others. In the second place, these primary symptoms have been observed to be followed after an interval of time by secondary symptoms. It is true that in practice the nature of the case precludes us from obtaining full proof of these points in every individual instance, and we are forced to determine the treatment on probable conjecture rather than on certainty. But they have been ascertained to be generally true of the class of symptoms which is called venereal. It is on their truth that the received opinions of the pathology of the disorder rest, and in a medical argument, unless one or both of them is satisfactorily ascertained, it cannot be denied that we have no adequate proof of the existence of any virus at all.

The mode in which the disease has been derived, if it exists alone, may mislead, since there may be irritating qualities in the secretions of diseased parts, which may affect the parts to which they are applied, without the existence of any distinct morbid poison capable of generating a specific malady. Unless, therefore, the exact identity of the symptoms in the party which communicates and the party which receives the infection is fully shown, or unless the infection can be traced through several successive individuals, some uncertainty affects the conclusion. But where the regular sequence of secondary on primary symptoms is undoubtedly established, it is difficult to avoid the inference that there exists a distinct virus, which is received into the circulating fluids, and carries the seeds of the disease to the remoter parts of the body. It is observable, that the passages which have been so frequently quoted from Celsus and others, as proofs of the existence of the venereal disease in Europe before the close of the fifteenth century, refer only to the local injury sustained by those who come in contact with the diseased, and are entirely silent as to any constitutional affection being the consequence of the local malady.

But where the existence of a poison is proved, it may still be questioned whether this poison is the same with that of lues venerea ; and this question can only be answered by a comparison of the mode of communication, the character of the symptoms

Although the venereal disease keeps its specific properties distinct in its several forms, yet its symptoms are in appearance common to many

---

the course and progress of the disease, and the mode of cure. Where these are the same as are found in syphilis, we can searcely doubt the identity of the virus; where there is a decided and uniform difference under similar circumstances, we must naturally infer a diversity.

Hence any error or inaccuracy in our notions of the venereal disease itself will infallibly affect our discrimination of the diseases which resemble it, and lead, according to the prepossessions and bias of the individual, either to the undue extension or the undue limitation of the term. Of late years the most frequent error seems to have been the exclusion of cases which are manifestly syphilitic, on account of some difference from the preconceived opinions which have been formed of lues venerea. Writers on this subject seem scarcely to have been aware how various are the appearances of venereal symptoms, and how different at different times is the effect of remedies. A primary sore, in which the characters of a chancre as given by Mr. Hunter are not obviously visible, may nevertheless be venereal. It may be derived from a venereal sore, and may produce constitutional symptoms which have every character of genuine syphilis. In secondary affections the variety is still greater. Symptoms of a doubtful character are frequently so intermixed with others, which it is impossible to mistake, as to be certainly attributable to the same cause.

Hence when we meet with deviations from those forms of the disease which are most peculiar and most characteristic, we are not warranted in inferring a diversity of cause, or ascribing the symptoms to the existence of a different virus from that of genuine syphilis. Yet many histories have been given to the world as pseudo-syphilitic in which the appearances exactly accord with some forms of the lues venerea.

Again, the notions which have prevailed as to the mode of cure have been a still more fertile source of error. Mercury has been considered as the only cure of syphilis, and its action has been taken as the test of the nature of the malady. Where on the one hand mercury has disagreed, or where on the other the patient has recovered without resorting to its use, it has been inferred that the disease has not been venereal.

Yet it has been fully established by the experience of former ages, confirmed as it has been by a long series of experiments which have been recently instituted, that most if not all venereal symptoms, whether primary or secondary, may be subdued without the use of mercury. It is not necessary to refer to these experiments in detail. They are well known; and the conclusion which has been drawn from them is irresistible, or at least there are no sources of error which can materially impeach its general truth. On the other hand, the unfavourable action of mercury is no proof that the disease is not venereal. Many circumstances may interfere with its effect as an anti-syphilitic, and render it inert or injurious in cases which are truly venereal. When it produces no sensible effect on the system, it frequently has no action also on the venereal symptoms. When it produces vomiting, or dysentery, or erethismus, or materially deranges in any way the health, venereal symptoms will usually spread under its use. Cases are daily occurring in which the subsequent progress of the malady proves the truth of this view; in which the ultimate cure is effected by means of mercury, though at one time it has seriously aggravated the affections it was employed to cure. In such cases a practical knowledge of the course and aspect of lues venerea can alone guide the judgement. If the practitioner has not this knowledge, he will be staggered in his belief as to the nature of the disease on the occurrence of any untoward symptoms, and will usually abandon the mercurial treatment altogether. If he has such an acquaintance with the malady as to give him confidence in the accuracy of his opinion, he will inquire whether there

other diseases, and in that light it cannot be said to have any one symptom peculiar to itself.   For instance, every symptom of the venereal disease, in form of a gonorrhœa, may be produced by any other visible irritating cause, and often without any cause that can be assigned; even buboes and swelled testicles, which are symptoms of this disease, have followed both stimulating injections and bougies when applied to the urethra of a sound person; and indeed these two symptoms, when they do arise from a venereal cause, in many cases are only symptomatic, not specific, but more especially the swelled testicle.

Sores on the glans penis, prepuce, &c., in form of chancres, may, and do arise without any venereal infection, although we may observe that they are in general a consequence of former venereal sores which have been perfectly cured.

The symptoms produced from the infection, when in the constitution, are such as are common to many other diseases, viz. blotches on the skin are common to what is called scorbutic habits; pains common to rheumatism, swellings of the bones, periosteum, fasciæ, &c. to many bad habits, perhaps of the scrofulous and rheumatic kind.   Thus most of the symptoms of the venereal disease, in all its forms, are to be found in many other diseases; therefore we are led back to the original cause, to a number of leading circumstances, as dates, and its effects upon others from connexion when only local, joined with the present appearances and symptoms before we can determine absolutely what the disease truly is; for all these taken together may be such as can attend no other disease.   However, with all our knowledge, and with all the application of that knowledge to suspicious symptoms of this disease, we

---

has been no obstacle to the beneficial effects of the remedy which will account for its failure.   He will suspend it for a time, with the intention of resorting to it again at a subsequent period when he can employ it with greater precaution and under more favourable circumstances.

If then the points of distinction on which reliance has been usually placed are deceptive, it may be asked what other grounds of discrimination can be substituted.   The answer is plain.   Where there is a difference of virus, the difference of effects is not accidental or occasional, but constant and uniform.   No doubt can arise as to the diversity of measles and smallpox, though these diseases were formerly confounded, because the distinction, when once pointed out, is confirmed by daily experience.   The yaws of Africa and the West Indies, the sibbens of Scotland and Canada, the scherlievo of. the Illyrian coast, the effects of the poison of glanders on the human subject, cannot be confounded with syphilis, because the symptoms are different; and this difference, which may be traced uniformly through a series of individuals affected by these maladies, prevents the possibility of attributing them to the same cause.   The peculiarities which have been supposed to take the cases described as pseudo-syphilitic out of the class of syphilitic diseases are uncertain and variable, and can never constitute the distinctive characters of a separate and independent malady.]

are often mistaken, often calling it venereal when it is not; and sometimes supposing it to be some other disease when it is venereal.

Rheumatism, in many of its symptoms, in some constitutions, resembles the lues venerea; the nocturnal pains, swelling of the tendons, ligaments, and periosteum, and pain in those swellings, are symptoms
both of the rheumatism and the venereal disease when it attacks those
parts : I do not know that I ever saw the lues venerea attack the joints,
though many rheumatic complaints of those parts are cured by mercury,
and therefore supposed to be venereal[a].

Mercury, given without caution, often produces the same symptoms
as rheumatism; and I have seen even such supposed to be venereal, and
the medicine continued.

Other diseases shall not only resemble the venereal in appearance,
but in the mode of contamination, proving themselves to be poisons by
affecting the part of contact, and from thence producing immediate consequences similar to buboes; also remote consequences similar to the
lues venerea.

As errors in forming a judgment of a disease lead to errors in the cure,
it becomes almost of as much consequence to avoid a mistake in the one
as in the other; for it is nearly as dangerous in many constitutions to
give mercury where the disease is not venereal as to omit it in those
which are; for we may observe, that many of the constitutions which
put on some of the venereal symptoms, when the disease is not present,
are those with which mercury seldom agrees, and commonly does harm.
I have seen mercury, given in a supposed venereal ulcer of the tonsils,
produce a mortification of those glands, and the patient has been nearly
destroyed.

When treating of the lues venerea, and giving the symptoms and general appearances of the disease, I related some cases which appeared
to be venereal, though they really were not, and I shall now refer the
reader to these, as it will be unnecessary to give them again here, al-

---

[a] [The statement seems to be too general. Cases occasionally, though rarely, occur
where inflammation of the synovial membrane of the joints shall take place in union
with secondary symptoms of lues venerea of an undoubted character; shall increase in
severity during the increase of the other symptoms; and shall subside as soon as mercury is efficiently used, and the eruption or sore throat are controlled by its exhibition.
In such cases the synovial inflammation has an acute character; and is attended with a
degree of pain and tension and superficial redness, which sufficiently distinguishes it
from that languid form of the same affection which is common under circumstances of
general cachexia, whether that cachexia has been produced by mercury acting as a poison,
or by the long duration of the venereal disease itself, which has been allowed to continue
till every function necessary for the maintenance of nutrition and of health has become
deranged, and the patient has been reduced to a state which closely resembles scrofula.]

though if they had not been formerly taken notice of, this would have been a very proper place.

As the diseases in question are various, and not to be reduced to any system or order that I am acquainted with, I shall content myself with relating the cases, and thereby put it in the power of others to judge for themselves, if they should not be inclined to adopt the conclusions I have drawn from them.

On the 28th of July, 1776, a gentleman, then in the West Indies, scratched the end of his finger with a thorn. On the 31st he opened an abscess on the shoulder of a negro woman who had the yaws, and had been long subject to such abscesses in different parts of the body, and to incurable ulcerations afterwards. At the instant after the operation he perceived a little of the matter upon the scratch, and exclaimed that he was inoculated. On the 2nd of August he amputated a boy's finger, of thirteen years of age, for a sore resembling wormeaten wood. The scratch on his finger did not heal, but from time to time threw off whitish scales : this appearance alarmed him, and he rubbed in mercurial ointment very freely. Notwithstanding this, in the month of September, a painful inflamed tumor appeared on the second joint of the finger, which was soon followed by several others on the back of the hand, in the course of the metacarpal bone of the forefinger. He still continued the mercurial friction, but without effect, for the tumors daily multiplied, and by the month of November extended to within a small distance of the axilla. They did not go on to suppuration at this time. About the end of November he began to be affected with severe nocturnal pains in different parts of the body, but especially along the tibia and fibula, with frequent severe headaches, which continued to increase to an almost intolerable degree for five months, though he used mercurial friction, with decoction of sarsaparilla, every day in great quantity.

In the month of May, 1777, a scabby eruption appeared in different parts of the body, especially the legs and thighs, and the before-mentioned tumors ulcerated ; but this was followed by a remission of the nocturnal pains.

He never could bring on a salivation, though his mouth was constantly tender, even for months. The ulcerations became daily worse, and a voyage to England was thought the only resource. He arrived in London the first of August, and by the advice of Dr. William Hunter and Sir John Pringle, he began again a course of mercury and sarsaparilla, with a milk diet. I was called in, and judging that two thirds of a grain of mercurius calcinatus, every day, was too small a dose, if it were judged to be venereal, it was ordered to be gradually increased to five grains ; and he continued this course till November, when all the sores were perfectly healed.

He now discontinued the mercury, and remained free from all symptoms of the disorder, except some nodes on the tibia, and rheumatic pains on exposure to cold, until about twelve months ago[a], when he began to have an uneasiness in swallowing, a rawness in the throat, and a discharge of viscid mucus from that and the posterior nostrils, all of which still continue.

The following observations may be made on the above case :

There can be little doubt that the disease was the yaws. The yaws are a disease that resembles the venereal in several of its symptoms, as well as in the manner in which it is most commonly communicated. It differs, however, in some essential particulars. The yaws have a regular progress, after going through which they leave the constitution in a healthy state, at least free from that disease, it being sufficient for the cure that the patient be put in a state favourable to general health. Thus, a negro labouring under the disease must do little or no work, be kept clean, and have a better diet than usual. Under these circumstances, he commonly gets well in from four to nine months, although the unfavourable cases will continue much longer. Various medicines are given for the cure, but it is not clear that any of them do good. Mercury has considerable power over the disease, without being a specific for it. If given early it will either check the progress of the disease, or perhaps even heal up all the sores on the skin ; but nothing is gained by this, for the disease soon breaks out anew. Some practitioners of medicine in the West Indies are of opinion that interrupting the course of the disease by mercury is productive of no other evils than those of loss of time and an imperfect cure ; others affirm that it is often the cause of what they call the boneache. Towards the end of the disease it is generally allowed that mercury may be given safely, and even with advantage. It is probable the long continuance of the disease, being above fourteen months, and also the pains in the bones in the present case, were owing to the very early and free use of mercury. It may be allowable to add, that the yaws do not differ more from the venereal disease in curing themselves than in this circumstance, that, like the small-pox, they affect none a second time[b].

A gentleman applied to me for the cure of chancres, seated on the attachment of the prepuce to the penis, and also on the frænum. Mer-

---

[a] [The first edition of the work was published in 1786, consequently it would appear that a considerable interval elapsed between the healing of the ulcerations and the occurrence of the sore throat.]

[b] [The earliest and best description of the yaws is given in the fifth volume of the Edinburgh Medical Essays, and has been attributed to a gentleman of the name of Home. The case related by Dr. Adams, in his work on morbid poisons, as occurring at Madeira seems not to have been a case of yaws at all.]

cury was used chiefly by friction, in order to affect the constitution; it was also applied to the sores, in order to affect them locally. The cure of the chancres went on gradually and without interruption; and in about five weeks they were perfectly healed. He almost immediately had connexion with a woman, and long before we could suppose the mercury had all got out of his constitution. In a very few days after the first connection, the prepuce began to be chopped all round on the edge of its reflection. He continued his connection, and upon its growing worse he applied to me, and I found the chops very deep, and the prepuce there so tight and sore that he could not bring it back upon the penis. The question now was, whether this was venereal or not? The sores themselves did not appear to be so; but more was to be taken into the account than simply appearances. It was first to be considered whether it might possibly be a return of his former complaint. This could not be the case, because the sores were not in the same parts. It was next to be questioned, was it possible for this part of the prepuce to have been contaminated at the same time with the former, and the poison not to have come into action till now, having been prevented by the course of mercury, which had not cured the disposition? This could not be well answered, although not probable, because the poison appeared to come too soon into action after the leaving off of the medicine; for I did suppose there was still a great deal of mercury in the constitution. Was it then possible for him to have caught it from the woman? This, I supposed, could not have been the cause of these chops, whatever effect this connexion might have to render them venereal hereafter; for they appeared too soon after it, especially as he had mercury in his constitution at the time, and as the parts had been accustomed to the application of venereal matter but a very little time before. Although, from all circumstances taken together, I was convinced the case was not venereal, yet an apprehension arose in his mind concerning the possibility of having given it to the lady, as he had connection after the first appearance of the sores. I was equally convinced of the impossibility of the one as of the other, therefore desired him to rest easy on that head. He went immediately into the country, and nothing being done for those chops, they got perfectly well. In less than a fortnight after this connection, the lady became a little indisposed with a slight fever, and a swelling came in one of her groins. I watched the progress of this swelling, which was slow, and I did not believe it to be venereal. It at last formed matter and broke, and a poultice was applied to it. Instead of ulcerating or spreading, it rather had a healing disposition, and in about six weeks it was perfectly well. While it was healing, scurfy eruptions came out on the skin, some on the face and thighs, but more especially on the hands and feet, where the cuticle peeled off. Upon the first appearance of these I was a little staggered; but, as the sore was healing, I was unwilling to give credit to the appearance, and therefore begged that nothing might be done; and they all got well.

From the general outline of these cases, one would naturally have said they were venereal; but the particular circumstances being all investigated, and the whole taken together, led me to suppose that they were not, and the event proved that to be the case.

The following case was communicated by Mr. French, of Harpur-street.

" June the 9th, 1782, a gentleman applied to me for an ulcer which was seated on the glans penis, attended with excessive pain. Knowing him to be an intemperate man, and learning from himself that during a state of intoxication he had been connected with a woman, I judged the complaint to be venereal. He was now in a feverish state, and unfit for the exhibition of mercury : I therefore prescribed for him decoction of bark, with elixir of vitriol and tinctura thebäica, proportioned to his pain. I directed him to abstain from every kind of fermented liquor; to live chiefly upon milk, and to wash the ulcer with a liniment composed of equal parts of oil of almonds and aqua sapphirina.

" About the 17th of the same month, some check having been given to the fever, the sore looking cleaner, and his pain having abated, I ordered him small doses of argentum vivum and extract of hemlock.

" July the 4th, finding the mercurial course to disagree, I ordered three grains of the extract of hemlock to be taken two or three times a day, and the decoction of bark to be taken as before, with twenty drops of tinctura thebäica, which was gradually increased to sixty, at bed-time.

" The ulcer had spread very much during the mercurial course, and had now destroyed half the glans penis.

" October 1st, Mr. Hunter was consulted, and ordered the patient to add the powder of sarsaparilla to the decoction of bark, to take laudanum freely, and wash the sores with tinctura thebäica. Soon after beginning this course the remainder of the glans penis sloughed off, the parts gradually healed, and health was restored.

" There were two other symptoms in this case which deserve to be taken notice of: a considerable enlargement of the scalp on the right side of the os frontis, and on the left parietal bone, attended with excessive pain, and vibices resembling the sea-scurvy on the inside of the left tibia, both of which disappeared in the course of the cure.

" Some months after, the tumor in the head returned, and several abscesses were formed, which were opened, and the cranium found carious to a great extent. On account of the pain, he has for some months past taken two hundred and forty drops of laudanum and six grains of opium daily. These sores healed up, and others broke out in different parts of the head, which also got well; and in June, 1785, there was only one large ulcer in the angle of the right eye."

A lady was delivered of a child on the 30th of September, 1776. The infant being weakly, and the quantity of milk in the mother's breasts abundant, it was judged proper to procure the child of a person in the neighbourhood to assist in keeping the breasts in a proper state. It is worthy of remark that the lady kept her own child to the right breast, the stranger to the left. In about six weeks the nipple of the left breast began to inflame, and the glands of the axilla to swell. A few days after, several small ulcers were formed about the nipple, which, spreading rapidly, soon communicated and became one ulcer, and at last the whole nipple was destroyed. The tumour in the axilla subsided, and the ulcer in the breast healed in about three months from its first appearance. On inquiry, about this time, the child of the stranger was found to be short-breathed, had the thrush, and died tabid, with many sores on different parts of the body. The patient now complained of shooting pains in different parts of the body, which were succeeded by an eruption on the arms, legs, and thighs, many of which became ulcers.

She was now put under a mercurial course, with a decoction of sarsaparilla. Mercury was tried in a variety of forms: in solution, in pills internally, and externally in the form of ointment. It could not be continued above a few days at a time, as it always brought on fever or purging, with extreme pain in the bowels. In this state she remained till March 16, 1779, when she was delivered of another child in a diseased state. This child was committed to the care of a wetnurse, and lived about nine weeks; the cuticle peeling off in various parts, and a scabby eruption covering the whole body. The child died.

Soon after the death of the child, the nurse complained of headache and sore throat, together with ulceration of the breasts. Various remedies were given to her, but she determined to go into a public hospital, where she was salivated, and after some months she was discharged, but not cured of the disease. The bones of the nose and palate exfoliated, and in a few months she also died tabid.

Of the various remedies tried by the lady herself, none succeeded so well as sea-bathing. About the month of May she began a course of the Lisbon diet-drink, and continued it with regularity about a month, dressing the sores with laudanum, by which treatment the sores healed up; and in September she was delivered of another child, free from external marks of disease, but very sickly; and it died in the course of the month.

About a twelvemonth after, the sores broke out again, and, although mercurial dressings and internal medicines were given, remained for a twelvemonth, when they began again to heal up[a].

---

[a] [The author is evidently of opinion that these and similar cases are not venereal, and he elsewhere denies it to be possible that an infant can be contaminated by its parent before its birth.   Whether he is right in this opinion must be judged by the following statement of the facts, which are sufficiently frequent and peculiar to be given with confidence in their truth.

When a mother suffers during the period of pregnancy from a constitutional venereal affection, she seems to be particularly disposed to miscarry.   The abortion seems to be caused by the death of the infant, which is very generally born dead, and has usually ceased to show signs of vitality for some days before its ejection.

If, however, miscarriage does not take place, it is most usual that the infant at birth shows no signs of disease.   But at a variable period, generally from three to five weeks after birth, it becomes slightly indisposed.   Then eruptions appear about the thighs and the groins, between the nates, or on the pudenda.   They wear the aspect of discoloured patches, generally affecting a circular form, with a shining surface, and some slight desquamation, but without the least tubercular thickening.   As the disease proceeds these patches enlarge, and eventually occupy almost the whole body ; and in the folds they sometimes slightly excoriate, and even, near the anus, at the umbilicus, or on the female pudenda, form small condylomatous excrescences.   Then ulcers in many cases take place in the interior of the mouth, and in the throat; the nostrils are partially obstructed by an increase of their secretion, and the voice becomes weak and hoarse.   With all this there is much general indisposition.   From the first appearance of the symptoms the child does not thrive, and as they continue it becomes very weak and emaciated.   If the case be neglected it often terminates fatally, but under the use of mercury all the symptoms are readily subdued, and perfect health may be restored.

Those who come into close contact with a child thus diseased may be contaminated in consequence.   If such a child has sores in the interior of the mouth, and in this state sucks the breast of a healthy woman, it is very common that the nipple should become ulcerated; and the ulcer will not resemble the fissures which are so common on the nipples of women who give suck, and which usually occasion no loss of substance, but will be a corroding ulcer, and will destroy the whole or the greater part of the nipple before it is healed.   It also produces in general an enlarged gland in the axilla, which, however, rarely passes into suppuration.   At an interval of some weeks sore throat, eruptions, or nodes arise, which are in no respect distinguishable from the common forms of lues venerea.

If a woman, who has been thus infected by a child which she has suckled, suckles also another child which is healthy, no infection will be communicated, provided the sound child is kept carefully to the opposite breast, and is never allowed to take into its mouth the nipple to which the diseased child is applied.   But if this precaution is not taken, and the children are applied indiscriminately to either breast, the sound child will contract sores in the interior of the lips, and these will be followed by scaly eruptions on the skin, exactly resembling those which are seen in an infant which has received the infection from its mother.

It would be easy to substantiate what has been stated by the recital of cases.   The results are tolerably uniform ; at least the deviations from the ordinary course are not greater than those which occur when the venereal disease is communicated in the usual way by sexual connection.

It is difficult, in the face of these facts, to deny that such cases are the effects of the

The following cases, being all derived from one stock, show as much as possible that new poisons are rising up every day, and those very similar to the venereal in many respects, although not in all: therefore it is the want of similarity that becomes the criterion to judge by, and not the similarity.

The parents of the child who is the subject of the following history were and are to all appearance healthy people. The child was weakly when born; and the mother having little or no milk, when it was three weeks old she gave it to a nurse whose milk was then seven months old and was giving suck to her own child. The foster mother allowed her own to suck the right breast, while the other sucked the left.

The nurse observed that the skin of the foster child began to peel off; but no rawness or soreness took place except about the anus, where it looked as if scalded. The same kind of peeling took place on the lips, but they did not appear to be sore, although the people in the country said it was the thrush. The inner surface of the mouth and tongue appeared sound. In a fortnight after her receiving the child it died, and then she allowed her own child to suck both breasts for three weeks; at the end of which she came to town to nurse a gentleman's child.

She gave suck to this second child; but after being in town about ten or eleven days, she did not feel herself perfectly well: which made them suppose that the new mode of life, confinement in town, and probably better living, might not agree with her, and she went into the country and took the gentleman's child with her. About three or four days after she went to the country, for instance, about a fortnight after she took this child, and five weeks after the death of the first child, her left nipple, which the first-nursed child had always sucked, began to be sore, so that she could not let the child suck it. This ulcer on the nipple became extremely painful; in a day or two eruptions came out on her face, and soon after all over her body, but most on her legs and thighs. They continued coming out for about a fortnight, and had at first very much the appearance of the eruptions of the smallpox, and on the third

---

venereal virus. It is true that the symptoms in children are not precisely the same either in course or appearance with the most usual symptoms of the venereal disease in adults. Diseases of the bones or periosteum seem never to occur, nor are the eruptions tubercular. Yet as the symptoms in the adult from whom the disease is received, and the adult to whom it is communicated, are exactly identical with those of common syphilis, it must be inferred that the difference is to be ascribed to the age and circumstances of an infant, and not to a diversity of virus.

It is impossible to admit the argument used by the author, that secondary symptoms never contaminate, and therefore these cases must be mistaken. The facts are so well established that it is more easy to question the principle which he has laid down than to doubt the facts.]

day of their eruption were attended with fever, universal uneasiness, and great pain.

Two or three days after the eruption on the skin appeared, one of the glands of the armpit began to swell, and formed matter, and was opened within a fortnight after its first appearance, and healed almost directly. Some of the eruptions increased fast and became very broad sores, nearly of the size of a half-crown, especially on the legs and thighs, and were covered with a broad scab; many remained small, and only appeared like pimples. About a fortnight after the first appearance of the eruption, some began to die away; and in four weeks more after this appearance, a foul ulcer attacked the left tonsil.

The surgeon in the country, from all these circumstances, finding he could not get any ground by the before-mentioned treatment, determined to give her the solution of the corrosive sublimate, of which he gave half a grain in solution night and morning; in about a week there seemed to be a stop put to the swelling of the ulcers, and the discharge to be somewhat lessened, the ulcer in the throat putting on a better appearance.

It was at this period I first saw her, which was about six weeks after the first appearance of the eruption, and a fortnight after the appearance of the ulcer in the tonsil. The eruptions were then very much as before described, but the ulcer in the tonsil was clean and healing. From the history of the case I did conceive it not to be venereal; I therefore desired that all medicines might be left off, which medicines could only have been taken for a fortnight at most, because it was after the appearance of the ulcer on the tonsil the mercury was given, which was only of a fortnight's standing when I saw her. She soon after recovered.

After being well for some time she again applied to the surgeon in the country, an abscess having formed where the complaint first began in the breast, attended with fresh eruptions on the face.

The abscess was opened, and it healed up in a few days, and upon taking some cooling physic the eruptions disappeared. She has continued very well ever since, without any other bad effect than the total loss of her nipple. This case was certainly understood to be venereal.

About five days after the appearance of the eruption on the nurse, the gentleman's child was taken away and given to a healthy woman of a florid complexion, aged twenty-four years, and who had lain in with her first child eleven months when she became wetnurse to this child. After a few days she observed eruptions on the child's head, not unlike those already described on the first nurse which it had sucked. Its mouth soon after became excoriated, so that it sucked with difficulty. After a short time those eruptions on the head became dry and peeled off, others appeared on the face, knees, and feet, but wholly unlike the former, as the first maturated, while the latter appeared only cutaneous, peeling off and leaving a circumscribed spot of a light dun colour, which continued increasing for five weeks. These eruptions continued nearly three months from their commencement, at which period the child was extremely emaciated; but no particular treatment was indicated, so no medicine was exhibited, and in a few weeks after it came to London and got perfectly well.

The second nurse, a few days after giving suck to the child, had blotches appear on her left breast, precisely the same with those on the first nurse, with this difference only, that they were fewer in number, and attended with a greater degree of phlegmonous inflammation. They continued, and increased in size for seven or eight days; then the nipple of the same breast became ulcerated, the ulceration spreading so much as to endanger the loss of it: her thighs now became diseased, and afterwards her legs.

She suckled this child about twelve weeks. The disease seemed no longer to increase, and in twelve or fourteen days after this entirely disappeared, without her taking any medicine, except a few ounces of the decoction of the bark. The only application to the breast was unguentum simplex.

The milk at this time became so small in quantity that they were under the necessity of providing a third wetnurse for the child, and the second returned to the country. Her own child being weaned, she had no further occasion for the milk, and in a few days it wholly disappeared; but by way of amusing the child when peevish, she allowed it to take the nipple which had been diseased in its mouth; the consequence was, that in a few days this child also became diseased in like manner with the former. She now applied to an eminent surgeon for assistance, who, not being acquainted with the history, supposed it venereal, and ordered a colourless medicine, supposed, from circumstances, to be the solution of sublimate, sixteen grains to half a pint of water; the dose a table-spoonful. She took this medicine as directed, and also gave it to her husband and child; the child a tea-spoonful only at a time. While taking this medicine she got well.

The third wetnurse, like the former, was in a short time affected; but the blotches in this case were still fewer in number, the disease appearing to lose considerably in its power, as each fresh infection became less malignant than the former. She got well without taking any medicine*.

* Added: "The following case shows the effect of the state of the mind upon the body, and the bad consequences attending the patient's being indulged in his own

opinions respecting the nature of a disease.   It is given as drawn up by himself for my
opinion.

" ' In May, 1789, when in London, I was unhappy enough to have connection with
a woman of the town.   Five days after I took more than usual exercise, and the day
being warm I perspired profusely.   This affected my head, more particularly my forehead.   In this situation I went into the country, and while on the road the sweating
increased ; when it went off it left a burning heat about the forehead, so that I could
not wear my hat.   This heat continued all night, attended with an external pain round
the forehead.   The next day it increased, but the day after its violence seemed to lessen ;
but it continued more or less for several weeks.   On my return home I was connected
with my wife.

" ' My mind became so much agitated that I found it impossible to be at peace till I
unfolded my situation to a surgeon and apothecary.

" ' I began to fear that those affections of the head might arise from disease.   The
surgeon seemed to apprehend no danger.   I pressed him to give me some opening
draughts, to carry off the inflammation about the head, and flattered myself that they
would also carry off any virus that I had contracted.   Notwithstanding this, I still,
however, found some of those disagreeable sensations, together with an uneasiness in
the throat and teeth.

" ' All this time there was nothing more than usual in the genital parts, but a degree
of heat not felt or observed before.

" ' I now conceived that this heat was increasing.   By a constant and minute inspection, I found the size of the penis at times to diminish ; the nut assumed a pale
yellowish colour, and the glands behind the nut seemed to be covered with mucus.
The heat about the head diminished ; the throat and teeth felt more uneasy.

" ' In the course of a fortnight after my return I persuaded my apothecary to give
me small doses of calomel.   For the first few days they worked me very violently.   The
quantity of calomel was then lessened.   All this time I felt no discharge of any kind,
but after taking those medicines a few days I felt some heat and pain in the groin, and
the penis seemed at times hot, and I felt some shooting pains about the head.

" ' A fortnight completed this course, and now I entered upon some alteratives.
While taking them my throat seemed to get worse and worse, but more so towards night.

" ' Six weeks after the connection I was pronounced well, and left off all medicines.

" ' Soon after this, in the mornings, prior to my making water, I perceived a small
quantity of a whitish discharge on the opening of the lips of the urethra ; never in quantity so large as a pea, and never but in the morning.   I was induced to try what stain
this would give to clean linen : it left a greenish spot.   This was immediately communicated to the surgeon, who bid me think nothing of it, assuring me it was of no consequence.

" ' My mind was too unhappy to remain satisfied in this state, or with those assu-
rances ; I therefore had the advice of a physician.

" ' He said if I was affected it was in a very small degree, and that there was no possibility of my injuring my wife.   Notwithstanding which, he thought I had better take
some medicines, which he would prescribe, for a fortnight, and then go on with strengthening remedies.   I now began taking these medicines.   I took a large tea-spoonful of
an electuary three times a day ; my throat soon began to feel better ; after the fortnight the strengthening plan was begun.

" ' Those medicines being left off, my throat became uneasy, as before ; once or twice
I discovered a discharge from the urethra, which was quite clear, and more glutinous
than my water.   This I always found was after erections.

" ' The strengthening medicines were continued about a fortnight.   My throat felt very sore at night, and looked red all round.   A hard reddish pimple now appeared in the roof of the mouth.   Those circumstances made me very unhappy.

" ' I now began taking an alectuary, like the former, and drank a pint of decoction of the woods every day.   This plan was adhered to for six weeks.

" ' I took strengthening medicines for about a fortnight, and then left them off.

" ' I used a variety of things for my mouth and throat; one time an electuary, and gargled with port wine; another time I gargled with a decoction of roses, honey, &c.

" ' I now find myself in a much worse situation than ever; for although I have never been disabled from pursuing my business, I have some additional disagreeable sensations; very unpleasant feelings in the shin-bones, which affect me more after walking or standing, as if pins were pricking me.   They are not violent, but disagreeable.   My legs sometimes seem uncommonly stiff; there is a soreness in the knee, and in the hollow under the knee; a pain in the small of the back, sometimes in my arm.   I think my corns, which are often troublesome, have been more so, especially in damp weather.

" ' About three months ago I discovered a spot on the inside of the right thigh, the size of a shilling, which at times assumed a copper colour, but in common the colour of the skin; but whenever heated it assumed this colour.   On the other side several more, of a lighter kind, have appeared.   There are several small ones, of the size of a large pin's head, about different parts of the body, rising above the skin.   There is no particular pain attends them.

" ' Within this week some very large spots have appeared about the neck, and the right side of the neck feels sore at times.   For some time past my nose and forehead have felt different from what they used to do.   There has been a heat, attended at times with a pricking and throbbing pain, with a stiffness that I cannot describe.   The skin about the nose seems red.   This instant there is a pain and stiffness felt in it.   My eyes seem weaker than they used to be and sometimes look red.   My mouth has been affected; the membrane appears pale, and broken in some places.   The saliva is very disagreeable: the breath is not offensive.   Whenever I have wind in the stomach, my throat is very sore indeed.

" ' It is necessary that I should observe that I am of a scorbutic habit, which has always thrown out pimples betwixt my shoulders, down my arms, and sometimes some few in my face.

" ' When I returned home in May, I found my wife looking pale and weak.   This I concluded to be the effect of breeding.   It appears since, that on my return, she must have been advanced about six weeks in her pregnancy.   I prayed the surgeon to tell me if he thought there was any danger of my injuring her, and that if there was, I would fling myself at her feet and inform her of what had happened.   This I also told the doctor; both assured me there was no danger.   Towards the latter end of June she seemed to have a slow fever.   The apothecary attended her.   She appeared very weak.   By degrees she got better.   In July she received a terrible fright, so that she became very poorly again; was very weak, and complained of an unusual discharge from the vagina.   For this, through much persuasion, I got her to consent to have the doctor's advice.   This I pressed very much, as he was acquainted with all the circumstances that had attended me.   I was very apprehensive that her complaints were now the effect of an injury received from me.   I told the doctor of the discharge, prayed him to give her symptoms due consideration, and pressed him to prescribe such medicines as would effectually remove the complaint.   He attended her, and assured me that there was not the smallest appearance of her complaints arising from such a cause.   He said they were the effects of weakness and pregnancy.   She never complained of any pain in the parts, nor of any heat in making water.   At this time she was troubled with an almost unremitting pain in her teeth, gums, &c.   The doctor prescribed some strengthening cordial medicines, which she continued to take for some time.   She grew better, but was almost continually affected with pains in her teeth. This discharge lessened by degrees. Her habit was always disposed to be costive, but more so when with child. This the doctor accounted for from her habit, her being with child, &c., and assured me that everything was perfectly natural, and that there was not the smallest appearance of anything arising from disease. About a month or more before she was brought to bed, those complaints in her teeth, ears, and head seemed to increase, a redness appeared over her eyebrows, where there was great pain, &c.

" ' At this time I observed some little spots about her face, of a yellowish colour, one in her forehead, two or three less near her ears, &c., and some few on her arms.

" ' At length she was brought to bed; had a fine child, perfectly healthy. Her teeth were still sore, the right side of her cheek so much so, that she could not bear it to be touched. Her left breast began now to be very troublesome, and the more so as the milk advanced. (In this breast she always complained of a pain from her first child, and sometimes she fancied she could feel a hard lump.) Both her nipples were very sore, were surrounded with little ulcerations; but the left was by far the worst. It was very painful to her to give suck; she was obliged to have her breasts drawn now and then. Her nipples got better by degrees, and she now tells me they are well. There was early after she had children a redness betwixt the breasts; but this also went off.

" ' There now seems a little redness on each side of her nose near her eyes, and sometimes the tip and sides of her nostrils appear red. She says there is no pain. Her pain is now in the left gums, and extends through to the cheek. Her water is frequently very thick, and there is, very soon after it is discharged, an evident sediment in it.

" ' The infant is free from all appearances of disease, but at present is afflicted with the snuffles to a degree that exceeds anything of the kind that I ever saw in any of our other children. I am always disposed to anticipate the worst, and it pains me very much, lest it should arise from this general source of evil. The child is hearty, thrives very well, sleeps well. Two children that are at home have now and then been poorly : in the corners of their mouths there was, for weeks, an evident excoriation, assuming a whitish colour. This, I think, is now gone. There seem some small pimples about the neck, very small, and there are two or three of these small spots about each of them; and sometimes their noses are red and sore. Indeed my mind has been afflicted with an idea that I have by this unguarded act injured my whole house. My situation is truly wretched. I had made up my mind to take time by the forelock, to attack this disorder very early; but, alas! I am afraid, I have fallen into bad hands.

" ' This business involves a great variety of questions of the first importance to me. The questions, with their answers, must be referred to your better judgement: I will state two or three for our satisfaction.

" ' If my complaints arise from lues, is it possible for me to have injured my children by kissing them, sleeping, &c. ?

" ' If my wife's discharge was venereal, would it not most likely have produced a similar one in me? or, would not my having received the lues into my habit prevent it ?

" Are those pains in the head, teeth, ears, &c. likely to arise from this cause? If my wife's nipples had been affected from the complaint, would the person that drew her breast be infected? and if so, how long, and in what manner would her infection appear? Would the nipples have got well had this been the case? Can the child's snuffles arise from this cause? Can any part be injured by this complaint, without manifest inflammation, swelling, and discharge?

" ' I have only to add, that I pray you, Sir, to be good enough to give this complex and unhappy case every necessary attention. I should wish for effectual relief.' "— Home.

§. 1. *Of Diseases supposed to be Venereal produced by Trans-planted Teeth.*

Since the operation of transplanting teeth has been practised in London, some cases have occurred in which the venereal infection has been supposed to be communicated in this way, and they have been treated accordingly; nor has the method of cure tended to weaken the suspicion: yet when all the circumstances attending them, both in the mode of catching the disease, and in the cure when they have been treated as venereal, are considered, there is something in them all which is not exactly similar to the usual appearance of the venereal disease when caught in the common way; especially too when it is considered that some of the cases were not treated as venereal, and yet were cured, and therefore the cures of the others, which appeared to be from mercury, are not clear proofs of their having been venereal*.

I believe that I have seen most, if not all, the cases of this kind which have occurred, and have attended some of them. In all of them the time of local affection, after the insertion of the tooth, has been almost regularly a month, which is too long for the venereal to take effect at a medium; and where they have produced constitutional symptoms, those again have either followed the local too close for the venereal, or too regular as to time. But it may be advanced, that a disease has been produced probably as bad in its consequences as the venereal. That a disease has been formed in this way is certain.

The first case of this kind which came under my care was a lady who had one of the bicuspidati transplanted. The transplanted tooth fastened very well. About a month after she danced till five or six o'clock in the morning, caught cold, and had a fever in consequence, which lasted near six weeks. In this time ulceration in the gum and jaw took place, though it was then not known. And when she was beginning to recover it was found that not only the gum and socket of this tooth were diseased, but also those of the teeth next to it. The two teeth were taken out, and the sockets of both afterwards exfoliated; but the parts were very backward in healing.

This backwardness gave rise to various opinions, the principal of which was, that it was venereal. In the mean time a rising appeared upon one of the legs, which was of the indolent node kind; this was also suspected by some to be venereal, or rather was a corroborating circum-

---

* It is to be remarked here that I do not, in the present case, lay any stress at all on my opinion of the lues venerea not having the power of contamination; and I believe we must allow, if the disease were venereal, it must have been contracted from a lues venerea in the person from whom the tooth was taken; for chancres are not common in the mouth, and they would be seen on examination. I believe few discharges similar to gonorrhœa take place there.

stance of the former opinion; but I gave it as my opinion that it was not. I desired she might go to the sea and bathe, which she did, and got perfectly well, both in the jaw and leg, and has continued so ever since.

The second case of this kind I have seen was also in a young lady: the transplanted tooth fastened extremely well, and continued so for about a month, when the gum began to ulcerate, leaving the tooth and socket bare. The ulcer continued, and blotches appeared upon the skin, and ulcers also in the throat. The disease was treated as venereal, the complaints gave way to this course, but they recurred several times after very severe courses of mercury: however, she at last got well.

The only observation I can make on this case is, that the symptoms recurred after continued courses of mercury much oftener than is usual in venereal cases, and I had my suspicions all along that it was scrofulous.

The third case was of a gentleman, where the transplanted tooth remained, without giving the least disturbance, for about a month, when the edge of the gum began to ulcerate, and the ulceration went on till the tooth dropped out. Some time after, spots appeared almost everywhere on the skin; they had not the truly venereal appearance, but were redder or more transparent, and more circumscribed. He had also a tendency to a hectic fever, such as restlessness, want of sleep, loss of appetite, and headache. After trying several things, and not finding relief, he was put under a course of mercury, and all disease disappeared according to the common course of the cure of the venereal disease, and we thought him well; but some time after the same appearances returned, with the addition of swelling in the bones of the metacarpus. He was now put under another course of mercury more severe than the former, and in the usual time all the symptoms again disappeared. Several months after the same eruptions came out again, but not in so great a degree as before, and without any other attendant symptoms. He a third time took mercury, but it was only ten grains of corrosive sublimate in the whole, and he got quite well. The time between his first taking mercury and his being cured was a space of three years.

Query: Could this case be venereal? The two first courses of mercury removing the eruptions would seem to prove it was; but the third course also removing them, which consisted of only ten grains of corrosive sublimate, would seem to prove that it could not be venereal; for if it had, the appearances which returned after the second course, in which a considerable quantity of mercury had been given, would not have yielded to ten grains.

The fourth case was that of a young lady who had a tooth transplanted, and about the same distance of time after it, as mentioned in the former cases, the gum began to ulcerate, and the ulceration was making considerable progress. The surgeon who was first consulted desired mercury to be given immediately. I was afterwards desired to see her, and advised that mercury should not be had recourse to, that we might ascertain the nature of the case; for if she took mercury and got well, it would be adding one more to the number of the supposed venereal cases arising from such a cause. I recommended drawing the tooth, that we might see what effects would be produced by the removal of the first cause. The tooth was drawn, and the gum healed up as fast as any common ulcer, and has ever since continued well.

This case requires no comment. I may, however, be allowed to observe, that if the lady had gone through a course of mercury, she would have, in all probability, also got well; for the tooth, in the time necessary for completing the course of mercury, would have dropped out; and if this had really happened, we need not hesitate in affirming that it would have been considered as venereal.

The fifth case was that of a young lady, eighteen years of age, who had one of the incisores transplanted, which fastened very well; but six or seven weeks after the operation, an ulceration of the gum took place, the tooth was immediately ordered to be removed, and the bark was given without any other medicine, and she got well in a few weeks.

The sixth case was that of a gentleman, aged twenty-three, a native of one of the West India islands, who had the two front incisors transplanted; and about the same time after the operation, as in the former cases, an ulceration of the gums took place, which increased to a very great degree, and the edges of the gum sloughed off. An eminent surgeon was consulted, who ordered the bark; and the patient, without taking any other medicine, got well, in nearly the same time as the ladies in cases four and five, who had the teeth taken out. The gums recovered themselves perfectly, but were considerably shorter.

If we take some of the above cases, and consider them as they at first appeared, we shall almost pronounce them to have been venereal. If we take the others, we shall pronounce them absolutely not to be venereal. And if we consider every circumstance relating to those probably venereal, we shall, as far as reasoning goes, conclude that they were not venereal. The first case that appeared at the time to be venereal is the second of those before related; but, as I did not attend the lady through the whole of the cure, I can say less upon it. She certainly had the symptoms recur oftener than they do in venereal cases in common, where the disease is attended with no ambiguity, and took more than the usual quantity of mercury. There is therefore in this case something not clearly understood, because it does not exactly agree with venereal cases in general in all its parts.

The fourth case was similar in its recurring, and in the quantity of mercury that appeared to be necessary to remove the symptoms.

The most serious effects of transplanting a tooth happened to a young lady, and are related, in the Medical Transactions, iii. 25, by the late Sir William Watson.

The dentist, being alarmed at the first appearance, desired me to visit her upon his own account. The edge of the gum had just then begun to ulcerate. As I did not know well what was best to be done, I desired him to make a strong solution of corrosive sublimate, and let the mouth be often washed with it, and also to apply some lint, soaked in it, to the part; but as this did not stop its progress, she applied to Sir William Watson, to whose account of the case I must refer the reader, and from that account I must take my materials to reason upon. However, I may remark, that the case appears to have been supposed at last to have been venereal, whatever might have been the first opinion, and for the two following reasons: first, from the mode of catching the disease being possible; and, secondly, from its not giving way to medicines which are of no service in the venereal disease; and this opinion appears to have been confirmed by the disease giving way to mercury. But the case itself, abstracted from the mode of catching it, and even the mode of cure, does not perfectly agree with the common attending circumstances of the venereal; nor has that attention been paid to the necessary circumstances sufficient to determine it to be venereal.

The progress of the ulceration in the mouth, which was the first symptom, was by much too rapid for a venereal ulcer in common: for it must be considered, if venereal, simply as a chancre or local affection.

Now let us trace the progress of the disease into the constitution. "About this time," viz. when the local disease was making such rapid progress, "blotches appeared in her face, neck, and various parts of the body: several of these became ulcerated painful sores." Now this date of the constitutional affections following the local is by much too soon to be venereal: we know if a lues venerea arises either from a gonorrhœa or chancre, it does not appear in common till about six weeks, often much later, but seldom sooner. I do not count much upon the circumstance of there being no swelling of the lymphatic glands of the neck, forming buboes, as that is not a constant symptom attending the venereal matter getting into the circulation, although it should be allowed to have some weight, especially where other circumstances do not perfectly agree. The appearances from the constitution, when they did take place, were much more violent and rapid in their progress than any venereal blotches I ever saw. We know in the lues venerea that they are months before they arrive at the stage of scabs; also the pain attending those sores did not in the least correspond with the lues venerea. Venereal blotches hardly give any sensation, or at least very little; but after all, mercury cured this disease, whatever it was. Twenty-eight grains of calomel, made into fourteen pills, were taken, probably in ten or twelve days. for it was directed she should take one or two each day, as the bowels would allow; but although tinctura thebäica was given, they purged so much as made it necessary to give no more in this way. But although so little mercury was taken, and had also run off considerably by the bowels, yet "the ulceration of her mouth and cheeks did not spread, but was less painful and of a milder appearance; the blotches in her face and body grew paler, and such of them as had ulcerated healed apace and no new ones appeared. Unguentum cœruleum fortius" was therefore directed "to be well rubbed into her legs and thighs twice a day, in small doses," lest it should be determined to the bowels. "In about ten or twelve days her griping and purging returned with violence, the ointment was therefore discontinued. At this time the blotches were all gone; the ulceration in her face and body were completely healed, and those of her mouth nearly so."—[*Op. cit.*, p. 328.]

The only remark I have to make on the cure is, that the quantity of mercury was not sufficient to cure chancres on the penis, making such rapid progress as those did in her mouth; nor could the same quantity of mercury cure venereal sores on the skin, which had made such rapid progress as they did in this case; and if we take in the effect this had upon her health, with the termination of the whole, I think we should pronounce it not venereal: for the specific circumstances, if it was venereal, were just as uncommon as the mode of catching it.

Many of these cases, suspected of being venereal, I have seen occasionally; and although the patients recovered while under a course of mercury, yet on account of the want of attention in the practitioners to the very circumstances that would decide the disease to be either venereal or not, I pass them over unnoticed.

After having considered the cases themselves of those who had the teeth transplanted, let us also consider the persons from whom the teeth were taken; for I cannot help thinking that this will throw some light upon the subject. Let me suppose that the young girls from whom the teeth were taken really had the lues venerea, and that the teeth were of course also infected, which is a supposition most unfavourable to my real opinion, it appears to me that even in this case there can be no difference between the gums of the girl from whom the tooth was taken, and the gums of the person who received it. If the ulceration took place in the last from contamination would not the socket in the girl from whom the tooth was taken likewise have ulcerated? But this did not happen in any of them. I have here supposed the teeth capable of being contaminated; although I believe we have never yet seen them have this disease primarily, but only in consequence of its breaking out somewhere else, in the mouth, throat, or nose, and spreading to them.

But still, if they are capable of having the disease, and communicating it to others, it becomes very extraordinary that those people should have hit upon the few teeth that probably were ever so contaminated.

When we consider that the girls from whom the teeth were taken had not the least appearance of disease at the time, and had none when the disease broke out in the person who received the teeth, it becomes strange that it should break out in the receivers and not in the giver.

It is also singular that an ambiguity should follow this disease in all its stages : in the mode of its being caught, the appearance, and the cure.

Let us sum up all the arguments in favour of the disease not being venereal. First, two patients, whose cases were similar to the others in their origin, recovered without medicine. Secondly, they who seemed to be cured by mercury had not a treatment exactly similar to those who were indisputably poxed. Thirdly, I consider it as impossible for parts to have the power of contaminating which are not themselves diseased. Fourthly, the parts contaminating were never known to have been contaminated themselves. But it must be nearly the same thing to those who want to have teeth transplanted, whether my reasoning is just or not ; for a disease in consequence of the operation most certainly has taken place ; and in some cases this has been worse, or cured with more difficulty, than the lues venerea in common; and whatever the disease may be, I yet know of no mode of prevention, except the drawing of the tooth early, and that has been tried in one case only, and in that case was successful.

From this account many may be deterred from having this operation performed. In that light no evil can arise, except the mortification which arises from a reflection that no relief is to be had in cases of bad teeth. But it is to be remembered that this is a publication of all the unsuccessful cases, which is the very reverse of what is generally practised in medical books; and they are mentioned upon no other principle than that the disease, when it happens, may not be improperly managed.

It may be asked, what is this disease ? There is more difficulty in answering what it is than what it is not. I should say that a sound tooth transplanted may occasion such an irritation as shall produce a species of disease which may be followed by the local complaints above mentioned.

I cannot conclude without intimating that undescribed diseases, resembling the venereal, are very numerous ; and that what I have said is rather to be considered as hints for others to prosecute this inquiry further, than as a complete account of the subject.

END OF THE SECOND VOLUME.

Printed by Richard Taylor, Red Lion Court, Fleet Street.

Printed in the United States
By Bookmasters